BLADDER CANCER

CURRENT CLINICAL UROLOGY

Eric A. Klein, SERIES EDITOR

BLADDER CANCER

CURRENT DIAGNOSIS AND TREATMENT

Edited by

MICHAEL J. DROLLER, MD

Mount Sinai School of Medicine,
New York, NY

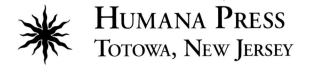

HUMANA PRESS
TOTOWA, NEW JERSEY

© 2001 Humana Press Inc.
999 Riverview Drive, Suite 208
Totowa, New Jersey 07512
Visit our Website at http://humanapress.com

For additional copies, pricing for bulk purchases, and/or information about other Humana titles, contact Humana at the above address or at any of the following numbers: Tel: 973-256-1699; Fax: 973-256-8341; E-mail: humana@humanapr.com

Due diligence has been taken by the publishers, editors, and authors of this book to ensure the accuracy of the information published and to describe generally accepted practices. The contributors herein have carefully checked to ensure that the drug selections and dosages set forth in this text are accurate in accord with the standards accepted at the time of publication. Notwithstanding, as new research, changes in government regulations, and knowledge from clinical experience relating to drug therapy and drug reactions constantly occurs, the reader is advised to check the product information provided by the manufacturer of each drug for any change in dosages or for additional warnings and contraindications. This is of utmost importance when the recommended drug herein is a new or infrequently used drug. It is the responsibility of the health care provider to ascertain the Food and Drug Administration status of each drug or device used in their clinical practice. The publisher, editors, and authors are not responsible for errors or omissions or for any consequences from the application of the information presented in this book and make no warranty, express or implied, with respect to the contents in this publication.

This publication is printed on acid-free paper. ∞

ANSI Z39.48-1984 (American National Standards Institute)
Permanence of Paper for Printed Library Materials.

Cover design by Patricia F. Cleary.
Cover illustration: From Droller MJ. Current Problems in Surgery. In: *Bladder Cancer,* Ravitch MM and Steichen FM (eds.). Year Book Medical Publishers, Inc., 1981; XVII(4): p. 219.
Production Editor: Kim Hoather-Potter.

Photocopy Authorization Policy:
Authorization to photocopy items for internal or personal use, or the internal or personal use of specific clients, is granted by Humana Press Inc., provided that the base fee of US $8.00 per copy, plus US $00.25 per page, is paid directly to the Copyright Clearance Center at 222 Rosewood Drive, Danvers, MA 01923. For those organizations that have been granted a photocopy license from the CCC, a separate system of payment has been arranged and is acceptable to Humana Press Inc. The fee code for users of the Transactional Reporting Service is: [0-89603-818-1/01 $10.00 + $00.25].

Printed in the United States of America. 10 9 8 7 6 5 4 3 2 1

Library of Congress Cataloging-in-Publication Data
Bladder cancer : current diagnosis and treatment/edited by Michael J. Droller.
    p. ; cm. – (Current clinical urology)
  Includes bibliographical references and index.
  ISBN 0-89603-818-1 (alk. paper)
    1. Bladder–Cancer. I. Droller, Michael J. II. Series.
    [DNLM: 1. Bladder Neoplasms–diagnosis. 2. Bladder Neoplasms–therapy. WJ 504
  B63185 2000]
  RC280.B5 B637 2000
  616.99'462–dc21
                                     00-033523

PREFACE

Bladder Cancer: Current Diagnosis and Treatment has been designed to present state-of-the-art information on and understanding of the many aspects of bladder cancer that factor into decisions regarding its assessment and treatment. The guiding byword in this is the term *"understanding,"* and the authors were thus asked to encapsulate their comprehensive knowledge of their specific topics, offer their critical perspectives on the ever increasing amount of fresh data, and provide their insights regarding precisely what meaningfully advances our knowledge and understanding of bladder cancer.

The critical task in working toward this objective was to identify those who could provide all of these attributes—knowledge, perspective, and insight—in addressing the various areas that comprise this volume. In addition, because a substantial number of issues might still be unresolved, or in many instances be controversial, an attempt was made to recruit contributors who might offer differing perspectives on a given topic. This permitted an exposition on both sides of a given issue. Although this made the draft of each chapter a more onerous undertaking, the final result was a more complete compendium of reliably and objectively presented information.

I am indebted to each of our contributors for having undertaken their assignments with enthusiasm and with a productive application of their uniquely valuable knowledge and perspectives. To those who tired of my frequent calls and obsessive editing, I apologize. I do hope, however, that the final product reflects the focused attention and tremendous effort that was invested.

I am grateful to each contributor for having educated me to an extent that I had not anticipated. It is now time to share this with our readership with the hope that the information contained in *Bladder Cancer: Current Diagnosis and Treatment* will prove useful both as an information base and as a stimulant for further study.

Finally, I am grateful to Dr. Eric Klein of the Department of Urology, the Cleveland Clinic Foundation, for having permitted me to organize and edit this monograph; and to Mr. Paul Dolgert, Craig Adams, and the Humana Press for all of their assistance in bringing this project to fruition.

Michael J. Droller, MD

CONTENTS

Contributors

WILLIAM C. BAKER, MD • *Department of Urology, University of California, Davis School of Medicine, Sacramento, CA*

GEORG BARTSCH, MD • *Department of Urology, University of Innsbruck Medical School, Innsbruck A-6020, Austria*

VINCENT G. BIRD, MD • *Department of Urology, University of Miami School of Medicine, Miami, FL*

CHRISTER BUSCH, MD, PhD • *Department of Pathology, University Hospital, N9038 Tromsø, Norway*

CARLOS CORDON-CARDO, MD, PhD • *Department of Pathology, Memorial Sloan Kettering Cancer Center, New York, NY*

RICHARD J. COTE, MD • *Department of Pathology, University of Southern California, Kenneth Norris Jr. Cancer Hospital and Research Institute, Los Angeles, CA*

GUIDO DALBAGNI, MD • *Department of Urology, Memorial Sloan Kettering Cancer Center, New York, NY*

ARLINE D. DEITCH, PhD • *Department of Urology, University of California, Davis School of Medicine, Sacramento, CA*

RALPH W. DEVERE WHITE, MD • *Department of Urology, University of California, Davis School of Medicine, Sacramento, CA*

MICHAEL J. DROLLER, MD • *Department of Urology, Mount Sinai School of Medicine, New York, NY*

YVES FRADET, MD • *Laval University Cancer Research Center, Québec, Canada*

MARY K. GOSPODAROWICZ, MD • *Department of Radiation Oncology, Princess Margaret Hospital, University Health Network, Toronto, Canada*

H. BARTON GROSSMAN, MD • *Department of Urology, The University of Texas MD Anderson Cancer Center, Houston, TX*

SIMON J. HALL, MD • *Department of Urology, The Mount Sinai Medical Center, New York, NY*

DEBRA HAWES, MD • *Department of Pathology, Keck School of Medicine, University of Southern California, Los Angeles, CA*

COURTNEY M. P. HOLLOWELL, MD • *Section of Urology, University of Chicago Hospitals, Chicago, IL*

SONNY L. JOHANSSON, MD, PhD • *Department of Pathology and Microbiology, University of Nebraska Medical Center, Omaha, NE*

ICHABOD JUNG, MD • *Department of Urology, University of Rochester Medical Center, Rochester, New York*

LYNN LADETSKY, MD • *Department of Radiology, State University of New York, Health Care Center at Brooklyn, Brooklyn, NY*

SETH P. LERNER, MD • *Scott Department of Urology, Baylor College of Medicine, Houston, TX*

PER-UNO MALMSTRÖM, MD, PhD • *Department of Urology, Uppsala University Hospital, Akademiska Sjukhuset, Sweden*

EDWARD M. MESSING, MD • *Department of Urology, University of Rochester Medical Center, Rochester, NY*

RANDALL MILLIKAN, MD, PhD • *Department of Genitourinary Medical Oncology, University of Texas MD Anderson Cancer Center, Houston, TX*

MICHAEL F. MILOSEVIC, MD • *Department of Radiation Oncology, Princess Margaret Hospital, University Health Network, Toronto, Canada*

HAROLD MITTY, MD • *Department of Radiology, Mount Sinai School of Medicine, New York, NY*

JAMES E. MONTIE, MD • *Department of Urology, University of Michigan School of Medicine, Ann Arbor, MI*

MICHAEL A. O'DONNELL, MD • *Department of Urology, University of Iowa Hospitals and Clinics, Iowa City, IA*

ROSALEEN B. PARSONS, MD • *Department of Radiology, Fox Chase Cancer Center, Philadelphia, PA*

ARTHUR T. PORTER, MD • *Department of Radiation Oncology, Detroit Medical Center, Detroit, MI*

DEREK RAGHAVAN, MD, PhD • *USC Norris Comprehensive Cancer Center, University of Southern California, Los Angeles, CA*

RANDALL G. ROWLAND, MD, PhD • *Department of Surgery, Division of Urology, University of Kentucky, Chandler Medical Center, Lexington, KY*

WILLIAM A. SEE, MD • *Department of Urology, University of Wisconsin at Milwaukee School of Medicine, Milwaukee, WI*

JOEL SHEINFELD, MD • *Memorial Sloan-Kettering Cancer Center, New York, NY*

DONALD G. SKINNER, MD • *Department of Urology, USC Norris Comprehensive Cancer Center, University of Southern California, Los Angeles, CA*

MARK S. SOLOWAY, MD • *Department of Urology, University of Miami School of Medicine, Miami, FL*

JOHN P. STEIN, MD • *Department of Urology, USC Norris Comprehensive Cancer Center, University of Southern California, Los Angeles, CA*

GARY D. STEINBERG, MD • *University of Chicago Hospitals, Section of Urology, Chicago, IL*

GUNNAR STEINECK, MD • *Clinical Epidemiology, Division of Epidemiology, Karolinska Hospital, Stockholm*

ARNULF STENZL, MD • *Department of Urology, University of Innsbruck Medical School, Austria*

PETER F. THALL, PhD • *Department of Biostatistics, University of Texas MD Anderson Cancer Center, Houston, TX*

DAN THEODORESCU, MD, PhD • *Department of Urology, University of Virginia Health Sciences Center, Charlottesville, VA*

PADRAIQ WARDE, MD • *Department of Radiation Oncology, Princess Margaret Hospital, University Health Network, Toronto, Canada*

HANS WIJKSTRÖM, MD, PhD • *Department of Urology, Huddinge University Hospital, Karolinska Institute, Stockholm, Sweden*

1 Demographic and Epidemiologic Aspects of Bladder Cancer

Gunnar Steineck, MD

CONTENTS

INTRODUCTION

Urothelial bladder cancer is the ninth most frequent cancer, accounting for 3.2% of the 8.1 million new cancer cases estimated to have occurred in the world in 1990. Approximately 261,000 new cases of bladder cancer (202,000 among men and 50,000 among females) occurred in 1990 *(1)*, and 114,000 subjects (86,000 males and 28,000 females) died the same year of the disease *(2)*.

In Europe and the United States, almost all urinary bladder tumors have a transitional cell histology originating from the urothelium, that lines the cavity of the renal pelvis, ureter, urinary bladder and urethra. This urothelial cancer (synonym: transitional cell carcinoma) sometimes contains areas of squamous cell carcinoma and (more rarely) adenocarcinoma. Pure squamous cell carcinoma is found in approx 1–3% of cases, and pure adenocarcinoma (many probably developing from the urachus) are typically found in less than 1% of patients. Some rare bladder cancers include malignant melanomas and sarcomas. In areas

From: *Current Clinical Urology: Bladder Cancer: Current Diagnosis and Treatment*
Edited by: M. J. Droller © Humana Press Inc., Totowa, NJ

1

where the parasite Schistosomia Haematobium is endemic, pure squamous cell carcinomas are common. The descriptive and etiologic information given below refers mainly to urothelial cancers.

DESCRIPTIVE EPIDEMIOLOGY

International Variation

The highest age-standardized incidence rates among men of urinary bladder cancer are found in North America (23.3 per 100,000 person years), Northern Africa (23.3) and Southern Europe (22.0) *(1)*. The corresponding figures for women are 5.4 per 100,000 person-years in North America, 4.8 in Northern Africa and 3.2 in Southern Europe. The lowest frequencies Parkin and coworkers estimated for Melanesia (2.7 among men and 0.6 among women) and Middle Africa (2.8 among men and 0.5 among women). Thus, the ratio between highest and lowest incidence rates is close to 10 for both genders. The quality of the information varies considerably between the areas and probably account for some of the variation. Still, undoubtedly the frequency varies around the world, which strongly suggests that life habits and environmental factors may determine the disease incidence. In the United States, urinary bladder cancer is the fourth most common cancer in men (39,500 estimated new cases in 1998) and the tenth most common in women (14,900 cases in 1998) *(3)*. The same year approximately 8400 men and 4100 women in the United States died of the disease.

Age, Sex, and Race

The age specific incidence of bladder cancer increases sharply with age, and peaks at 80 yr of age or older. Bladder cancer is predominantly a tumor among males, the gender ratio typically is about 3:1. In the United States, the incidence rate of bladder cancer is higher in whites than in blacks, with an incidence ratio close to 2 *(4)*. The situation is thus different than that found, for example, for prostate cancer, a disease more common among blacks.

Time Trends

From 1990 to 1996, the incidence of bladder cancer in the United States has been decreasing at a rate of 0.8% per year (1.2% among men and 0.4% among women) *(4)*. Up to 1990, the incidence was rising, but the mortality decreasing. In Sweden, urinary bladder cancer incidence among men has decreased since a few years, while women still faces an increasing occurrence. In Europe and the United States, urinary bladder cancer incidence typically is higher in urban than in rural areas.

ANALYTICAL EPIDEMIOLOGY

A full smorgasbord of exposures and risk groups has been reported to increase the urothelial cancer risk (transitional cell carcinoma in the renal pelvis, ureter, urinary bladder or urethra). With a few exceptions, however, we do not know which carcinogenic agent, if any, increases the urinary bladder cancer incidence in the reported populations. Strong associations and observation of subjects with a clear-cut one agent exposure (a pseudoexperimental situation) makes it possible to say that some chemicals (beyond reasonable doubt) are carcinogenic to the human urothelium. These agents include certain aromatic amines (2-naphthylamine, 4-aminobiphenyl, benzidine, ortho-tolouidine), two pharmacological substances (phenacetin and chlornaphazin) and ionizing radiation. No one doubts that inhalation of tobacco smoke, containing at least 40 candidate carcinogens, influences the disease incidence. Combustion gases are another source of mixed exposures that have been related convincingly to urinary bladder cancer. Ongoing discussions include whether the disease can be prevented by a high fluid intake, ingestion of vitamin A supplements, intake of acetyl salicylic acid, avoidance of acetaminophen or by a low intake of beef and pork. We also have good evidence that several specific chemicals other than aromatic amines cause urinary bladder cancer.

Concerning squamous cell carcinoma in the urinary bladder, subjects with a history of many urinary tract infections have an increased risk, as do individuals living in areas where the parasite Schistosoma Haematobium is endemic.

Tobacco Smoking

The link between the proportion of tobacco smokers in a population and urinary bladder cancer incidence has been clear for more than three decades *(5)*. In the United States, Sweden and many other Western countries, about half the bladder cancer cases occurring today among men, and about one third of those in women, would have been avoided if our societies had been tobacco-free.

Dose-Effect

The excess risk of urinary bladder cancer probably relates in a nonlinear way to the amount of tobacco smoked—a different situation than that for lung cancer. Concerning daily consumption, available data indicate an initial sharp increase in risk levels with a two to threefold increase in bladder cancer risk for subjects smoking at least 10 cigarettes per day. The risk does not further increase until the daily consumption rises above 40–60 cigarettes per day. In most western countries, the urinary bladder cancer incidence is two to three times higher among cigarette smokers as compared with those who have never smoked *(5)*.

Type of Tobacco and Smoking Device

One can prepare tobacco to be black or white; Danish smokers frequently consume black tobacco and in France the cigarette Gauloise mainly contains this type of tobacco. On the average, users of black tobacco have a two to three times higher risk of urinary bladder cancer than those who choose blond tobacco *(6)*. Smokers of low-tar and low-nicotine ("light") cigarettes have a reduced risk compared to smokers of high-tar and high-nicotine cigarettes. Individuals who smoke unfiltered cigarettes seem to have a 50% increased risk of bladder cancer compared with those who smoke filtered cigarettes. Switching from unfiltered to filtered cigarettes does not reduce the risk according to some studies *(7)*. A possible mechanism is that filters protect from early, but not late, stages of carcinogenesis. In USA, a typical pipe smoker has a lower risk of contracting urinary bladder cancer than an average cigarette smoker. The difference depends to a large extent, if not entirely, on smaller tobacco consumption and less inhaling among pipe smokers; when smoking characteristics are accounted for, pipe and cigarette smoking elevate the risk to a similar degree *(8–10)*. Cigar smoking, snuff and chewing tobacco probably do not influence urinary bladder cancer risk.

Other Smoking Characteristics

Available data indicate that an early start of smoking increases urinary bladder cancer risk as compared to a late start, even after adjustment for the total amount of tobacco consumed during life. If these findings are confirmed, humans would be more susceptible to the carcinogenic agents in tobacco smoke at a young age, as compared to an old age. Starting to smoke early in life, however, also implies that one can stop before the ages when cancer or cardiac problems usually occur. Former smokers have an increased risk compared with never-smokers up to 10 yr after smoking cessation *(5)*, and it is unclear if one ever gets back to the background risk of urinary bladder cancer after smoking cessation. A possible mechanism would be that certain carcinogens in tobacco are involved in early stages of carcinogenesis and that the changes persist in the urothelium. However, former smokers have a reduced risk as compared with current smokers, and tobacco smoke probably also contains carcinogens that operate during late stages in urothelial neoplastic development.

Tobacco-Related Carcinogens

Candidate urothelial carcinogens in tobacco smoke include the aromatic amines 2-naphthylamine, 4-aminobiphenyl, and ortho-tolouidine, the heterocyclic amine Trp-P-2 and one of the many polycyclic aromatic hydrocarbons *(5,11)*. Adducts between DNA and 4-aminobiphenyl have been found in tumor samples from smokers indicating that this agent may be responsible for some carcinogenicity of tobacco smoke *(12)*. No such DNA-adducts could be found 5 yr after smoking cessation.

Industry-Related Carcinogens

A large number of occupations and occupational chemicals have been found to have an excess incidence of urinary bladder cancer. Many of the increased relative risks depend on background variability (chance); typically, more than 100 jobs and chemicals are analysed in a study. Selective reporting of positive associations (publication bias) certainly is an issue in this literature. To sort out real hazards in the abundant epidemiological data, one needs to have consistent findings. Also, a simplistic exposure pattern, high relative risks and supportive evidence from animal studies can assist to this judgment. With stringent criteria, we can be sure that certain aromatic amines cause urinary bladder cancer. There is also no doubt that exposure to combustion gases, probably including engine exhausts, increases the risk to contract the disease. Combustion gases contains a plenitude of chemicals, for example, small amounts of aromatic amines, nitroarenes and several different polycyclic aromatic hydrocarbons.

The suggestions that nearly 25% of white male cases *(13)* and above 10% of white female cases *(14)* in United States during the 1980s could be attributed to occupational exposures probably was a gross overestimation since chance findings were included as causal *(15,16)*. On the other hand, if we only consider aromatic amines and combustion gases when the attributable proportion of cases is calculated, we probably make an underestimation since some of the candidate urothelial carcinogens probably influence disease incidence. However, we have not been able to prove this with current epidemiological tools.

Aromatic Amines

During the nineteenth century the German dye industry expanded, and new chemicals were used to dye textiles instead of the natural products from the middle East that had been used previously. At the end of the nineteenth century, the German surgeon Rehn reported three cases of urinary bladder cancer among dye industry workers and suggested that these workers had an excess risk *(17)*. Aniline was for long suspected to be the responsible carcinogenic agent. In Sweden, schoolchildren were forbidden to lick their aniline-pencils. However, in 1938 Hueper found that dogs contracted urinary bladder cancer after exposure to 2-naphthylamine but not aniline *(18)*. Later on, Case demonstrated a strong carcinogenic potential of 2-naphthylamine in humans. Fifteen men who worked with distilling this agent all developed bladder tumors *(19)*. His pioneer and epidemiological work was done in English dye and rubber industry, and he was one of the first authors to calculate person-years to obtain a denominator for the incidence of a disease *(20,21)*.

The action of 2-naphthylamine is remarkably organ specific; all species (mouse, rat, rabbit, guinea pig, dog) given the carcinogen develop bladder tumors *(22)*. We have uncertain data, however, on the induction-latency period (the time between the start of exposure to 2-naphthylamine and the diagnosis of bladder cancer), the combined data reported by Case from England suggest about 20 yr, with a range of at least 12–41 yr *(19)*. Possibly 2-naphthylamine may be active in both early and late stages of carcinogenesis, but efforts to link exposure to specific DNA-changes in tumors have not been successful *(23)*.

Later reports mainly from the dye and rubber industry linked the aromatic amines 4-aminobiphenyl and benzidine to urinary bladder cancer. Data are also persuasive for linking ortho-tolouidine (found during rubber manufacturing) to the disease incidence. In rubber manufacturing one uses the aromatic amine (2-chloroaniline) (MBOCA) and it probably is one of the causative agents for observed urinary bladder cancer risk in the industry *(24)*.

There are no data indicating that workers previously exposed to aromatic amines ever will return to the background incidence for urinary bladder cancer. Thus, just as for former cigarette smokers, an excess risk may persist through life. Therefore, as long as members of industrial cohorts exposed to aromatic amines are alive we will probably encounter bladder tumors related to these agents. Screening such workers may be worthwhile, for example, to diminish the amount of treatment needed to control the disease.

Polycyclic Aromatic Hydrocarbons

Employees in the aluminum industry, gas production workers and chimney sweeps have excess risks of urinary bladder cancer *(9,25–27)*. Consistent findings from different work places, and relations between the accumulated exposure to combustion gases and risk elevation, provide convincing evidence for a causal link. Combustion gases contain high levels of polycyclic aromatic hydrocarbons, and one or several chemicals in this group may be the responsible carcinogen. However, several aromatic amines, including 2-naphthylamine, and other impurities, e.g., nitroarenes, can also be found in these mixtures. Which agent(s) acting on the urothelium is unknown.

Truck drivers, chauffeurs, delivery men and garage/gas station are workers with an elevated bladder cancer incidence that are exposed to diesel exhausts *(9,13,28–30)*. The data strongly indicate a causal link and diesel exhausts partly contain the same chemicals as combustion gases from coal. However, some authors propose that deviating dietary habits and abnormal voiding patterns explain the increased urinary bladder cancer risk among drivers, and not exhaust exposure.

Other Industry-Related Agents

Benzene is an organic solvent linked to leukemia. Swedish data indicate that this agent also causes bladder cancer *(28)*. However, in a Chinese cohort of workers exposed to benzene no risk elevation was found *(31)*. Chlorinated aliphatic hydrocarbons are used in dry cleaning, shoemaking and repair, and have long been suspected to be bladder carcinogens *(29)*. High relative risks, and the simple exposure pattern in some processes used in dry cleaning, provide good evidence for a causal link to urinary bladder cancer. Creosote has been used to preserve wood in telephone poles. This mixture contains similar chemicals as combustion gases. Line workers are exposed to creosote and have an increased risk of bladder cancer *(29)* and there is good evidence for a causal link. Machinists and machine manufacturing workers in the metal industry are exposed to cutting fluids and oils. The excess risk of bladder cancer reported for these groups may be explained by the presence of aromatic amines, nitrosamines or polycyclic aromatic hydrocarbons in cutting fluids and oils *(29)*. Polychlorinated biphenyls are found in hydraulic oil and in oils used for insulation in high power electrical devices. Electricians may get in contact with these agents, as do some drivers of electrical trains working in cabins where engine oil containing polychlorinated biphenyls are dispersed in the air. Electricians and train drivers typically suffer an increased risk of urinary bladder cancer, and polychlorinated biphenyls are probably the responsible agents *(9,29)*. Apart from the above-mentioned factors, additional carcinogens may be searched for in risk groups such as chemical workers, miners, pesticide applicators and cooks.

Food and Drinks

Strong data has been presented indicating that high fluid consumption decreases the risk of urinary bladder cancer. It has been suggested that consumption of beef and pork, or animal fat, influences an increased disease incidence. However, we do not know if we can modify our bladder risk by changing diet. We can say, however, that coffee drinking or intake of artificial sweeteners (saccharine, cyclamate) explain few or no cases.

Fluid

No one would be surprised to learn that a diluted urine caused less damage to the urothelium than a concentrated one. Still, epidemiological evidence for a long time said the opposite. Early Danish *(32)* and German *(33)* studies for example, obtained increased relative risks of urinary bladder cancer in subjects with a high fluid intake. Recently, however, data from the Physicians Health Study showed a decreased urinary bladder cancer risk in men with high fluid intake *(34)*. In this particular analysis, 47,909 men were followed, generating 435,458 person-years. In the highest quintile (an intake of more than 2.5 L fluid a day), 36 cases occurred per 100,000 person-years, while the corresponding figure in the lowest quintile was 68. Smoking was more common in the highest quintile, and could not explain the difference. After adjusting for age, smoking and some other potential confounders, the relative risk (with 95% confidence interval) was 0.5 (0.3–0.8). A gradient was seen in going from quintile one to five; the relative risks were 1.0, 0.8, 0.9, 0.7 and 0.5. Reasonable methodological flaws cannot explain the protective effect seen, and the precision in the estimate was high. Possibly the studies from Denmark and Germany were biased. Another explanation would be that beer, frequently consumed by those with a high fluid intake in Denmark and Germany, may increase urinary bladder cancer risk. Beer, containing nitrosamines, probably influences rectal cancer incidence *(35,36)*. The American data, however, indicate that beer consumed in the USA do not influence the urinary bladder cancer risk. There is no indication that consumption of alcoholic beverages other than beer influences the occurrence of urinary bladder tumors.

The complexity concerning the effects by fluid intake is further highlighted by the reports that chlorination of tap water may cause an increased risk of urinary bladder cancer *(37,38)*. Chlorinated products, with some chemical resemblance to those dry cleaners are exposed to, can be found in the water. Although major efforts have been made, the epidemiological data for this association are not conclusive. If a high fluid intake by itself prevents urinary bladder cancer, investigating whether a component in tap water increases the risk certainly provides methodological challenges. The findings from the Physician Health study can be seen as an average for the United States *(34)*, and the relative risks were consistent among all regions—contradicting that chlorinated water alters the risk.

An epidemiological study that documents a tenfold risk increase is by itself nearly conclusive. Such a urinary bladder cancer risk was found among those on the southwestern coast of Taiwan drinking artesian well water *(39–41)*. This water contains arsenic, and arsenic is thus a strong candidate for being carcinogen to the urothelium.

Coffee was initially included as a dummy variable in a case-control study of urinary bladder cancer. The investigator wanted to calibrate his method by a coffee variable, thinking it would not be related to the disease under study. Instead they unexpectedly obtained a high relative risk, and it was reported as an important observation *(42)*. More than 35 subsequent studies addressed the issue; when Viscolic and coworkers 22 yr later summarized the evidence, they obtained an estimate just above unity. This deviation could probably be explained by an unaccounted effect by tobacco smoking, a habit closely related to coffee drinking in many populations *(43)*. Thus, drinking coffee probably does not influence urinary bladder cancer risk. If one considers the large data amount investigating whether there is an association, future studies probably will not change this judgment. A relative risk of 0.8 was seen in Physicians Health Study among high consumers of coffee *(34)*. On the other hand, there is good evidence that coffee drinking is protective for colorectal cancer, possibly by diminishing the fecal transit time *(44)*.

Meat and Heterocyclic Amines

Beef, pork or animal fat consumption may alter the incidence of urinary bladder cancer *(10,45)*. Available data are far from conclusive, but there is good evidence that consumers of such foods have an increased risk. Heterocyclic amines are formed when we fry meat, especially under high temperatures. Sugar and creatinine are utilized in a chemical reaction, known as Maillard, producing heterocyclic amines *(46)*. They are mutagenic, and all studied heterocyclic amines are carcinogenic when given to rodents or monkeys. An excess risk of urinary bladder tumors was found when the heterocyclic amines Trp-P-2 was fed to rats *(47,48)*. This substance has some structural similarities to the strong bladder carcinogen 2-naphthylamine.

In informative case-control studies of urinary bladder cancer, subjects with a high consumption of beef or pork typically have an increased risk. In a study from Stockholm, a high consumption of fried meat gave a higher risk than if the meat was boiled *(45)*. A second study, including 1565 subjects focused on the question as to whether intake of heterocyclic amines causes cancer. A method was developed in which survey data and laboratory findings were combined to estimate the daily intake of heterocyclic amines *(49–52)*. Diet was assessed by means of a semi-quantitative food frequency questionnaire comprising a total of 188 food and drink items. The amount and type of dish ingested, frequency of consumption, cooking method and frying temperature were considered. In addition twenty-four color photos showed six dishes fried at four different temperatures. Each photo corresponded to a specific frying temperature, resulting in varying degree of surface browning. Altogether 19 dishes were fried at 150, 175, 200, and 225°C and three were baked/roasted at 150 and/or 200°C. The heterocyclic amine content was detected with HPLC in lyophilized meat and pan residues. Except for fried eggs, heterocyclic amines were found in all investigated dishes, either in the dish or in the corresponding gravy.

An inverse-U relation was found between the amount of ingested meat and urinary bladder cancer risk (53). A twofold increase in risk was found in the fourth intake quintile, as compared with the first, but in the fifth quintile the relative risk was below unity. Heterocyclic amine intake gave a similar risk pattern, but the relative risk in the fourth intake quintile was lower (1.4, 95% confidence interval 0.8–2.4). Thus, the study adds evidence to the notion that the amount of beef and pork in the diet may influence urinary bladder cancer incidence, but it could not show that the risk depends on cooking methods.

Unrecognized methodological problems may explain the inverse-U relation found between meat intake (mainly beef and pork) and urinary bladder cancer risk. If further data supports the relation, we must search for protective systems that are activated during a high intake and that balance the increased risk seen for a moderate meat intake. Messing has suggested that urinary pH may be of interest; a high meat intake may lower the urinary pH, and acid urine may inhibit certain growth factors that are important for tumor development (54).

The intake of heterocyclic amines, in the doses typically ingested by the study population, was not found to be related to colorectal or kidney cancer risk (53). However, findings were consistent with increased cancer risk when the heterocyclic amine intake was very high (1900 ng/day, or more). Due to the limited number of exposed subjects, the precision was very low at these doses. Adjustment for potential confounding factors (age, sex, smoking, energy, fat, protein, fiber, fruits, vegetables, physical activity) had little or no effect on relative risks.

Other Dietary Constituents

In several studies total fat intake, or animal fat intake, has been related to urinary bladder cancer risk (45). Also, total energy intake has been identified as a risk factor, especially in case-control studies. A major methodological problem is to disentangle the actions of beef and pork, animal fat, total fat and energy intake, all variables that are closely related: meat contains animal fat, fat energy, and high consumers of beef also tend to eat nonmeat fat more frequently than others. Also, a mechanism as to how fat may induce urinary bladder cancer is unclear.

One case-control study showed a protective effect of on urinary bladder cancer by supplements containing synthetic vitamin A, a substance that resembles retinol (dietary vitamin A from animal sources) *(45)*. Other vitamin-A analogues, synthetic retinoids, have been suggested as protective for recurrence of Ta-tumors after transurethral resection *(55,56)*. Data describing the effect on urinary bladder cancer risk by natural vitamins and minerals, that is, the effect of a high intake of fruits, roots, vegetables and berries, are, however, conflicting. Although vitamin A, natural or synthetic, as well as cruciferous vegetables *(57)*, may be of interest for the development and growth of urinary bladder cancer, no conclusive data exists as yet.

Rodents that are fed cyclamate, an artificial sweetener, contract urinary bladder cancer more often than do other rodents. A large American case-control study was primarily devoted to investigate if the risk also pertains to humans provided no support *(58)*. The combined evidence from this, and a number of subsequent studies from other populations, gives no support for the notion that artificial sweeteners influence urinary bladder cancer incidence in humans *(59)*. Thus, again, we have a large data pile, and although an absence of association stringently never can be definitely proved, it is safe to say that few or no of today's urinary bladder cancer cases are related to intake of artificial sweeteners. A varying metabolism may explain species differences.

Bracken Fern

In Balkan a nephropathy was endemic among cattle and humans. A high incidence of urinary bladder cancer has been concomitant with this disorder *(60,61)*. The ubiquitous bracken fern (genus Pteridium) was the responsible agent. After ingestion, it causes thiamin deficiency, acute hemorrhage associated with myeloid aplasia, blindness due to retinal degeneration and urinary bladder cancer. The major carcinogen (and the cause of the retinal degeneration and the myeloid aplasia) has been shown to be ptaquiloside, a norsesquiterpene glycoside that can be present in bracken fern in extraordinary concentrations. The highest concentrations were found in the crosiers and young unfolding fronds. Ptaquiloside has been found in the milk of cows fed on bracken fern experimentally and the milk of bracken-fed cows has been shown to cause cancer in rats.

DRUGS AND DISEASES

Due to simplistic exposure patterns, high exposure levels and strong associations certain drugs have been identified as urothelial carcinogens. Also, some diseases may initiate or promote bladder carcinogenesis.

Drugs

In a Swedish weapon factory the workers were offered free analgesics to prevent head ache from machine noise. Mainly one substance, phenacetin, was taken. It was consumed before work, put on the sandwiches during lunch breaks, and the total consumption added up to several kilograms. After some years evidence accumulated that the workers had an increased incidence of kidney failure due to papillary necrosis as well as urothelial tumors situated in the renal pelvis *(62)*. Phenacetin increases urinary bladder incidence by implantation of cancer cells from the renal pelvis. Phenacetin may also act directly on the bladder urothelium *(63)*, but the urinary bladder cancer risk (if any) is lower than the risk of renal pelvic cancer; possibly the responsible carcinogen (phenacetin or a metabolite) is quickly inactivated in the urine.

Acetaminophen and phenacetin resemble each other chemically, and share metabolic pathways. In one study, rodents contracted urinary bladder tumors after being fed acetaminophen. During the 1980s phenacetin consumption was succeeded by intake of acetaminophen in many populations. The median induction-latency time between exposure to acetaminophen and urinary bladder cancer risk may be more than a decade. Consumers of analgesics typically consume more than one brand, and some pills contain mixtures of phenacetin, acetaminophen and aspirin, or at least two of the drugs. These facts, and the difficulties in measuring former drug intake with interview data, have made it impossible to estimate the effect (if any) of acetaminophen on urinary bladder cancer incidence. In one study, a significantly increased risk was found, after adjustment for age, smoking, and consumption of other analgesics *(64)*.

Acetyl salicylic acid, chemically unrelated to acetaminophen and phenacetin, is a prostaglandin inhibitor preventing colon cancer *(65)*. A study from Stockholm gave a relative risk of urinary bladder cancer of 0.7 after adjusting for age, gender, smoking and consumption of other analgesics *(64)*. However, in summarizing the observational epidemiological studies, the methodological issues are as challenging as for acetaminophen. The randomized studies comparing acetyl salicylic acid with placebo do not yet have sufficient power to illustrate a possible effect on urinary bladder cancer risk. Thus, we must have more data before we can evaluate whether acetyl salicylic acid protects against urinary bladder cancer.

Chlornaphazine, closely related chemically to 2-naphthylamine, was used for a short time to treat polycytemia verae. In a Danish cohort a very high urinary bladder cancer incidence was documented *(66)*. Despite some methodological shortcomings, the data were conclusive for a causal relation. A short induction-latency time (less than five yr) was found for some patients. The drug has since been withdrawn from the market.

Cyclophosphamide is used by oncologists to treat certain tumors. The drug is toxic to the urinary bladder mucosa, and probably increases urinary bladder cancer risk *(67)*. The evidence is primarily based on a summary of case reports, but there is some evidence that bladder cancer risk increases with the cumulated total dose of cyclophosphamide.

There is no doubt that ionizing radiation influences urinary bladder cancer incidence. Patients having undergone external beam radiation therapy of organs in the pelvic region, with fields that have included the urinary bladder, contract the disease more often than other subjects. The increased risk is best documented after radiotherapy for cervical cancer *(68)*.

Diseases

Undoubtedly an indwelling catheter predisposes for squamous cell carcinoma of the urinary bladder *(69)*. The high relative risk seen in historical cohorts may not be representative for today's situation; repeat urinary tract infections probably explain the risk, and the frequency of such to some part depends on preventive efforts. If subjects having had many urinary tract infections in addition suffer an increased urothelial cancer risk is unclear.

In the Middle East and parts of Africa infection with the *Schistosoma haematobium* (Bilharzia) is endemic and squamous cell carcinoma of the urinary bladder cancer a common malignancy. For example, the disease is the most common malignancy in Egyptians, accounting for 27.6% of all cases, 38.5% of cancers in the male and 11.3% in the female *(70)*. Causality has not definitely been proven, but the geographical correlation between the two conditions, the common predominant occurrence in young males, the clinicopathological identity of Bilharzia-associated bladder cancer, and evidence in experimentally infected animals are facts supporting an association *(71)*. Tissue damage induced by the parasite may lead to a chronic inflammation predisposing for malignancy; an increased cell proliferation due to a chronic inflammation may imply an increased frequency of random mutations promoting carcinogenesis. Also, in a bladder infected with *Schistosoma haematobium* N-nitroso compounds are formed and these may be the responsible agents for an increased cancer risk. Secondary to Bilharzia bacteria may infect the bladder; various strains of bacteria can mediate reactions leading to the formation of *N*-nitrosamines. Inflammatory cells, stimulated as a result of the infection, may induce the endogenous synthesis of *N*-nitrosamines as well as generating oxygen radicals. In addition, some evidence suggests that a disturbed tryptophan metabolism, possibly by liver involvement of the parasite, causes excretion of carcinogenic metabolites *(71,72)*.

Inherited Effect-Modification

Two distinct genes, NAT1 and NAT2, code for acetyltransferase activity in humans. Expression of NAT2 determines whether individuals have slow or rapid N-acetylating metabolism. Some data indicate that this expression modifies the urinary bladder cancer risk after exposure to aromatic amines. Formation of adducts between benzpyrene and hemoglobin may be related to DNA-damage. Among cigarette smokers, relatively slow acetylators have significantly higher levels of such adducts than relatively fast acetylators and acetylation may modify the bladder cancer risk after smoking *(73,74)*. However, we have only sparse data on this issue, and no definitive conclusions can be drawn.

Genetics

Subjects with a family history of urinary bladder cancer have an increased disease risk. However, these findings are probably largely explained by shared life habits (e.g., smoking or a specific diet) rather than by inherited mutations. The rarity of the disease compromises the possibility to find inherited genetic alterations (like an altered *BRCA-2* in breast cancer or *p16* in malignant melanoma). Current data indicate that such inherited alterations, if they exist, explain fewer urinary bladder cases than inherited changes in prostate or breast cancer *(75)*.

Relevance of Micropathology

From epidemiological data we can draw causal inferences concerning the association between exposure distribution in a population and disease incidence when the same population is followed over time. We start with a statistically documented association, determine the possibility that it occurred by chance, and finally judge if the total effect of systematic errors (confounding and bias) explain the increased relative risk or not *(76)*. In doing so, we find, for example, that the distribution of exposure to 2-naphthylamine or smoking in a population influences urinary bladder cancer incidence when the population is followed. A causal relation is documented beyond any reasonably doubt. We also know the cell cycle regulation is disturbed in all investigated tumors.

One invariably finds mutations, or signs of allele deletion or methylation in at least one of the genes *p16*, *p53* and *Rb*, which are involved in cell cycle regulation. However, it is uncertain if etiological insights from population data can, at this point, contribute to an understanding of how carcinogens start and maintain tumor development in an individual. The notion that a specific carcinogen may cause a specific mutations in a specific tumor suppressor gene initially was supported from data on aflatoxin exposure and liver cancer as well as ultraviolet radiation and malignant melanoma. For urinary bladder cancer, efforts to find such associations have so far not provided conclusive evidence.

PREVENTION

Obviously elimination of agents (specific chemicals or mixed exposures) causally linked to urinary bladder cancer lowers disease incidence. If one has been exposed to a specific bladder carcinogen (such as beta-naphthylamine or chlornaphazine) primary prevention of urinary bladder cancer only (to reduce concomitant risk factors) may be motivated. Otherwise, few of us, however, try specifically to prevent urinary bladder cancer: when thinking in preventive terms, we want to hinder any disease that induces distressful symptoms or shortens life. There are situations where contradictory effects imply a real challenge. Consider, for example, estrogenic supplementation after the menopause, giving symptom relief and diminished risk of osteoporosis but creating a small increased breast cancer risk. Such is not the case for the prevention of urinary bladder cancer; there is no doubt that elimination of bladder cancer risks would also promote health in general.

Smokers have an increased risk of about 40 diseases, and a decreased risk of another ten; tobacco smoke contains a plenitude of chemicals with divergent effects. However, the lowered risk of Alzheimer's disease among tobacco users—a fact known by many—is balanced by an increased incidence of stroke. Smokers of middle age have a threefold increased risk in dying from any cause. If fewer young subjects than we see today start to smoke certainly future population health would improve. One can have an optimistic view on this matter. Scientifically, the relation between cancer risk and smoking was convincingly documented during the 1950s by Sir Richard Doll. In some populations smoking prevalence peaked in 1960s or 1970s. In USA, per capita consumption increased from approximately 54 cigarettes per adult in 1900 to 4345 cigarettes per adult in 1963 *(4)*. Many more environments (public transportation, restaurants, schools, family homes) are tobacco-free today than three decades ago. The incidence of some smoking related tumors in many countries, including USA and Sweden, is decreasing. Producing and documenting knowledge such as this can affect personal decisions, community life, legislation and price policies.

A less optimistic view can also be put forward; the number of adults currently smoking cigarettes in the USA has changed little between 1993 and 1997, increasing trends in tobacco smoking among adolescents during the 1990s are worrying, and the regained acceptance of cigar use among better educated men and women increases tobacco use *(4)*. In many developing countries cigarettes are heavily marketed. The rapid increase in cigarette smoking that occurred during the first half of this century, and the resulting epidemic of tobacco-related deaths (first among men and later among women) has stopped. However, we are far from completely eradicating tobacco use from our society.

Should a physician advise a patient with urinary bladder cancer to stop smoking? If patients do not raise the issue, such unwanted information may cause harm by inducing guilt, the afflicted patient experience that he or she is blamed for causing his or her disease. If the patient raises the issue, without hesitation a physician can inform that stopping smoking would improve future expected health. Already after 3 yr the cardiac infarction mortality *(77)*, and possibly also the excess incidence of some other cardio-vascular events *(78)*, has returned to unity—at least for most patients with superficial tumors this reduced mortality risk by far outweighs the mortality risk from urinary bladder cancer. After 10 yr the lung cancer risk is near unity. In addition, smoking cessation may diminish the **recurrence** risk of bladder tumors, although such an effect has not convincingly been documented.

Fewer workers today than some decades ago are significantly exposed to hazardous chemicals due to, for example, technological development, labor market agreements on exposure levels or legislation regulating work environment. Aromatic amines, for example, have been abolished from most work places. However, many subjects are continuously exposed to combustion gases, implying that work-related exposures still are an issue. Also, although chemical hazards have a limited public health impact, the risk of contracting urinary bladder cancer—and other diseases (lung cancer, chronic pulmonary obstruction, allergy) related to the same agents—may be material for workers in some environments. Moreover, in developing countries not being able to afford modern technology, exposure levels probably are higher than in Western countries. Preventing health risks from work-related chemicals is theoretically simple—avoidance of exposure—but in practice a balance between economic realities and health aspects ultimately supervening.

In Western countries, authorities regulate the sales of pharmaceutical substances. When the bladder carcinogenicity of phenacetin and chlornaphazine was recognized, the drugs were withdrawn from the market. Acetaminophen is currently sold as a safe analgesic. Data concerning its possible carcinogenicity are not strong enough to suggest taking regulatory actions. Some regard aspirin (or another drug with acetyl salicylic acid) as an alternative: this drug may in the short run give adverse effects (risk of serious bleeding, risk of life threatening aggravation of bronchial asthma). On the other hand, in the long run it prevents cardiac infarction *(79)*, colon cancer *(65)* and possibly also urinary bladder cancer *(64)*.

Should we recommend an increased fluid intake to prevent urinary bladder cancer? If one drinks more fluid, within reasonable limits and restricted to nonalcoholic beverages, typically no adverse health effects can be expected (except in, for example, individuals with heart failure). Drinking more may prevent kidney stones, in addition to preventing urinary bladder cancer. However, the Physician Health Study indicates that we need to drink 2 L every day to obtain a preventive effect *(34)*.

Concerning intake of beef and pork, two different official committees in England and the USA recently declared that these food items constitute a health hazard - still, this position is controversial. What can be said today is that those who eat fish **instead of** beef and pork diminishes their cardiac infarction risk (fish is protective) and may also avoid urinary bladder, as well as colo-rectal cancer. Also, we have no indication that chicken or turkey negatively influences health, and it may be beneficial to choose these items **instead of** beef or pork. Finally, today the combined epidemiological data does not suggest that frying fish, chicken or turkey in the pan results in substances that affect health when consumed in typical doses. Data on grilling are sparse, and no conclusions can be drawn.

If one considers total health impact, there is no doubt that high fat intake predisposes for overweight or obesity, factors related to an increased overall mortality *(80)*. However, a high total fat intake by itself does not necessarily imply a health hazard. Likewise, diminishing **animal** fat in general is probably beneficial in terms of a reduced cardiovascular morbidity, and may also diminish urinary bladder cancer incidence.

The entire field of diet and health is unfortunate. Official campaigns based on weak scientific evidence were put forward in the beginning of the 1980s; the public's notion to "avoid fat" (with no further specification) will probably lead to a back-lash to the spread of solid nutritional epidemiological evidence especially if, for example, fatty acids in olive oil turns out even to promote health.

There is no doubt that we increase our probability of a long life without distressful symptoms if we have a high intake (possibly more than 400 g per day) of fruits, roots, vegetables and berries. However, a randomized, placebo-controlled chemoprevention study failed to show that intake of beta-carotene decreases lung cancer incidence; smokers comprised the study population, and the mortality was, unexpectedly, higher among those randomized to beta-carotene. Beta-carotene is a vegetabilic precursor to Vitamin A, but it is one of probably more than a hundred carotenoids in our diet. Supraphysiological doses of one of these may, for example, block a combined beneficial effect. It is uncertain if we will ever be able to identify single chemicals in a vegetable rich diet that are the preventive agents. For prevention of urinary bladder cancer, we cannot today give any specific recommendations.

For health in general, a high physical activity level has a substantial effect. However, we have as yet no data to judge if such can prevent urinary bladder cancer incidence.

SCREENING

We lack controlled studies and thereby have no definite scientific evidence for recommending a search for asymptomatic urinary bladder cancer. Some criteria for accepting a screening program in the general population have been put forward. They include that the disease must be an important health problem, the means for screening should have adequate sensitivity and specificity, latent or early symptomatic stages of the disease must be recognizable, and interventions must lead to a decrease in morbidity and mortality (81). Possibly many muscle invasive urinary bladder tumors have an undetected carcinoma in situ for some time before the cancer (by an additional genetic event?) invades. Also, primary cancer in situ can be cured by instillation of BCG or a cytostatic drug in the bladder—a therapy with less long term effects than a cystectomy. Available tests (for microscopic hematuria or malignant cells) have a high sensitivity and a reasonable specificity. Tumors detected in asymptomatic individuals on the average have a lower stage than tumors in subjects seeking health care for bladder symptoms (82, 83). Also, the course of tumors detected in asymptomatic individuals seems to be similar, adjusted for stage and grade, as in sporadic cases. This fact can be put forward as an argument that some tumors would later on have invaded muscle but that they were detected at an earlier stage with a more favorable prognosis. An early detection not altering disease course (lead time) only adds frustration—the patients are aware of their tumor for an extended time but have no benefit from the knowledge.

Thus, the low disease incidence is the only strong argument against investigating whether screening for urinary bladder cancer would be beneficial; the expected gain in overall mortality is low, and one can question if it will outweigh the negative effects, for example, the risk of an unnecessary cystoscopy. Urinary bladder tumors are rarely an incidental finding at autopsy, and it is unlikely that screening in a population would harm by the diagnosis of clinically unimportant tumors.

In certain groups, however, urothelial cancer may be a significant health problem, for example, among workers exposed to high level of aromatic amines or combustion gases and subjects exposed to high levels of phenacetin. Despite the lack of comparative trials addressing if a decreased morbidity or mortality can be achieved, some argue that we have a good rationale for screening for urinary bladder cancer in such populations. The high incidence of squamous cell carcinoma of the urinary bladder in endemic areas with Schistosoma Haematobium may also justify screening. Screening can be performed with a test for detecting microscopic hematuria, malignant cells (cytology) or detection of certain antigens. In the absence of knowledge on inherited genes, genetic screening for urinary bladder cancer is a nonissue.

Uncontrolled screening constitutes a challenging practical problem for the urologic community. Depending on the age, the prevalence of urinary bladder cancer among reported subjects with microscopic hematuria (who agrees to be cystoscopized) varies between 0 and 16% *(84,85)*. Thus, once the hematuria has been found, one can argue against a diagnostic cystoscopy to subjects in whom the hematuria cause is obvious and the disease rare (e.g., in young females with a urinary tract infection) only. Otherwise, it probably should be carried through. Subjects with macroscopic hematuria of unknown cause (and no known contamination of menstrual bleeding) have a high prevalence of urinary bladder cancer.

REFERENCES

1. Parkin DM, Pisani P, Ferlay J. Estimates of the worldwide incidence of 25 major cancers in 1990. Int J Cancer 1999; 80: 827–841.
2. Pisani P, Parkin DM, Bray F, Ferlay J. Estimates of the worldwide mortality from 25 cancers in 1990. Int J Cancer 1999; 83: 18–29.
3. Landis SH, Murray T, Bolden S, Wingo PA. Cancer statistics, 1998 [Published Errata appear in CA Cancer J Clin 1998, 48, 192 and 1998, 48, 329]. Ca Cancer J Clin 1998; 48: 6–29.
4. Wingo PA, Ries LA, Giovino GA, Miller DS, Rosenberg HM, Shopland DR, et al. Annual report to the nation on the status of cancer, 1973–1996, with a special section on lung cancer and tobacco smoking. J Natl Cancer Inst 1999; 91: 675–690.

5. IARC Tobacco Smoking. IARC Monographs on the Evaluation of the Carcinogenic Risk of Chemicals to Humans, Vol 38, IARC, Lyon, 1985, 244–268.

6. Lopez-Abente G, Gonzalez CA, Errezola M. Tobacco smoke inhalation pattern, tobacco type, and bladder cancer in Spain. Am J Epidemiol 1991; 134: 830.

7. Hartge P, Silverman D, Hoover R, et al. Changing cigarette habits and bladder cancer risk: a case-control study. J Natl Cancer Inst 1987; 78: 1119–1125.

8. Hartge P, Hoover R, Kantor AF. Bladder cancer risk and pipes, cigars and smokeless tobacco. Cancer 1985; 55: 901.

9. Steineck G, Plato N, Alfredsson L, Norell SE. Industry-related urothelial carcinogens: application of a job-exposure matrix to census data. Am J Ind Med 1989; 16: 209–224.

10. Steineck G, Norell SE, Feychting M. Diet, tobacco, and urothelial cancer: a 14-year follow-up of 16,477 subjects. Acta Oncol 1988; 77: 323–327.

11. IARC Overall Evaluations of Carcinogenicity: an Updating of IARC Monographs Volumes 1 to 42. IARC Monographs on the Evaluation of the Carcinogenic Risk of Chemicals to Humans, Supplement 7; IARC, Lyon, 1987.

12. Talaska G, Schamer M, Skipper P, Tannerbaum S, Caporaso N, Unruh L, et al. Detection of carcinogen-DNA adducts in exfoliated urothelial cells of cigarette smokers: association with smoking, hemoglobin adducts, and urinary mutagenicity. Cancer Epidemiol Biom Prev 1991; 1: 61–66.

13. Silverman DT, Levin LI, Hoover RN, et al. Occupational risks of bladder cancer in the United States. I. White men. J Natl Cancer Inst 1989; 81: 1472–1480.

14. Silverman DT, Levin LI, Hoover RN. Occupational risks of bladder cancer among white women in the United States. Am J Epidemiol 1990; 132: 453.

15. Mannetje A, Kogevinas M, Chang-Claude J, Cordier S, Gonzalez CA, Hours M, et al. Occupation and bladder cancer in European women. Cancer Causes and Control 1999; 10: 209–217.

16. Mannetje A, Kogevinas M, Chang-Claude J, Cordier S, Gonzalez CA, Hours M, et al. Smoking as a confounder in case-control studies of occupational bladder cancer in women. Am J Ind Med 1999; 36: 75–82.

17. Rehn L. Blasengeschwülste bei fuchsin-arbeitern. Arch Family Med 1895; 50: 588–600.

18. Hueper WC, Wiley FH, Wolfe HD. Experimental production of bladder tumours in dogs by administration of beta-naphthylamine. J Indust Hyg Toxicol 1938; 20: 46–81.

19. Case RAM. Tumours of the urinary tract as an occupational disease in several industries. Ann R Coll Surg Engl 1966; 39: 213–235.

20. Case RAM, Pearson JT. Tumours of the urinary bladder in workers engaged in the manufacture and use of certain dyestuff intermediates in the Brittish chemical industry. Part II. Further consideration of the role of aniline and of the manufacture of auramine and magenta (fuchsine) as possible causative agents. Br J Ind Med 1954; 11: 213–216.

21. Case RAM, Hosker ME, Mcdonald DB, Pearson JT. Tumours of the urinary bladder in workers engaged in the manufacture and use of certain dyestuff intermediates in the Brittish chemical industry. Part I.The role of aniline, benzidine, alpha-naphthylamine and beta-naphthylamine. Br J Ind Med 1954; 11: 75–104.

22. Hicks RM, Wright R, Wakefield JSJ. The induction of rat bladder cancer by 2-naphthylamine. Br J Cancer 1982; 46: 646–661.

23. He MRJA, Mason T, Mettlin C, Vogler WJ, Maygarden S, Liu E. P53 mutations in bladder tumors from arylamine-exposed workers. Cancer Res 1996; 56: 294–298.

24. Ward E, Smith AB, Halperin W. 4,4'-methylenebis (2-chloroaniline): an unregulated carcinogen. Am J Ind Med 1987; 12: 537–549.

25. Thériault G, Tremblay C, Cordier S, Gingras S. Bladder cancer in the aluminum industry. Lancet 1984; i: 947–950.

26. Henry SA, Kennaway NM, Kennaway EL. Incidence of cancer of bladder and prostate in certain occupations. J Hyg 1931; 31: 125–137.
27. Gustavsson P, Gustavsson A, Hogstedt C. Excess of cancer among Swedish chimney sweeps. Br J Ind Med 1988; 45: 777–781.
28. Steineck G, Plato N, Gerhardsson M, Norell SE, Hogstedt C. Increased risk of urothelial cancer in Stockholm during 1985–87 after exposure to benzene and exhausts. Int J Cancer 1990; 45: 1012–1017.
29. Steineck G, Plato N, Norell SE, Hogstedt C. Urothelial cancer and some industry-related chemicals, an evaluation of the epidemiologic evidence. Am J Ind Med 1990; 17: 371–391.
30. Silverman DT, Hoover RN, Mason TJ, Swanson GM. Motor exhausts-related occupations and bladder cancer. Cancer Res 1986; 46: 2113–2116.
31. Yin SN, Hayes RB, Linet MS, Li GL, Dosemeci M, Travis LB, Zhang ZN, et al. An expanded cohort of cancer among benzene-exposed workers in China. Benzine Study Group. Environ Health Perspect 1996; 104: 1339–1341.
32. Jensen OM, Wahrendorf J, Knudsen JB, Sorensen BL. The Copenhagen case-control study of bladder cancer. II. Effect of coffee and other beverages. Int J Cancer 1986; 37: 651–657.
33. Kunze E, Chang-Claude J, Frentzel-Beyme R. Life style and occupational risk factors for bladder cancer in Germany. Cancer 1992; 69: 1776–1790.
34. Michaud DS, Spiegelman D, Clinton SK, Rimm EB, Curhan GC, Willett WC, Giovannucci EL. Fluid intake and the risk of bladder cancer in men. N Engl J Med 1999; 340: 1390–1397.
35. Hsing AW, McLaughlin JK, Chow WH, Schuman LM, Co Chien HT, Gridley G, et al. Risk factors for colorectal cancer in a prospective study among U.S. white men. Int J Cancer 1998; 77: 549–553.
36. Carstensen JM, Bygren LO, Hatschek T. Cancer incidence among Swedish brewery workers. Int J Cancer 1990; 45: 393–396.
37. Cantor KP, Lynch CF, Hildesheim ME, Dosemeci M, Lubin J, Alavanja M, Craun G. Drinking water source and chlorination byproducts. I. Risk of bladder cancer. Epidemiol 1998; 9: 21–28.
38. Cantor KP, Hoover R, Hartge P, Mason TJ, Silverman DT, Altman R, et al. Bladder cancer, drinking water source, and tap water consumption: a case-control study. J Natl Cancer Inst 1987; 79: 1269–1279.
39. Chiang HS, Guo HR, Hong CL, Lin SM, Lee EF. The incidence of bladder cancer in the black foot disease endemic area in Taiwan. Br J Urol 1993; 71: 274–278.
40. Chen CJ, Chen CW, Wu MM, Kuo TL. Cancer potential in liver, lung, bladder and kidney due to ingested inorganic arsenic in drinking water. Br J Cancer 1992; 66: 888–892.
41. Brown KG, Chen CJ. Significance of exposure assessment to analysis of cancer risk from inorganic arsenic in drinking water in Taiwan. Risk Analysis 1995; 15: 475–484.
42. Cole P. Coffee-drinking and cancer of the lower urinary tract. Lancet 1971; i: 1335–1337.
43. Viscoli CM, Lachs MS, Horwitz RI. Bladder cancer and coffee drinking: a summary of case-control research. Lancet 1993; 341: 1432–1437.
44. Reddy BS. Chemoprevention of colon cancer by dietary administration of naturally-occurring and related synthetic agents. Adv Exp Med Biol 1997; 400B: 931–936.
45. Steineck G, Hagman U, Gerhardsson M, Norell SE. Vitamin A supplements, fried foods, fat and urothelial cancer. a case-referent study in Stockholm in 1985–87. Int J Cancer 1990; 45: 1006–1011.

46. Jägerstad M, Laser Reuterswärd A, Öste R, Dahlqvist A. Creatine and Maillard products as precursors of mutagenic compounds formed in fried beef. In: *The Maillard Reaction in Foods and Nutrition* (Waller GR, Feather MS, eds.). ACS Symposium series 215, American Chemical Society, Washington, DC, 1983, pp. 507–519.

47. Takahashi M, Toyoda K, Aze Y, Furuta K, Mitsumori K, Hayashi Y. The rat urinary bladder as a new target of heterocyclic amine carcinogenicity: tumor induction by 3-amino-1-methyl-5h-pyrido[4,3-b]indole acetate. Jap J Cancer Res 1993; 84: 852–858.

48. Hashida C, Nagayama K, Takemura N. Induction of bladder cancer in mice by implanting pellets containing tryptophan pyrolysis products. Cancer Lett 1982; 17: 101–105.

49. Augustsson K, Skog K, Jagerstad M, Steineck G. Assessment of the human exposure to heterocyclic amines. Carcinogenesis 1997; 18: 1931–1935.

50. Skog K, Augustsson K, Steineck G, Stenberg M, Jägerstad, M. Polar and non-polar heterocyclic amines in cooked fish and meat products and their corresponding pan residues. Food Chem Toxicol 1997; 35: 555–565.

51. Augustsson K, Lindblad J, Övervik E, Steineck G. A population-based dietary inventory of cooked meat and assessment of the daily intake of food mutagens. Food Addit Contam 1999; 16: 215–225.

52. Skog K, Steineck G, Augustsson K, Jagerstad M. Effect of cooking temperature on the formation of heterocyclic amines in fried meat products and pan residues. Carcinogenesis 1995; 16: 861–867.

53. Augustsson K, Skog K, Jagerstad M, Dickman PW, Steineck G. Dietary heterocyclic amines and cancer of the colon, rectum, bladder, and kidney: a population-based study. Lancet 1999; 353: 703–707.

54. Messing EM. Growth factors and bladder cancer: clinical implications of the interactions between growth factors and their urothelial receptors. Semin Surg Oncol 1992; 8: 285–292.

55. Whelan P. Retinoids in chemoprevention. Eur Urol 1999; 35: 424–428.

56. Alfthan O, Tarkkanen J, Gröhn P, Heinonen E, Pyrhönen S, Säilä K. Tigason (etretinate) in prevention of recurrence of superficial bladder tumors. a double-blind clinical trial. Eur Urol 1983; 9: 6–9.

57. Michaud DS, Spiegelman D, Clinton SK, Rimm EB, Willett WC, Giovannucci EL. Fruit and vegetable intake and incidence of bladder cancer in a male prospective cohort. J Natl Cancer Inst 1999; 91: 605–613.

58. Hoover RN, Hartge P. Artificial sweeteners and human bladder cancer. Lancet 1980; I: 837–840.

59. Silverman DT, Hartge P, Morrison AS, Devesa SS. Epidemiology of bladder cancer. Hematol Oncol Clin North Am 1992; 6: 1–30.

60. Shahin M, Smith BL, Worral S, Moore MR, Seawright AA, Prakash AS. Bracken fern carcinogenesis: multiple intravenous doses of activated ptaquiloside induce DNA adducts, monocytosis, increased TNF alpha levels, and mammary gland carcinoma in rats. Biochem Biophys Res Commun 1998; 244: 192–197.

61. IARC bracken fern (pteridium aquilinum) and some of its constituents. IARC monographs on the evaluation of the carcinogenic risk of chemicals to humans. 1986; 40: 47–65.

62. Hultengren N, Lagergren C, Ljungqvist A. Carcinoma of the renal pelvis in renal papillary necrosis. Acta Chir Scand 1965; 3: 314–320.

63. Piper JM, Matanoski GM, Tonascia J. Bladder cancer in young women. Am J Epidemiol 1986; 123: 1033–1042.

64. Steineck G, Gerhardsson de Verdier M, Wiholm B-E. Acetaminophen, some other drugs, some diseases, and the risk of transitional cell carcinoma. Acta Oncol 1995; 34: 741–748.

65. Marnett LJ. Aspirin and related nonsteroidal anti-inflammatory drugs as chemopreventive agents against colon cancer. Prev Med 1995; 24: 103–106.

66. Thiede T, Christensen BC. Bladder tumors induced by chlornaphazine. A five-year follow-up study of chlornaphazine-treated patients with polycythaemia. Acta Med Scand 1969; 185: 133–137.

67. Khan MA, Travis LB, Lynch CF, Soini Y, Hruszkewycz AM, Delgado RM, et al. P53 mutations in cyclophosphamide-associated bladder cancer. Cancer Epidemiol Biom Prev 1998; 7: 397–403.

68. Kleinerman RA, Boice JDJ, Storm HH, Sparen P, Andersen A, Pukkala E, et al. Second primary cancer after treatment for cervical cancer. An International Cancer Registries Study. Cancer 1995; 76: 442–452.

69. Kantor AF, Hartge P, Hoover RN, Fraumeni JF. Epidemiological characteristics of squamous cell carcinoma and adenocarcinoma of the bladder. Cancer Res 1988; 48: 3853–3855.

70. Tawfik HN. Carcinoma of the urinary bladder associated with schistosomiasis in Egypt: the possible causal relationship. Princess Takamatsu Symp 1987; 18: 197–209.

71. Mostafa MH, Sheweita SA, O'Connor PJ. Relationship between schistosomiasis and bladder cancer. Clin Microbiol Rev 1999; 12: 97–111.

72. Tricker AR, Mostafa MH, Spiegelhalder B, Preussmann R. Urinary excretion of nitrate, nitrite and n-nitroso compounds in schistosomiasis and bilharzia bladder cancer patients. Carcinogenesis 1989; 10: 547–552.

73. Bartsch H, Caporaso N, Coda M, Kadlubar F, Malaveille C, Skipper P, et al. Carcinogen hemoglobin adducts, urinary mutagenicity, and metabolic phenotype in active and passive cigarette smokers. J Natl Cancer Inst 1990; 82: 1826–1831.

74. Vineis P, Caporaso N, Tannenbaum SR, Skipper PL, Glogowski J, Bartsch H, et al. Acetylation phenotype, carcinogen-hemoglobin adducts, and cigarette smoking. Cancer Res 1990; 50: 3002–3004.

75. Hemminki K, Vaittinen P. National database of familial cancer in Sweden. Genet Epidemiol 1998; 15: 225–236.

76. Steineck G, Kass P, Ahlbom A. A comprehensive clinical epidemiological theory for bias recognizing four distinct study stages. Acta Oncol 1998; 154: 15–23.

77. Kawachi I, Colditz GA, Stampfer MJ, Willett WC, Manson JE, Rosner B, et al. Smoking cessation and time course of decreased risks of coronary heart disease in middle-aged women. Arch Int Med 1994; 154: 169–175.

78. Kawachi I, Colditz GA, Stampfer MJ, Willett WC, Manson JE, Rosner B, et al. Smoking cessation and decreased risk of stroke in women. JAMA 1993; 269: 232–236.

79. Hennekens CH. Update on aspirin in the treatment and prevention of cardiovascular disease. Am Heart J 1999; 137: S9–S13.

80. Calle EE, Thun MJ, Petrelli JM, Rodriguez C, Heath CW Jr. Body-mass index and mortality in a prospective cohort of U.S. adults. N Engl J Med 1999; 341: 1097–1105.

81. Cadman D, Chambers L, Feldman W, Sackett D. Assessing the effectiveness of community screening programs. JAMA 1984; 251: 1580–1585.

82. Mayfield MP, Whelan P. Bladder tumours detected on screening: results at 7 years. Br J Urol 1998; 82: 825–828.

83. Kryger JV, Messing E. Bladder cancer screening. Semin Oncol 1996; 23: 585–597.

84. Froom P, Froom J, Ribak J. Asymptomatic microscopic hematuria—is investigation necessary? J Clin Epidemiol 1997; 50: 1197–1200.

85. Messing EM, Young TB, Hunt VB, Emoto SE, Wehbie JM. The significance of asymptomatic microhematuria in men 50 or more years old. Findings of a home screening study using urinary dipsticks. J Urol 1989; 137: 919–925.

2

Biology and Molecular Aspects of Development and Progression of Bladder Cancer

Dan Theodorescu, MD, PHD
and William A. See, MD

CONTENTS

INTRODUCTION AND OBJECTIVES

Carcinoma of the urinary bladder is the second most common urologic malignancy *(1)*. Not only are neoplasms of the urinary bladder of high clinical relevance, but they represent one of the best understood of the genito-urinary (GU) neoplasms. Relative to other tumors, the etiology, natural history, tumor biology, treatment options and outcome for the spectrum of bladder malignancies are well defined. This level of understanding arises as a consequence of multiple factors and represents a convergence of knowledge from diverse scientific disciplines. Insight provided by these disciplines, coupled with unique features of this neoplasm which make it assessable for detection, monitoring and treatment, combine to make this disease a model system for modern oncology.

From: *Current Clinical Urology: Bladder Cancer: Current Diagnosis and Treatment*
Edited by: M. J. Droller © Humana Press Inc., Totowa, NJ

The intent of this chapter is to provide the reader an overview of our current understanding of this tumor from the standpoint of its clinical and molecular biology. To this end, a brief review of the clinical biology will be provided to serve as a backdrop against which our molecular understanding of this tumor has proceeded. Indeed the process through which our insights into this neoplasm have evolved, "hypothesis generating" clinical observation followed by scientific investigation, can serve as a paradigm for our work in other GU tumors.

Proceeding from a brief review of the clinical biology it is the author's intent to present our current understanding of the molecular basis for the biology of this disease. Finally in closing, we will provide a brief consideration of what relevance these molecular insights may hold for the future clinical management of patients with bladder neoplasms in terms of detection, monitoring, treatment and prognosis.

CLINICAL BIOLOGY AND NATURAL HISTORY

Histologic Types of Bladder Cancer

Neoplasms involving the urinary bladder encompass a spectrum of histologic types (2). Any of the cellular elements composing the bladder wall and its lining can undergo malignant transformation. Furthermore, specific elements may de-differentiate into more primitive phenotypes under the influence of specific etiologic factors. In order of prevalence, the histologic variants comprising bladder neoplasms are transitional, squamous cell, adenocarcinoma, and finally sarcoma. While there are significant geographic variations in the relative incidence of these different histologic types, particularly as it pertains to squamous cell carcinoma, in the United States, transitional cell carcinoma in its variants are by far the most common type (2). In addition to marked differences in their incidence, squamous cell carcinoma and adenocarcinomas involving the urinary bladder are distinct from transitional cell carcinomas in multiple respects including their etiology, epidemiology, and clinical biology. It is beyond the scope of this chapter to attempt to exhaustively deal with these differences. Consequently this work will focus exclusively on transitional cell carcinoma of the urinary bladder.

As a point of histologic clarification it is important to understand that it is not uncommon for transitional cell malignancies to have minor elements which have dedifferentiated along adenomatous or squamous cell lines. However, from the clinical management standpoint, urinary neoplasms with minor components of these two histologic types are treated for their primary component. The clinical relevance of these minor components or the percentage at which a minor component becomes clinically significant is poorly defined at this time.

Clinical Biology: Superficial Tumors

In the transformation pathway which leads to the development of superficial transitional carcinoma the most striking biologic feature is the propensity for tumor recurrence. Recurrence polychronotropism (multiple in space and time) in superficial bladder tumors is uniquely high relative to any other organ site. Up to 70% of patients ultimately suffer disease recurrence *(3,4)*. While in the absence of progression recurrence per se is not life threatening, this phenomenon nonetheless constitutes a cause of significant morbidity and treatment expense. While less common, the progression of superficial tumors to muscle invasion has potential mortal consequence. Progression risks vary widely by stage, and grade ranging from less than 5% for TA grade 1 up to 50% for T1 lesions with associated carcinoma *in situ (5)*.

Clinical Biology: Invasive Tumors

For tumors in the invasive pathway, the pivotal issue dictating patient survival is tumor metastasis. The propensity for invasive TCC to disseminate by both lymphatic and hematogenous routes is clearly established. At some point in their disease history 40–50% of patients in this group will manifest metastatic disease *(6,7)*. Liver, lung, and regional lymph nodes represent the sites most commonly involved by metastatic disease.

Predictors of Clinical Behavior

The management of urothelial neoplasms is undergoing a period of transition where a number of new markers are being assessed for their clinical utility relative to the conventional prognostic benchmarks of tumor stage and grade. As an example, there is an active phase III trial which stratifies patient management according to *P53* status *(8)*. However, at this juncture, the "historic" parameters remain the proven and widely utilized prognosticators upon which clinical decision making is based. Even so, the current classification system has shortcomings. The staging system for superficial bladder tumors illustrates some of these limitations.

Superficial bladder tumors are defined as limited to the bladder layers above the muscularis propria. While not a surprising consequence of the "superficial" vs "invasive" categorization, the tendency of some clinicians to view so called superficial disease as a single entity represents a serious shortcoming of the present staging system. In reality, tumors within the superficial category are far more complex and represent a spectrum of malignancy encompassing no less than 7 stage/grade categories. Each of these has a potentially different relevant clinical endpoint. Despite this seeming complexity, these seven categories can be broadly divided into two subcategories based upon their relevant clinical endpoints of either recurrence or progression. As a high recurrence risk is a common feature of all categories of superficial bladder cancer it is progression risk that primarily distinguishes them. We propose that for the purpose of clinical decision making, superficial bladder cancer should therefore be divided into low and high risk categories based upon progression risk. Low risk tumors would encompass grade 1 and 2 Ta lesions with high risk tumors including carcinoma *in situ*, T1, and any grade 3 tumor. The above proposal is not intended to supplant the need for TNM staging but rather to be complimentary and highlight to the clinician the distinct biology of the different stage/grade classifications of so called superficial tumors.

The current stage and grading system works well for clinical management of the invasive categories of bladder neoplasms. In general, the staging system distinguishes organ confined vs metastatic neoplasms. These categorizations provide good correlation with prognosis and treatment outcome. The recognition that extravesical tumor spread, and node positivity portend poorer outcome, are currently being used as the basis for patient stratification into studies of adjuvant chemotherapy.

Stage and grade have been and remain important clinical tools for patient management. However, the current system functions best at the extremes of the neoplastic process, specifically low grade/stage tumors and high grade/stage tumors. Regrettably, a significant portion of patients will fall between these boundaries. For these patients stage and grade classification remain relatively crude indicators of individual tumor biology. The next section will discuss exciting work, which is making progress towards a more sophisticated understanding of the molecular level cellular functions, which constitute the very soul of tumor biology.

TUMOR DEVELOPMENT

The first insight into the etiology of transitional cell carcinomas of the urinary bladder began with the observation of an increased incidence associated with industrial development. Workers in the aniline dye industry in Germany were noted to be at increased risk for the development of this tumor *(9)*. This association made bladder neoplasms the first of what would subsequently be recognized as many chemically induced tumors. Subsequent understanding has come to identify the process of uroepithelial transformation as one of contact carcinogenesis. Carcinogens ingested by one of multiple routes, either inhaled, consumed, or absorbed through the skin, are concentrated in the urine and subsequently come in contact with the lining of the urinary tract. This diffuse exposure predisposes to what has come to be known as field change. Thus the entire uroepithelium to which urine has been exposed may have multiple areas of frank or preneoplastic transformation.

Early clinical observations regarding the biology of the "at risk" field suggested that sites of preneoplastic changes could follow several distinct clinical courses. It is possible that areas of dysplasia remain simply dysplastic. Alternatively, the urinary epithelium can progress either to superficial bladder neoplasms, characterized by recurrence but rare life threatening progression, or along the path towards invasion with its well recognized risk of mortality. Evidence in support of these disparate pathways comes from the low progression rate of the majority of superficial bladder tumors, coupled with the fact that many invasive neoplasms present as such initially. An example of a clinical evidence based pathway detailing these distinctions in tumor biology is illustrated in Fig. 1 *(10)*. Insight afforded by these clinical observations has played a central role in generating hypotheses, developing models, and directing basic research in bladder cancer. Not only have these clinical observations served as the basis for research undertakings, but these subsequent research activities have in turn provided strong evidence to support the validity of these clinical models.

Carcinogenesis

Models of molecular carcinogenesis must explain the relevant clinical natural history and aspects of tumor behavior such as uncontrolled cellular proliferation, neovascularization, and altered apoptosis. In addition, models of neoplastic transformation should account for other clinically relevant features of the neoplasm in question. For superficial and invasive transitional cell carcinomas of the urinary bladder, these would include tumor recurrence and tumor metastasis respectively.

The historic view of two stage carcinogenesis in which tumor initiation (mutation) is followed by tumor promotion (epigenetic changes) has been conceptually important but is currently thought to be too simplistic. It is now believed that there may be six or more independent mutational events *(11,12)* necessary for carcinogenesis. Furthermore,

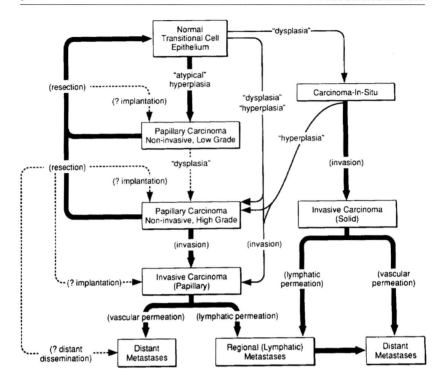

Fig. 1. Proposed pathway for bladder tumor development derived from clinical observation. Note that the superficial and invasive pathways are distinct, with divergence early in the process of tumorigenesis. (From Jones PA, Droller MJ. Pathways of development and progression in bladder cancer: new correlations between clinical observations and molecular mechanisms. Semin Urol 1993; 11: 177–192).

chemical carcinogens may be genotoxic, non-genotoxic (13) or induce epigenetic effects (14) with dose response relations being linear or non-linear (15,16). Endogenous mutagenic mechanisms such as DNA oxy-radical damage, de-purination and polymerase infidelity also contribute to carcinogenesis (12,17–19) leading to a debate regarding the relative importance of endogenous versus exogenous mutagenic events and the value of animal bioassays or short term mutagenic assays for assessment of human cancer risks (11,18,20,21). In the section below we will discuss two of the best characterized molecular paradigms leading to transitional cell carcinoma. Together, these will highlight how the effect of a chemical carcinogen may be altered by the characteristics of the host and serve as both a model system and framework for further research in this area.

Many different exposures and risk factors have been identified in bladder cancer. In the late nineteenth century, the German physician Rehn observed an association between the occurrence of bladder cancer and exposure of workers to aromatic amines (arylamines) and polycyclic aromatic hydrocarbons (PAH) compounds found in the dyestuff industry. In addition to these environmental exposures, tobacco smoking has also been associated with an elevated risk for multiple types of human cancers (22). Several of the chemicals identified in tobacco smoke have been shown to cause cancer in laboratory animals (23). The property that is common to all of the diverse types of chemical carcinogens is that they can form directly or are metabolized to highly reactive electrophilic forms (24). These electron deficient species can attack the many electron rich or nucleophilic sites in molecules such as proteins and nucleic acids to form covalent adducts or induce mutagenesis (25). There is considerable evidence to suggest that DNA is the molecular target of these agents. Damage to DNA induced by these adducts is hypothesized to lead to mutations in proto oncogenes and/or tumor suppressor genes. Two components of tobacco smoke, benzopyrene, a PAH, and 4-aminobiphenyl, an arylamine, form adducts with DNA, suggesting that these components may be direct mutagens contributing to the development of bladder cancer.

Interestingly, neither PAHs nor arylamines are direct carcinogens and therefore it would seem that additional steps are necessary for their activation and metabolism (Fig. 2A). The normal role of the host enzymes which act on chemical carcinogens is to convert these foreign lipophilic compounds into more hydrophilic forms that can be readily excreted. However, in attempting to create a hydrophilic product, these enzymes inadvertently form a reactive product. Most of these reactions are catalyzed by cytochrome P450 dependent mono oxygenases located predominantly in the liver. In the case of carcinogenic arylamines, the first step in this process is N-oxidation catalyzed by hepatic cytochrome P450 1A2 isoenzyme (CYP1A2) (26). This enzyme has been shown to be inducible by several environmental factors including cigarette smoke, which has resulted in significant individual and population variability when the activity of this enzyme is measured (27). Due to its critical role, it is not surprising to find indirect evidence that a phenotype associated with enhanced CYP1A2 activity, may be a risk factor for bladder cancer (28). These electrophilic metabolically active forms of arylamines or hydroxylamines can form adducts with hemoglobin or circulate freely as glucuronide conjugates and be excreted in the urine (29). Hydroxylamines are then hydrolyzed in the acidic urinary environment allowing formation of adducts with nucleophilic sites in the transitional bladder mucosa.

Fortunately, alternative processing of arylamines can occur by detoxi-fying pathways (Fig. 2A), with the most studied of these pathways being *N*-acetylation. Two isoenzymes of *N*-acetyltransferase (NAT 1 and NAT 2) have been identified in humans *(25)*. The NAT2 enzyme is encoded by a single polymorphic gene, with individuals having any two of several possible mutant alleles display a slow acetylator phenotype and hence exhibit impaired detoxification of carcinogenic arylamine *(30)* (Fig. 2B). Several recent case control studies have investigated the relationship of NAT2 phenotype or genotype and bladder cancer risk *(31–33)* and have demonstrated that "slow aceltylators", namely, individuals who detoxify arylamines slowly due to decreased activity of these pathways, have substantially higher risk of bladder cancer. On the other hand, NAT2 does not appear to play a role in bladder carcinogenesis induced by PAH *(34)*. In addition to NAT2, glutathione S transferase M1 (GST-M1), a family member of a class of enzymes which detoxify reactive chemicals by promoting their conjugation to glutathione *(35)* has also been studied in relation to bladder cancer risk. Metabolites of several PAH that are present in cigarette smoke as well as arylamines are known or potential substrates of GST-M1 *(35,36)*. Thus, NAT2 and GSTM1 likely play key roles in the risk for bladder cancer development in individuals exposed to similar doses/durations of carcinogens. In addition, the status of these enzymes may explain in part the wide variation in bladder cancer risk in different ethnic and racial groups *(37,38)*. Both NAT2 and GSTMI have shown racial/ethnic variations which may explain in part why similar smoking habits result in different risks of bladder cancer *(31,36,39)*.

A number of specific genes are known to be mutated by chemical car-cinogens. Two of the genes, *HRAS* and *P53*, have also been implicated in bladder tumorigenesis and progression. The *HRAS* gene codes for p21Ras, a small GTPase involved in signal transduction *(40)*, which was the first proto oncogene found to be mutated in the T24 bladder cancer cell line *(41)*. Evidence from clinical studies using immunohistochemi-cal techniques has demonstrated a correlation between the levels of the Ras protein and the degree of tumor invasiveness and that *HRAS* expres-sion is an independent prognostic variable for tumor invasion *(42)*. In addition, an in vivo *(43)* study has implicated this molecule in several of the steps involved in tumor invasion, supporting the notion that *HRAS* overexpression is causally related to tumor progression and not merely epiphenomenon. Detailed staining for *HRAS* in normal bladder tissue has revealed that the basal (progenitor) cells of the multilayered transi-tional epithelium stain with the highest intensity while more superficial (differentiated) compartments stain to a much lesser degree. Thus the level of normal *HRAS* protein diminishes considerably with differentia-

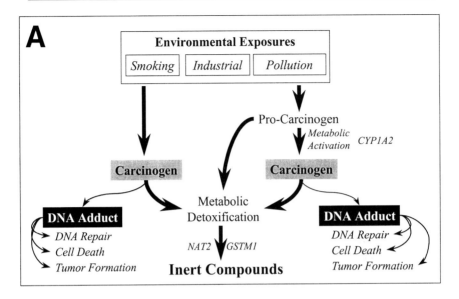

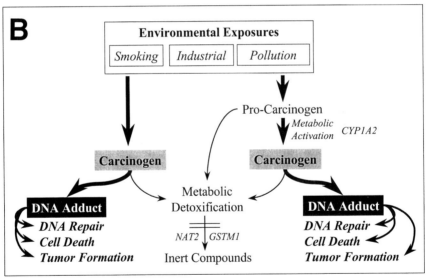

Fig. 2. Hypothetical model of carcinogen activation and detoxification and resulting cellular consequences in (**A**) patients with normal detoxification, and (**B**) in individuals with abnormal detoxification mechanisms. Abbreviations: CYP1A2, hepatic cytochrome P450 1A2; NAT 2, *N*-acetyltransferase 2; GST-M1, glutathione S transferase M1.

tion. However, *HRAS* overexpression per se is not restricted to the malignant state in bladder tissue. It is thus conceivable that a deregulation of *HRAS* gene expression *(42)* or expression of a mutant protein *(41)* can occur and result in the induction of bladder cancer. Support for this idea comes from results demonstrating that transfection of an *HRAS* gene will convert SV40 immortalized human urothelial cells into invasive transitional cell carcinomas *(44,45)*. Recent reports *(46,47)* utilizing PCR-based methods, revealed that approximately 40% of bladder tumors harbor *HRAS* codon 12 mutations.

For genotoxic carcinogens, the interaction with DNA is likely not to be random, and each class of agents reacts selectively with purine and pyrimidine targets *(48,49)*. In addition, targeting of carcinogens to particular sites in DNA is determined by the nucleic acid sequence *(50)*, by specific DNA repair processes and host cell type, making some genetic sequences more at risk than others. As expected from this chemistry, genotoxic carcinogens are potent mutagens, able to cause base mispairing or small deletions, leading to missense or nonsense mutations *(48)*, but the spectra of mutations seems to be dependent on the agent. For example, the mutations found in activated *RAS* protooncogenes associated with tumors of animals exposed to *N*-nitroso compounds are predominantly G:C to A:T base substitutions *(51)*. Although there are several guanine residues in *RAS* codons that would generate a transforming protein if substituted by adenine, these experiments have revealed that the mutations detected in tumors occur overwhelmingly at only one of the possible mutation sites. PAHs, on the other hand, produce a different mutation spectrum *(52)*, and other chemical classes, such as tobacco-specific nitrosamines, have yet other spectra *(53)*. In vitro studies using either prokaryotic or human cells, indicate that human exposure to mutagens may result in a narrow non-random spectrum of mutations *(54)*. Finally, adding another layer of complexity in humans, the spectra of *KRAS* gene mutations in adenocarcinomas vary according to tissue sites, indicating that mutational spectra may be dependent on the causal agent, the target gene and the tissue involved.

Another important genetic target for chemical carcinogenesis is the *P53* tumor suppressor. This gene is of particular relevance in bladder cancer because of its putative roles in both transformation *(55)* and progression *(8)*. Mutations in the *P53* tumor suppressor gene are a frequent event in both transitional cell and squamous cell carcinomas of the bladder *(56)* with up to 40% of bladder cancers harboring such lesions. Especially valuable have been studies of the timing of occurrence of these mutations during different stages of bladder cancer pathogenesis. Mutations are rare in low-grade papillary tumors but are common in CIS and more invasive high-grade bladder cancers, suggesting that *P53* may play a role in both transformation *(55)* and progression *(8)*. Recent immunohistochemical studies of patients with bladder TCC have revealed a significant correlation between the number of cigarettes smoked and the incidence of positive *P53* immunohistochemistry. Studies comparing cases of bladder cancer from smoking and nonsmoking patients showed an increased frequency of G:C to C:G transversions in both groups. While smokers did not have a different mutational spectrum than non-smokers, they did exhibit a higher frequency of double mutation events *(57,58)*. Mutations in *P53* are particularly detrimental due to this gene's multiple cellular regulatory and supervisory roles *(59)*.

Molecular Basis of Tumor Development

The molecular basis of urothelial transformation and progression can be deduced from numerous studies carried out over the last several years. Using cytogenetic, molecular genetic and immunohistochemical methods, a general pattern seems to be emerging as to which genes and/ or chromosomal locations are important for tumor development and progression. In this section we will highlight the genetic abnormalities associated with neoplastic transformation and focus on those associated with progression later on. Multistage carcinogenesis is regarded as a consequence of the accumulation of somatic genetic alterations which include activation of cellular proto oncogenes, and the inactivation of tumor suppressor genes. As outlined above for Ras and *P53*, environmental carcinogens can induce alterations of both gene types. In addition, to these studies, a large number of reports have surveyed the cytogenetic changes found in TCC *(60)*. Studies of TCC revealed consistently high incidence of chromosomal abnormalities in chromosome 9 *(61)* and 17p *(62)*.

Currently, it would appear that chromosome 9 *(63)* and *P53 (64)* changes may occur relatively early in the genesis of TCC while other changes such as EGFR and E-Cadherin are associated with progression. Chromosome 9 deletions are often found early in bladder tumor development, a finding also observed in other cancers such as lung *(65)*, ovary *(66)* and kidney *(67)*. A candidate tumor suppressor gene *CDKN2A*:p16 was recently identified in the 9p21 region *(68)*, an area commonly altered in bladder cancer *(60)*. *CDKN2A* encodes a protein which is part of a new group of cell cycle inhibitory molecules known as cyclin dependent protein kinases (CDK) *(69)*. Among these are also p15 (*INK4B/MTS2*) which together with p16 can inhibit the phosphorylation of the retinoblastoma protein (*RB*), thereby inhibiting the cell cycle. Loss of either of these genes may have profound implications on the cell cycle and result in uncontrolled growth and tumor formation. The loss of p16, often accompanied by p15 loss is a very frequent occurrence in bladder cancer, occurring in up to 40% of cases *(70)*. The importance of *P53* in bladder tumorigenesis was suggested by the high frequency of LOH of chromosome 17p where this gene is located (17p13.1). *P53* codes for a 53kDa phosphoprotein with DNA binding properties which is involved in multiple cell functions including gene transcription, monitoring the fidelity of DNA synthesis and apoptosis *(71)*. *P53* mutations may be induced by carcinogens as outlined above, resulting in a selective growth advantage of cells harboring these defects. The role of *P53* as a target for chemical carcinogenesis was discussed earlier. While there is significant evidence to support the role of *P53* in bladder tumor progression, the role of *P53* has only recently been clarified in tumorigenesis of TCC. Recent genetic evidence has suggested that different clinical forms of TCC may result from different genetic lesions *(55)*. A model has been recently proposed which hypothesizes two different pathways leading to the development of superficial bladder tumors including carcinoma in situ (Fig. 3). This model postulates that chromosome 9 alterations in normal cells lead to papillary superficial TCC while *P53* mutations lead to carcinoma *in situ* (CIS/Tis). Both *P53* and chromosome 9 losses can play a complimentary role further downstream in tumor progression in concert with other genetic changes.

In addition to these changes, microsatellite instability at loci on chromosome 9, was found in TCC *(72)*. Microsatellites are sequences of polymorphic nucleotide repeats found throughout the human genome *(73,74)*, which are routinely used in the analysis of loss of heterozygosity (LOH) in human cancers. In addition, abnormalities or instabilities consisting of alterations of the number of repeats of a specific microsatellite in tumor DNA when compared to normal tissue DNA, indicate that replication errors have occurred *(75)*. The persistence of these errors is an indication of the reduced ability of cancers to repair mutations. The greater the instability, the less the capacity of repair the greater the potential for the generation of heterogenous populations some of which exhibiting novel and more malignant attributes such as enhanced growth, growth factor independence and drug resistance among many others. In colon cancer, microsatellite instability has been linked to alterations in the *MSH2* gene, located on 2p16 *(76)*, which codes for an enzyme involved in DNA repair.

Since microsatellite abnormalities found in TCC appear to be early changes *(61,72,77)*, they may be reflecting severe deregulation of cellular DNA which if left unchecked may lead to unrepaired mutations in key regulatory genes such as p53. In addition, genes such as *MSH2* may themselves be targets of carcinogenic insults. Finally, a case study by Schoenberg et al. *(78)* describes a patient who developed TCC of the

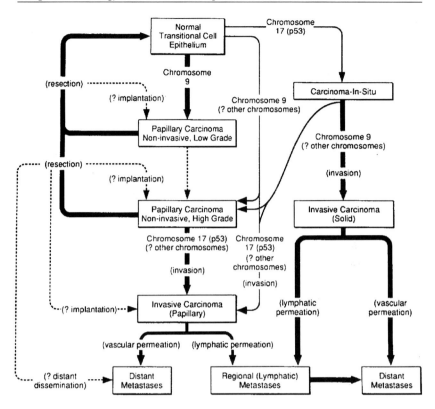

Fig. 3. Proposed pathway for bladder tumor development derived from molecular epidemiological data. The divergent, distinct pathways for superficial and invasive tumors parallels the model developed from observations of clinical biology (Fig. 1). (From Jones PA, Droller MJ. Pathways of development and progression in bladder cancer: new correlations between clinical observations and molecular mechanisms. Semin Urol 1993; 11: 177–192).

bladder and renal pelvis at an early age. The patient was found to have the germline translocation t(5;20)(p15;q11), which may have been an initiating factor in the disease. A recent literature review by Kiemeney and Schoenberg *(79)* examined case reports and epidemiological studies on TCC and concludes that there is evidence for a familial bladder cancer gene, which is a distinct entity from the known cancer predisposition syndromes.

MOLECULAR BASIS
OF SUPERFICIAL TUMOR RECURRENCE

A central feature of the clinical biology of superficial bladder cancer is its idiosyncratic rate of recurrence. Its uniquely high metachronous recurrence rate, distinguishing it from all other organ sites involved by contact carcinogenesis, has served as the basis for a longstanding debate in the urologic literature. While a number of theories have been proposed to account for this unique feature of superficial bladder cancer, two fundamental theories have received greatest attention. The concept of urothelial field change following exposure to a urinary carcinogen is both intuitively appealing and supported by multifocality and associated dysplasia in this disease *(80,81)*. Nonetheless other contact carcinogen induced tumors should have similar risks and yet fail to have metachronous recurrence rates approximating those associated with superficial bladder neoplasms. For this reason, and given the unique nature of the lower urinary tract, other authors have proposed intraepithelial tumor dissemination and or treatment induced implantation as a phenomenon accounting for the idiosyncrasy of superficial bladder cancer recurrence biology *(82–85)*. Anecdotal evidence in support of this concept in addition to the unusual recurrence rate include the temporality of recurrence in relation to surgical removal of a primary lesions and the location of recurrences in relation to the index lesion *(86)*.

Debate on this issue is traceable to the turn of the century when Albarran first proposed implantation as a mechanism accounting for bladder tumor recurrence *(87)*. The pendulum swung several times in the ensuing years. In the 1950s, Melicow, and Kaplan clearly demonstrated associated areas of dysplasia and pre-neoplasia in the urothelium intervening between sites of frank neoplasia *(80,81)*. However subsequent work by McDonald showed that urothelial malignancies could be implanted into and grow on sites of urothelial trauma even given relatively crude immunosuppression and understanding of transplant rejection in that era *(84)*. These observations were later expanded on by Soloway and the specific mechanisms involved in tumor implantation delineated by See *(85,88,89)*.

A definitive answer to the issue of the mechanism of bladder tumor recurrence was not provided until early in the 1990s. Using a molecular analysis of X chromosome inactivation in women with multifocal bladder tumors Sidransky et al. provided strong evidence to suggest that the multifocal tumors were clonal in origin *(90)*. Subsequently, Habuchi demonstrated that heterotopic urothelial recurrence was associated with identical mutations in *P53* at both the upper and lower track sites of occurrence *(91)*. Most recently this same group did microsatellite analysis on patients with multifocal metachronous tumor recurrence *(92)*. They found identical microsatellite alterations on multiple chromosomes in 80% of patients with multifocal recurrences. Overall this combination of data provides virtually conclusive evidence that the majority of superficial bladder recurrences are clonal in their etiology. Nonetheless some minor issues related to the precise mechanism of recurrence remain unresolved. Tsai found mosaicism in the human uroepithelium which suggested that clonal heterogeneity within the bladder was more limited than previously thought *(93)*. Indeed further evidence suggested that the bladder could develop from as few as 200 primordial cells and that the risk of tumor development and recurrence might be a consequence of limited diversity within the progenitor cell population.

While the etiologic debate regarding the mechanism of tumor recurrence has been largely resolved, the molecular mechanisms underlying the ability of superficial bladder tumors to implant and grow at sites different from the primary are largely undefined. See et al. outlined the requisite steps necessary for tumor implantation and or intraepithelial tumor dissemination to occur *(94)*. In the case of implantation the obvious first step is the presence of free floating tumor cells on the luminal surface of the bladder. These tumor cells must remain viable in the detached state and subsequently be able to adhere to sites on the urothelial surface. Following adherence, the local milieu must be conducive to the ultimate outgrowth of the adherent cell or cells. This would include an ability for the cells to divide, proliferate, and develop a vascular support structure.

Clinical observation and basic science research has provided some insight into factors associated with certain of the aforementioned steps. The mechanism of bladder tumor ablation, that is electrosurgical disruption into a fluid-filled medium, frees tumor cells from their underlying site of origin and effectively disseminates them throughout the luminal surface of the bladder. Surgical injury associated with the process of electrosurgical resection of bladder tumors results in sites of urothelial injury which selectively predisposes to tumor cell adherence via the formation of fibrin clots and effective entrapment/adherence of tumor cells at these sites. Given the central role of cellular adherence to clots at the site of urothelial injury, several studies have suggested that tumor intrinsic pericellular proteolysis through one of several fibrinolytic pathways may be a regulator of tumor cell adherence and ultimate outgrowth *(95–97)*. However, little work has been done to define whether specific molecular alterations in pericellular proteolysis might account for patterns of recurrence.

Other facets of the implantation process, such as proliferation and neovascularization, have been alluded to in other work. The epidermal growth factor/TGF alpha autocrine and paracrine loops have been suggested to predispose to recurrence *(98)*. Subsequently, cellular production of vascular endothelial growth factor, allowing for the establishment of a vascular support structure, has been suggested as a prognostic feature correlating with recurrence risk *(99)*. While a number of associated factors have been identified, these studies are at a very preliminary stage. The precise mechanisms responsible for dysregulation of cellular expression of these various proteins remain to be clarified.

MOLECULAR BASIS
OF BLADDER CANCER PROGRESSION

While less common than tumor recurrence, progression of superficial tumors to muscle invasion has profound consequences with respect to prognosis and treatment. In fact, tumor progression encompasses a spectrum of clinical and biological changes in both the tumor and the host *(100)* from early invasion of the basement membrane to widely metastatic disease. In this section we will focus and highlight the changes occurring when superficial bladder cancers become muscle invasive.

In general, organs are composed of a series of tissue compartments separated from each other by two types of extracellular matrix: basement membranes and interstitial stroma *(101)*. The extracellular matrix determines tissue architecture, has important biologic functions, and is a mechanical barrier to tumor cell invasion. The nuances of what is meant by invasive and superficial bladder cancer are worth mentioning here, since they are somewhat at odds with the pure definition of tumor invasion which is the penetration of normal tissue barriers such as the basement membrane. In the purest sense only stage Ta and CIS tumors are truly "superficial," thus not penetrating the basement membrane of the bladder wall. Historically however, urologists have also considered T1 tumors as superficial despite their invasion of the lamina propria. Tumors labeled as "invasive" on the other hand are those penetrating the true muscle of the bladder wall. As a group, most stage T1 lesions are more prone eventually to invade the detrusor during subsequent recurrences than are Ta tumors. Conversely, despite being truly superficial, CIS is more aggressive and behaves more akin to T1 than Ta tumors. This may be the result of the differing genetic lesions that led to its formation compared to those leading to Ta/T1 cancers *(102)*. Due to the significant drop in a patients' prognosis with any step in tumor progression, the genetic basis of this phenomenon is therefore a subject of considerable clinical importance. In the current section we will highlight the cytogenetic, molecular genetic and immunohistochemical evidence supporting the role of specific genetic changes in the progression of bladder cancer to muscle invasive disease.

Cytogenetic Changes
Associated with TCC Progression

Several recent studies have examined the common regions of deletion in human bladder tumors *(60,102)*. In a recent series, Knowles *(60)* and associates screened 83 cases of transitional cell carcinoma for loss of heterozygosity (LOH) on all autosomal chromosome arms. The most frequent losses were monosomies of chromosome 9 (57%), losses on chromosomes 11p (32%), 17p (32%), 8p (23%), 4p (22%), and 13q (15%). This series was composed of a majority of superficial low grade lesions and thus the incidence of the various losses would be reflective of the genetic alterations specifically present in this cohort of patients. Other groups have focused on identifying the common deletions specifically associated with tumor progression. In these cases, a somewhat different spectrum of abnormalities was observed, involving alterations at chromosomal locations 3p *(103)*, 4q *(104)*, 8p *(105)*, 18q *(106)*, 10 *(107, 108)*, 15 *(109,110)*, and 17p *(64)*. Some of these changes have also been observed in a recently characterized highly tumorigenic variant of the T24 human bladder cell line *(111)*.

Previous studies on predominantly superficial bladder cancer specimens *(60)* indicated an overall low frequency of chromosome 10 allele losses and deletions in bladder cancer. However when cohorts with significant proportions of invasive tumors were investigated *(108)*, the incidence of LOH on this chromosome was found in 40% of tumors for at least one locus. Remarkably, LOH on chromosome 10 was observed mainly in muscle-invasive or high grade tumors, the latter of which were most likely invasive or to have high chance of future progression to invasive disease. Confirming these findings, Kagan and colleagues *(107)* found LOH with at least one allele lost on the long arm of chromosome 10 in 9/20 (45%) invasive transitional cell carcinomas. Recently, LOH studies have also suggested that human chromosome 15 may harbor a novel putative tumor suppressor gene which appears to play a role during metastasis in breast and bladder *(110)* cancer. This observation supported other studies where fluorescence in situ hybridization (FISH) for chromosome 15 specific centromeric repeat sequences, revealed loss of this chromosome in 67% of specimens from patients with histologically confirmed transitional cell carcinoma *(109)*.

Molecular and Immunohistochemical
Changes Associated with TCC Progression

Studies utilizing immunohistochemical techniques (IHC) have suggested that overexpression of *HRAS* protein (discussed above) *(42)*, *P53*

(112) and the epidermal growth factor receptor *(EGFR) (113)* in bladder tumors may be related to bladder tumor progression. Loss of *RB (64)* and *E-Cadherin (114)* expression has also been related to this transition. Below, we will discuss the evidence suggesting roles for these genes in bladder cancer progression.

E-CADHERIN (CDH1)

The disruption of intercellular contacts, which accompanies cell dissociation and acquisition of motility, is correlated with a redistribution of *E-cadherin* over the entire cell surface and within the cytoplasm. Normal urothelium expresses E-cadherin, a Ca^{2+} dependent cell adhesion molecule, located on chromosome 16q22.1 and shown to behave like an invasion suppressor gene in vitro and in vivo in experimental systems *(115)*. This may explain the inverse relation between expression of *E-cadherin* and bladder tumor grade *(116)*. Several investigators further examined *E-cadherin* expression in bladder cancer samples and sought a correlation with tumor behavior. In an early study on 49 patient specimens (24 superficial and 25 invasive tumors), decreased *E-cadherin* expression correlated with both increased grade and stage of bladder cancer. More importantly, abnormal E-cadherin expression correlated with shorter patient survival *(117)*. These relationships to stage and grade were subsequently confirmed by other groups *(118,119)* while those to survival were sometimes *(119)* but not always *(120)* shown, despite a correlation with distant metastasis *(121)*. This latter apparent inconsistency may be due to a lack of statistical power in the various analyses to demonstrate an effect.

EPIDERMAL GROWTH FACTOR RECEPTOR (EGFR)

Similar to *HRAS*, *EGFR* expression levels in bladder cancer have been associated with increasing pathologic grade, stage *(122)* and higher rates of recurrence *(123)* and progression in superficial forms of the disease *(113)*. As such they may be causally related to the transition from superficial to invasive disease. Most importantly, patients with increased *EGFR* expression on their tumor cells did not survive as long as patients with normal *EGFR* expression. However, when the comparison of survival was limited to patients with invasive bladder cancer, no significant difference was found between patients with high levels of *EGFR* expression and those with low *EGFR* values *(124)*, suggesting that EGFR overexpression might be associated with the phenotypic transition from superficial to invasive forms of disease. Interestingly, gene amplification and gene rearrangement does not appear to be a common mechanism for *EGFR* overexpression in bladder cancer *(125)*. However, superficial human bladder cancer cells which were engineered to overexpress either mutated or normal *HRAS* also begin overexpressing *EGFR* at both the mRNA and protein levels, therefore HRAS might also play a role in transcriptional regulation of *EGFR* besides its role in *EGFR* signal transduction *(40,126)*.

Taken together, these data suggest that regulation of *EGFR* is altered in bladder cancer. In addition, since *EGF* is present in large quantities in urine *(127)*, with concentrations up to 10-fold greater per milliliter than those found in blood, this situation is likely to potentiate the consequences of EGFR overexpression since *EGFR's* in bladder cancer are functional *(128)*. Supporting the notion that *EGFR* overexpression is causally related to tumor progression and not merely an epiphenomenon are a number of in vitro *(126,129)* studies that have implicated this molecule in several of the steps involved in tumor invasion, such as cell motility.

RETINOBLASTOMA (*RB*)

Deletions of the long arm of chromosome 13, including the *RB* locus on 13q14, were found 28 of 94 cases, with 26 of these 28 lesions being present in muscle-invasive tumors *(130)*. *RB* alterations in bladder cancer as a function of stage was studied in 48 primary bladder tumors *(131)* where a spectrum of altered patterns of expression, from undetectable *RB* levels to heterogeneous expression of *RB*, was observed in 14 patients. Of the 38 patients diagnosed with muscle invasive tumors, 13 were categorized as *RB* altered, while only 1 of the 10 superficial carcinomas had the altered *RB* phenotype. Patient survival was decreased in *RB* altered patients compared with those with normal *RB* expression.

Two recent studies *(132,133)* have also shown that *RB* and *P53* alterations can further deregulate cell cycle control at the G1 checkpoint and produce tumor cells with reduced response to programmed cell death. The imbalance produced by an enhanced proliferative activity and a decreased apoptotic rate may further enhance the aggressive clinical course of the bladder tumors harboring both *P53* and *RB* alterations. A study focusing on the clinical progression of T1 tumors has demonstrated that patients with normal expression of both proteins have an excellent outcome, with no patient showing disease progression. Patients with abnormal expression of either or both proteins had a significant increase in progression *(134)*. These data indicate the clinical utility of stratification of T1 bladder cancer patients based on *P53* and *RB* nuclear protein status. They suggest that patients with normal protein expression for both genes may be managed conservatively, whereas patients with alterations in one and particularly both genes may require more aggressive treatment. Conversely, conflicting results have been obtained when *RB* status has been examined in patients with invasive tumors *(135,136)*, indicating perhaps that this gene may have its primary role in progression from superficial to muscle invasive disease rather than further downstream in the metastatic cascade.

P53

Genetic alterations of the *P53* gene, such as intragenic mutations, homozygous deletions, and structural rearrangements, are frequent events in bladder cancer *(137)*. Structural alterations of the *P53* gene were investigated using single strand conformation polymorphism (SSCP) in 25 bladder tumors and mutations in 6 of 12 invasive carcinomas were found, while only 1 of 13 superficial bladder tumors had such mutations *(138)*. Moreover, mutations were not identified in any of the 10 grade 1 and 2 lesions, while 8 of 15 grade 3 bladder carcinomas were found to have intragenic mutations. In another study *(139)*, IHC detectable *P53* protein was studied in 42 bladder carcinomas. One out of 11 grade 1 (9%), 12/22 grade 2 (55%) and 8/9 grade 3 (89%) tumors showed positivity for *P53*. There were significantly more *P53* positive cases in grade 2–3 tumors than in grade 1 tumors. There were significantly more *P53* positive cases in stage T2-T4 tumors than in stage T1 tumors. Another study *(140)* analyzed 42 specimens of transitional cell carcinoma by interphase cytogenetics with a fluorescence in situ hybridization technique (FISH) and found that *P53* deletion was significantly correlated with grade, stage, S-phase fraction, and DNA ploidy, while *P53* overexpression correlated only with grade. Moch et al. *(141)* studied the overexpression of *P53* by IHC in 179 patients and found that *P53* immunostaining to strongly correlate with tumor stage. In addition, this was driven by a marked difference in *P53* expression between pTa (37% positive) and pT1 (71%) tumors, while there was no difference between pT1 and pT2–4 tumors. Similarly, a strong overall association between *P53* expression and grade was driven by a marked difference between grade 1 (28%) and grade 2 tumors (71%), and there was no significant difference between grade 2 and grade 3 tumors.

Several groups *(142,143)* have investigated the possibility that altered patterns of *P53* expression correlated with tumor progression in patients with T1 bladder cancer. Patients with T1 tumors were retrospectively stratified into two groups with either <20% tumor cells (group A) with positive nuclear staining or >20% of cells with nuclear immunoreactivity for *P53* (group B) *(142)*. Disease progression rates were 20.5% per year for group B and 2.5% for Group A, with patients in group 2 having significantly shorter progression free intervals. Disease specific survival was also associated with altered patterns of *P53* expression. Another study *(143)* reported an analysis of T1 tumors using immunohistochemistry and 20% positive nuclear staining as the cutoff value. The mean follow-up time was greater than 10 yr. Progression and tumor grade were both significantly related to *P53* nuclear overexpression. However in this last study, *P53* expression was not an independent predictor of disease progression.

Other studies have attempted to clarify the role of *P53* as a prognostic marker in muscle-invasive tumors. In one study, *P53* was evaluated in 90 bladder tumors from 111 patients treated with neoadjuvant MVAC *(144)*. Patients with *P53* overexpression had a significantly higher proportion of cancer deaths. The long term survival in the *P53* overexpressors was 41% vs 77% in the nonexpressors independent of stage and grade. In another study, histologic specimens of transitional-cell carcinoma of the bladder, stages pTa to pT4 from 243 patients who were treated by radical cystectomy were examined for the IHC detection of *P53* protein *(8)*. Nuclear *P53* reactivity was then analyzed in relation to time to recurrence and overall survival. In patients with transitional-cell carcinoma confined to the bladder, an accumulation of *P53* in the tumor-cell nuclei predicted a significantly increased risk of recurrence and death, independently of tumor grade, stage, and lymph-node status. In a third study, IHC *P53* protein expression analysis was performed in 90 patients with transitional cell carcinoma of the urinary bladder *(145)*. Positive nuclear staining of tumor cells by the antibody to *P53* protein was detected in 32 cases, most of which were invasive and nonpapillary tumors and in high grade tumors. In addition, patients with tumors positive for *P53* staining had a significantly worse survival rate.

OTHER GENES

Early studies in bladder cancer have indicated a strong association of low level *MYC* (8q.24) gains with tumor grade, stage, chromosome polysomy, p53 protein expression, p53 deletion and tumor cell proliferation as assessed by Ki67 labeling index *(146)*. These data were consistent with a role of chromosome 8 alterations in bladder cancer progression *(105)*. However, subsequent studies have not found statistical significant correlation between the methylation, expression of *MYC* gene and clinical-histopathological parameters *(147)*, between the *MYC* methylation pattern and clinical stage *(148)*. Furthermore, *MYC* overexpression did not correlate with tumor grade or tumor progression *(149)*. Thus the role of this gene in bladder cancer development or progression is at present unclear.

Amplification and protein overexpression of the *ERBB2* gene located on 17q11.2-q12, has been suggested as a prognostic markers for patients with recurrent progressive bladder tumors *(150,151)*. However, other studies have failed to link *ERBB2* expression levels as an independent variable predicting disease progression *(152)*. Other studies have indicated a high level of expression of this gene in malignant as compared to benign bladder epithelium *(152)*. From these studies it would appear that the role of *ERBB2* as a diagnostic marker may outweigh its usefulness as a prognostic indicator.

The *MDM2* (mouse double minute 2, human homolog of p53-binding protein) gene is located at 12q13-14 and codes for a 90 Kd nuclear protein which is a negative regulator of *P53*. In urinary bladder, a strong statistical association between *MDM2* and *P53* overexpression was found in addition to an association between *MDM2* overexpression and low-stage, low-grade bladder tumors *(153)*. In addition, the simultaneous assessment of *MDM2* and *P53* was found to be independent factors for both disease progression and survival *(154)*. However, as with *MYC* and *ERBB2* not all studies have shown assessment of this gene product to be independently related to tumor progression *(155)*.

CONCLUSION

We have attempted to review the current understanding of both the molecular pathogenesis, and the molecular basis for the biology of transitional cell bladder neoplasms. This status results from an amalgam of scientific disciplines, ranging from molecular epidemiology to urologic oncology, combining "forces" to exact an exponential growth in our knowledge of bladder tumor biology. We may stand poised on the brink of a true revolution in cancer management. The ongoing molecular dissection of all phases of tumor biology promises unprecedented change in the way we assess and manage neoplastic processes.

The identification of heritable genetic mutations could possibly already allow the early, specific, identification of individuals at risk for certain tumors. The recognition that both the individual genotype and the environment may combine for the ultimate determination of risk may allow patients to adapt their lifestyles for risk modification. For those patients with neoplastic disease, therapy can be tailored to the specific biology of the individual tumor. The ongoing integration of molecular biology with clinical science promises to bring all of this within our reach.

REFERENCES

1. Johansson SL, Cohen SM. Epidemiology and etiology of bladder cancer. Seminars in Surgical Oncology 1997; 13(5): 291–298. Abstract.
2. Eble JN, Young RH. Carcinoma of the urinary bladder: a review of its diverse morphology. Seminars in Diagnostic Pathology 1997; 14(2): 98-108. Abstract.

3. Grossman HB. Superficial bladder cancer: decreasing the risk of recurrence. Oncology 1996; 10(11): 1617–1624; discussion 1624, 1627–1628. Abstract.
4. Lamm DL, Torti FM. Bladder cancer, 1996. Ca: a Cancer Journal for Clinicians 1996; 46(2): 93–112.
5. de Vere White RW, Stapp E. Predicting prognosis in patients with superficial bladder cancer. Oncology 1998; 12(12): 1717–1723; discussion 1724–1726.
6. Kakizoe T, Fair WR, Smith PH, Algaba F, Ferrari P, Grossman HB, et al. What is the biology of invasion and metastasis in bladder cancer? Intl J Urol 1995; 2(Suppl 2): 58–63.
7. See WA, Fuller JR. Staging of advanced bladder cancer. Current concepts and pitfalls. Urol Clin N Amer 1992; 19(4): 663–683.
8. Esrig D, Elmajian D, Groshen S, Freeman JA, Stein JP, Chen SC, et al. Accumulation of nuclear p53 and tumor progression in bladder cancer. N Engl J Med 1994; 331(19): 1259–1264.
9. Rehn L. Blasengeschwulste bei fuschsin-arbeitern. Arch Klin Chir 1895; 50: 588–600.
10. Droller MJ. Treatment of regionally advanced bladder cancer. An overview. Urol Clin N Amer 1992; 19(4): 685–693.
11. Hay A. Testing times for the tests [news]. Nature 1991; 350: 555–556.
12. Loeb LA. Mutator phenotype may be required for multistage carcinogenesis. Cancer Res 1991; 51: 3075–3079.
13. Melnick RL, Kohn MC, Portier CJ. Implications for risk assessment of suggested nongenotoxic mechanisms of chemical carcinogenesis. Environ Health Perspect 1996; 104: 123–134.
14. MacLeod MC. A possible role in chemical carcinogenesis for epigenetic, heritable changes in gene expression. Mol Carcinog 1996; 15: 241–250.
15. Lutz WK. Endogenous genotoxic agents and processes as a basis of spontaneous carcinogenesis. Mutat Res 1990; 238: 287–295.
16. Swenberg JA, Richardson FC, Boucheron JA, Deal FH, Belinsky SA, Charbonneau M, Short BG. High- to low-dose extrapolation: critical determinants involved in the dose response of carcinogenic substances. Environ Health Perspect 1987; 76: 57–63.
17. Lutz WK. Dose-response relationship and low dose extrapolation in chemical carcinogenesis. Carcinogenesis 1990; 11: 1243–1247.
18. Weinstein IB. Mitogenesis is only one factor in carcinogenesis [see comments]. Science 1991; 251: 387–388.
19. Breimer LH. Molecular mechanisms of oxygen radical carcinogenesis and mutagenesis: the role of DNA base damage. Mol Carcinog 1990; 3: 188–197.
20. Ames BN, Gold LS. Too many rodent carcinogens: mitogenesis increases mutagenesis. Science 1990; 249: 970–971.
21. Infante PF. Prevention versus chemophobia: a defence of rodent carcinogenicity tests [see comments]. Lancet 1991; 337: 538–540.
22. Shopland DR, Eyre HJ, Pechacek TF. Smoking-attributable cancer mortality in 1991: is lung cancer now the leading cause of death among smokers in the United States? [see comments]. J Natl Cancer Inst 1991; 83: 1142–1148.
23. Vineis P, Caporaso N. Tobacco and cancer: epidemiology and the laboratory. Environ Health Perspect 1995; 103: 156–160.
24. Talalay P. Mechanisms of induction of enzymes that protect against chemical carcinogenesis. Adv Enzyme Regul 1989; 28: 237–250.
25. Wormhoudt LW, Commandeur JN, Vermeulen NP. Genetic polymorphisms of human N-acetyltransferase, cytochrome P450, glutathione-S-transferase, and epox-

ide hydrolase enzymes: relevance to xenobiotic metabolism and toxicity. Crit Rev Toxicol 1999; 29: 59–124.

26. Butler MA, Iwasaki M, Guengerich FP, Kadlubar FF. Human cytochrome P-450PA (P-450IA2), the phenacetin O-deethylase, is primarily responsible for the hepatic 3-demethylation of caffeine and N-oxidation of carcinogenic arylamines. Proc Natl Acad Sci USA 1989; 86: 7696–7700.

27. Kalow W, Tang BK. Caffeine as a metabolic probe: exploration of the enzyme-inducing effect of cigarette smoking [see comments]. Clin Pharmacol Ther 1991; 49: 44–48.

28. Kaderlik KR, Kadlubar FF. Metabolic polymorphisms and carcinogen-DNA adduct formation in human populations. Pharmacogenetics 1995; 5: S108–S117.

29. Bryant MS, Vineis P, Skipper PL, Tannenbaum SR. Hemoglobin adducts of aromatic amines: associations with smoking status and type of tobacco. Proc Natl Acad Sci USA 1988; 85: 9788–9791.

30. Bell DA, Taylor JA, Butler MA, Stephens EA, Wiest J, Brubaker LH, et al. Genotype/phenotype discordance for human arylamine N-acetyltransferase (NAT2) reveals a new slow-acetylator allele common in African-Americans. Carcinogenesis 1993; 14: 1689–1692.

31. Branch RA, Chern HD, Adedoyin A, Romkes-Sparks M, Lesnick TG, Persad R, et al. The procarcinogen hypothesis for bladder cancer: activities of individual drug metabolizing enzymes as risk factors. Pharmacogenetics 1995; 5: S97–S102.

32. Hein DW. Acetylator genotype and arylamine-induced carcinogenesis. Biochim Biophys Acta 1988; 948: 37–66.

33. Risch A, Wallace DM, Bathers S, Sim E. Slow N-acetylation genotype is a susceptibility factor in occupational and smoking related bladder cancer. Hum Mol Genet 1995; 4: 231–236.

34. Hayes RB, Bi W, Rothman N, Broly F, Caporaso N, Feng P, et al. N-acetylation phenotype and genotype and risk of bladder cancer in benzidine-exposed workers. Carcinogenesis 1993; 14: 675–678.

35. Board P, Coggan M, Johnston P, Ross V, Suzuki T, Webb G. Genetic heterogeneity of the human glutathione transferases: a complex of gene families. Pharmacol Ther 1990; 48: 357–369.

36. Bell DA, Taylor JA, Paulson DF, Robertson CN, Mohler JL, Lucier GW. Genetic risk and carcinogen exposure: a common inherited defect of the carcinogen-metabolism gene glutathione S-transferase M1 (GSTM1) that increases susceptibility to bladder cancer. J Natl Cancer Inst 1993; 85: 1159–1164.

37. Foster F. New Zealand Cancer Registry report. Natl Cancer Inst Monogr 1979; 4: 77–80.

38. Case RA, Hosker ME, McDonald DB, Pearson JT. Tumours of the urinary bladder in workmen engaged in the manufacture and use of certain dyestuff intermediates in the British chemical industry. Part I. The role of aniline, benzidine, alpha-naphthylamine, and beta-naphthylamine. 1954 [classical article]. Br J Ind Med 1993; 50: 389–411.

39. Yu MC, Skipper PL, Taghizadeh K, Tannenbaum SR, Chan KK, Henderson BE, Ross RK. Acetylator phenotype, aminobiphenyl-hemoglobin adduct levels, and bladder cancer risk in white, black, and Asian men in Los Angeles, California. J Natl Cancer Inst 1994; 86: 712–716.

40. Bos JL. New insights and questions regarding interconnectivity of Ras, Rap1 and Ral. Embo J 1998; 17: 6776–6782.

41. Parada LF, Tabin CJ, Shih C, Weinberg RA. Human EJ bladder carcinoma oncogene is homologue of Harvey sarcoma virus ras gene. Nature 1982; 297: 474–478.

42. Fontana D, Bellina M, Scoffone C, Cagnazzi E, Cappia S, Cavallo F, et al. Evaluation of c-ras oncogene product (p21) in superficial bladder cancer. Eur Urol 1996; 29: 470–476.

43. Theodorescu D, Cornil I, Fernandez BJ, Kerbel RS. Overexpression of normal and mutated forms of HRAS induces orthotopic bladder invasion in a human transitional cell carcinoma. Proc Natl Acad Sci USA 1990; 87: 9047–9051.

44. Pratt CI, Kao CH, Wu SQ, Gilchrist KW, Oyasu R, Reznikoff CA. Neoplastic progression by EJ/ras at different steps of transformation in vitro of human uroepithelial cells. Cancer Res 1992; 52: 688–695.

45. Christian BJ, Kao CH, Wu SQ, Meisner LF, Reznikoff CA. EJ/ras neoplastic transformation of simian virus 40-immortalized human uroepithelial cells: a rare event. Cancer Res 1990; 50: 4779–4786.

46. Czerniak B, Cohen GL, Etkind P, Deitch D, Simmons H, Herz F, Koss LG. Concurrent mutations of coding and regulatory sequences of the Ha-ras gene in urinary bladder carcinomas. Hum Pathol 1992; 23: 1199–1204.

47. Czerniak B, Deitch D, Simmons H, Etkind P, Herz F, Koss LG. Ha-ras gene codon 12 mutation and DNA ploidy in urinary bladder carcinoma. Br J Cancer 1990; 62: 762–763.

48. Essigmann JM, Wood ML. The relationship between the chemical structures and mutagenic specificities of the DNA lesions formed by chemical and physical mutagens. Toxicol Lett 1993; 67: 29–39.

49. Dipple A. DNA adducts of chemical carcinogens. Carcinogenesis 1995; 16: 437–441.

50. Levy DD, Groopman JD, Lim SE, Seidman MM, Kraemer KH. Sequence specificity of aflatoxin B1-induced mutations in a plasmid replicated in xeroderma pigmentosum and DNA repair proficient human cells. Cancer Res 1992; 52: 5668–5673.

51. Loechler EL, Green CL, Essigmann JM. In vivo mutagenesis by O6-methylguanine built into a unique site in a viral genome. Proc Natl Acad Sci USA 1984; 81: 6271–6275.

52. Marshall CJ, Vousden KH, Phillips DH. Activation of c-Ha-ras-1 proto-oncogene by in vitro modification with a chemical carcinogen, benzo(a)pyrene diol-epoxide. Nature 1984; 310: 586–589.

53. Ronai ZA, Gradia S, Peterson LA, Hecht SS. G to A transitions and G to T transversions in codon 12 of the Ki-ras oncogene isolated from mouse lung tumors induced by 4-(methylnitrosamino)-1-(3-pyridyl)-1-butanone (NNK) and related DNA methylating and pyridyloxobutylating agents. Carcinogenesis 1993; 14: 2419–2422.

54. Greenblatt MS, Bennett WP, Hollstein M, Harris CC. Mutations in the p53 tumor suppressor gene: clues to cancer etiology and molecular pathogenesis. Cancer Res 1994; 54: 4855–4878.

55. Simoneau AR, Jones PA. Bladder cancer: the molecular progression to invasive disease. World J Urol 1994; 12: 89–95.

56. Sidransky D, Von Eschenbach A, Tsai YC, Jones P, Summerhayes I, Marshall F, et al. Identification of p53 gene mutations in bladder cancers and urine samples. Science 1991; 252: 706–709.

57. Habuchi T, Takahashi R, Yamada H, Ogawa O, Kakehi Y, Ogura K, et al. Influence of cigarette smoking and schistosomiasis on p53 gene mutation in urothelial cancer. Cancer Res 1993; 53: 3795–3799.

58. Spruck CHD, Rideout WMD, Olumi AF, Ohneseit PF, Yang AS, Tsai YC, et al. Distinct pattern of p53 mutations in bladder cancer: relationship to tobacco usage

[published erratum appears in Cancer Res 1993 May 15;53(10 Suppl):2427]. Cancer Res 1993; 53: 1162–1166.

59. Brown JM, Wouters BG. Apoptosis, p53, and tumor cell sensitivity to anticancer agents. Cancer Res 1999; 59: 1391–1399.

60. Knowles MA, Elder PA, Williamson M, Cairns JP, Shaw ME, Law MG. Allelotype of human bladder cancer. Cancer Res 1994; 54: 531–538.

61. Orlow I, Lianes P, Lacombe L, Dalbagni G, Reuter VE, Cordon-Cardo C. Chromosome 9 allelic losses and microsatellite alterations in human bladder tumors. Cancer Res 1994; 54: 2848–2851.

62. Dalbagni G, Presti JC Jr, Reuter VE, Zhang ZF, Sarkis AS, Fair WR, Cordon-Cardo C. Molecular genetic alterations of chromosome 17 and p53 nuclear overexpression in human bladder cancer. Diagn Mol Pathol 1993; 2: 4–13.

63. Simoneau AR, Spruck CH 3rd, Gonzalez-Zulueta M, Gonzalgo ML, Chan MF, Tsai YC, et al. Evidence for two tumor suppressor loci associated with proximal chromosome 9p to q and distal chromosome 9q in bladder cancer and the initial screening for GAS1 and PTC mutations. Cancer Res 1996; 56: 5039–5043.

64. Reznikoff CA, Belair CD, Yeager TR, Savelieva E, Blelloch RH, Puthenveettil JA, Cuthill S. A molecular genetic model of human bladder cancer pathogenesis. Semin Oncol 1996; 23: 571–584.

65. Merlo A, Gabrielson E, Mabry M, Vollmer R, Baylin SB, Sidransky D. Homozygous deletion on chromosome 9p and loss of heterozygosity on 9q, 6p, and 6q in primary human small cell lung cancer. Cancer Res 1994; 54: 2322–2326.

66. Schultz DC, Vanderveer L, Buetow KH, Boente MP, Ozols RF, Hamilton TC, Godwin AK. Characterization of chromosome 9 in human ovarian neoplasia identifies frequent genetic imbalance on 9q and rare alterations involving 9p, including CDKN2.Cancer Res 1995; 55: 2150–2157.

67. Cairns P, Tokino K, Eby Y, Sidransky D. Localization of tumor suppressor loci on chromosome 9 in primary human renal cell carcinomas. Cancer Res 1995; 55: 224–227.

68. Cairns P, Shaw ME, Knowles MA. Initiation of bladder cancer may involve deletion of a tumour-suppressor gene on chromosome 9. Oncogene 1993; 8: 1083–1085.

69. Serrano M, Hannon GJ, Beach D. A new regulatory motif in cell-cycle control causing specific inhibition of cyclin D/CDK4 [see comments]. Nature 1993; 366: 704–707.

70. Gruis NA, Weaver-Feldhaus J, Liu Q, Frye C, Eeles R, Orlow I, et al. Genetic evidence in melanoma and bladder cancers that p16 and p53 function in separate pathways of tumor suppression. Am J Pathol 1995; 146: 1199–1206.

71. Choisy-Rossi C, Reisdorf P, Yonish-Rouach E. The p53 tumor suppressor gene: structure, function and mechanism of action. Results Probl Cell Differ 1999;23: 145–172.

72. Gonzalez-Zulueta M, Ruppert JM, Tokino K, Tsai YC, Spruck CHD, Miyao N, et al. Microsatellite instability in bladder cancer. Cancer Res 1993; 53: 5620–5623.

73. Kwiatkowski DJ, Henske EP, Weimer K, Ozelius L, Gusella JF, Haines J. Construction of a GT polymorphism map of human 9q. Genomics 1992; 12: 229–240.

74. Weber JL. Informativeness of human (dC-dA)n.(dG-dT)n polymorphisms. Genomics 1990; 7: 524–530.

75. Peltomaki P, Aaltonen LA, Sistonen P, Pylkkanen L, Mecklin JP, Jarvinen H, et al. Genetic mapping of a locus predisposing to human colorectal cancer [see comments]. Science 1993; 260: 810–812.

76. Leach FS, Nicolaides NC, Papadopoulos N, Liu B, Jen J, Parsons R, et al. Mutations of a mutS homolog in hereditary nonpolyposis colorectal cancer. Cell 1993; 75: 1215–1225.
77. Linnenbach AJ, Robbins SL, Seng BA, Tomaszewski JE, Pressler LB, Malkowicz SB. Urothelial carcinogenesis [letter]. Nature 1994; 367: 419–420.
78. Schoenberg M, Kiemeney L, Walsh PC, Griffin CA, Sidransky D. Germline translocation t(5;20)(p15;q11) and familial transitional cell carcinoma. J Urol 1996; 155: 1035–1036.
79. Kiemeney LA, Schoenberg M. Familial transitional cell carcinoma [see comments]. J Urol 1996; 156: 867–872.
80. Melicow MM. Histologic study of vesical urothelium intervening between gross neoplasms in total cystectomy. J Urol 1952; 68: 261–273.
81. Kaplan JII, McDonald JR, Thompson GJ. Multicentric origin of papillary tumors of the urinary tract. J Urol 1951; 66: 792–804.
82. Hinman F. Recurrence of bladder tumor by surgical implantation. J Urol 1956; 75: 695.
83. Kiefer JH. Bladder tumor recurrence in the urethra: a warning. J Urol 1953; 69: 653.
84. McDonald DF, Thornson T. Clinical implications of transplantability of induced bladder tumors to intact transitional epithelium in dogs. J Urol 1956; 75: 960–964.
85. Soloway MS, Masters S. Urothelial susceptibility to tumor cell implantation: influence of cauterization. Cancer 1980; 46: 1158–1163.
86. Boyd PJR, Burnand KG. Site of bladder tumor recurrence. Lancet 1974; 1: 1290.
87. Albarran J, Imbert L. Les Tumeurs du rein. Paris: Masson et cie. 1903, pp. 452-459.
88. See WA, Miller JS, Williams RD. Pathophysiology of transitional tumor cell adherence to sites of urothelial injury in rats. Mechanisms mediating intravesical recurrence due to implantation. Cancer Res 1989; 49: 5414.
89. See WA, Chapman PH, Williams RD. Kinetics of transitional tumor cell line 4909 adherence to injured urothelial surfaces in (F-344) rats. Cancer Res 1990; 50: 2499–2504.
90. Sidransky D, Frost P, Von Eschenbach A, Oyasu R, Preisinger AC, Vogelstein B. Clonal origin bladder cancer. N Engl J Med 1992; 326(11): 737–740.
91. Habuchi T, Takahashi R, Yamada H, Kakehi Y, Sugiyama T, Yoshida O. Metachronous multifocal development of urothelial cancers by intraluminal seeding. Lancet 1993; 342(8879): 1087–1088.
92. Takahashi T, Habuchi T, Kakehi Y, Mitsumori K, Akao T, Terachi T, Yoshida O. Clonal and chronological genetic analysis of multifocal cancers of the bladder and upper urinary tract. Cancer Res 1998; 58(24): 5835–5841.
93. Tsai YC, Simoneau AR, Spruck CH 3rd, Nichols PW, Steven K, Buckley JD, Jones PA. Mosaicism in human epithelium: macroscopic monoclonal patches cover the urothelium. J Urol 1995; 153(5): 1697–1700.
94. See WA, Chapman WH. Tumor cell implantation following neodymium-YAG bladder injury: a comparison to electrocautery injury. J Urol 1987; 137: 1266–1269.
95. See WA, Williams RD. Urothelial injury and clotting cascade activation: common denominators in particulate adherence to urothelial surfaces. J Urol 1992; 147: 541–548.
96. See WA. Plasminogen activators: regulators of tumor cell adherence to sites of lower urinary tract surgical trauma. J Urol 1993; 150: 1024–1029.

97. See WA, Yong X, Crist S, Hedican S. Diversity and modulation of plasminogen activator activity in human transitional carcinoma cell lines. J Urol 1994; 151: 1691–1696.
98. Turkeri LN, Erton ML, Cevik I, Akdas A. Impact of the expression of epidermal growth factor, transforming growth factor alpha, and epidermal growth factor receptor on the prognosis of superficial bladder cancer. Urology 1998; 51(4): 645–649.
99. Crew JP, O'Brien T, Bicknell R, Fuggle S, Cranston D, Harris AL. Urinary vascular endothelial growth factor and its correlation with bladder cancer recurrence rates. J Urol 1999; 161(3): 799–804.
100. Mahadevan V, Hart IR. Metastasis and angiogenesis. Acta Oncol 1990; 29: 97–103.
101. Bernstein LR, Liotta LA. Molecular mediators of interactions with extracellular matrix components in metastasis and angiogenesis. Curr Opin Oncol 1994; 6: 106–113.
102. Rosin MP, Cairns P, Epstein JI, Schoenberg MP, Sidransky D. Partial allelotype of carcinoma in situ of the human bladder. Cancer Res 1995; 55: 5213–5216.
103. Li M, Zhang ZF, Reuter VE, Cordon-Cardo C. Chromosome 3 allelic losses and microsatellite alterations in transitional cell carcinoma of the urinary bladder. Am J Pathol 1996; 149: 229–235.
104. Polascik TJ, Cairns P, Chang WY, Schoenberg MP, Sidransky D. Distinct regions of allelic loss on chromosome 4 in human primary bladder carcinoma. Cancer Res 1995; 55: 5396–5399.
105. Wagner U, Bubendorf L, Gasser TC, Moch H, Gorog JP, Richter J, et al. Chromosome 8p deletions are associated with invasive tumor growth in urinary bladder cancer. Am J Pathol 1997; 151: 753–759.
106. Brewster SF, Gingell JC, Browne S, Brown KW. Loss of heterozygosity on chromosome 18q is associated with muscle-invasive transitional cell carcinoma of the bladder. Br J Cancer 1994; 70: 697–700.
107. Kagan J, Liu J, Stein JD, Wagner SS, Babkowski R, Grossman BH, Katz RL. Cluster of allele losses within a 2.5 cM region of chromosome 10 in high-grade invasive bladder cancer. Oncogene 1998; 16: 909–913.
108. Cappellen D, Gil Diez de Medina S, Chopin D, Thiery JP, Radvanyi F. Frequent loss of heterozygosity on chromosome 10q in muscle-invasive transitional cell carcinomas of the bladder. Oncogene 1997; 14: 3059–3066.
109. Wheeless LL, Reeder JE, Han R, MJ OC, Frank IN, Cockett AT, Hopman AH. Bladder irrigation specimens assayed by fluorescence in situ hybridization to interphase nuclei.Cytometry 1994; 17: 319–326.
110. Wick W, Petersen I, Schmutzler RK, Wolfarth B, Lenartz D, Bierhoff E, et al. Evidence for a novel tumor suppressor gene on chromosome 15 associated with progression to a metastatic stage in breast cancer. Oncogene 1996; 12: 973–978.
111. Gildea JJ, Harding MA, Gulding KM, Theodorescu D. Genetic and phenotypic changes associated with the acquisition of tumorigenicity in human bladder cancer. 1999 (in press).
112. Lacombe L, Dalbagni G, Zhang ZF, Cordon-Cardo C, Fair WR, Herr HW, Reuter VE. Overexpression of p53 protein in a high-risk population of patients with superficial bladder cancer before and after bacillus Calmette-Guerin therapy: correlation to clinical outcome. J Clin Oncol 1996; 14: 2646–2652.
113. Lipponen P, Eskelinen M. Expression of epidermal growth factor receptor in bladder cancer as related to established prognostic factors, oncoprotein (c-erbB-2, p53) expression and long-term prognosis. Br J Cancer 1994; 69: 1120–1125.

114. Schmitz-Drager BJ, Jankevicius F, Ackermann R. Molecular biology of dissemination in bladder cancer—laboratory findings and clinical significance. World J Urol 1996; 14: 190–196.

115. Mareel M, Boterberg T, Noe V, Van Hoorde L, Vermeulen S, Bruyneel E, Bracke M. E-cadherin/catenin/cytoskeleton complex: a regulator of cancer invasion. J Cell Physiol 1997; 173: 271–274.

116. Syrigos KN, Krausz T, Waxman J, Pandha H, Rowlinson-Busza G, Verne J, et al. E-cadherin expression in bladder cancer using formalin-fixed, paraffin-embedded tissues: correlation with histopathological grade, tumour stage and survival. Int J Cancer 1995; 64: 367–370.

117. Bringuier PP, Umbas R, Schaafsma HE, Karthaus HF, Debruyne FM, Schalken JA. Decreased E-cadherin immunoreactivity correlates with poor survival in patients with bladder tumors. Cancer Res 1993; 53: 3241 3245.

118. Griffiths TR, Brotherick I, Bishop RI, White MD, McKenna DM, Horne CH, et al. Cell adhesion molecules in bladder cancer: soluble serum E-cadherin correlates with predictors of recurrence. Br J Cancer 1996; 74: 579–584.

119. Shimazui T, Schalken JA, Giroldi LA, Jansen CF, Akaza H, Koiso K, et al. Prognostic value of cadherin-associated molecules (alpha-, beta-, and gamma-catenins and p120cas) in bladder tumors. Cancer Res 1996; 56: 4154–4158.

120. Lipponen PK, Eskelinen MJ. Reduced expression of E-cadherin is related to invasive disease and frequent recurrence in bladder cancer. J Cancer Res Clin Oncol 1995; 121: 303–308.

121. Mialhe A, Louis J, Montlevier S, Peoch M, Pasquier D, Bosson JL, et al. Expression of E-cadherin and alpha-,beta- and gamma-catenins in human bladder carcinomas: are they good prognostic factors? Invasion Metastasis 1997; 17: 124–137.

122. Gorgoulis VG, Barbatis C, Poulias I, Karameris AM. Molecular and immunohistochemical evaluation of epidermal growth factor receptor and c-erb-B-2 gene product in transitional cell carcinomas of the urinary bladder: a study in Greek patients. Mod Pathol 1995; 8: 758–764.

123. Chow NH, Liu HS, Lee EI, Chang CJ, Chan SH, Cheng HL, et al. Significance of urinary epidermal growth factor and its receptor expression in human bladder cancer. Anticancer Res 1997; 17: 1293–1296.

124. Nguyen PL, Swanson PE, Jaszcz W, Aeppli DM, Zhang G, Singleton TP, et al. Expression of epidermal growth factor receptor in invasive transitional cell carcinoma of the urinary bladder. A multivariate survival analysis. Am J Clin Pathol 1994; 101: 166–176.

125. Sauter G, Haley J, Chew K, Kerschmann R, Moore D, Carroll P, et al. Epidermal-growth-factor-receptor expression is associated with rapid tumor proliferation in bladder cancer. Int J Cancer 1994; 57: 508–514.

126. Theodorescu D, Cornil I, Sheehan C, Man MS, Kerbel RS. Ha-ras induction of the invasive phenotype results in up-regulation of epidermal growth factor receptors and altered responsiveness to epidermal growth factor in human papillary transitional cell carcinoma cells. Cancer Res 1991; 51: 4486–4491.

127. Chow NH, Tzai TS, Cheng PE, Chang CJ, Lin JS, Tang MJ. An assessment of immunoreactive epidermal growth factor in urine of patients with urological diseases. Urol Res 1994; 22: 221–225.

128. Messing EM, Reznikoff CA. Normal and malignant human urothelium: in vitro effects of epidermal growth factor. Cancer Res 1987; 47: 2230–2235.

129. Theodorescu D, Laderoute KR, Gulding KM. Epidermal growth factor receptor-regulated human bladder cancer motility is in part a phosphatidylinositol 3-kinase-mediated process. Cell Growth Differ 1998; 9: 919–928.

130. Cairns P, Proctor AJ, Knowles MA. Loss of heterozygosity at the RB locus is frequent and correlates with muscle invasion in bladder carcinoma. Oncogene 1991; 6: 2305–2309.
131. Cordon-Cardo C, Wartinger D, Petrylak D, Dalbagni G, Fair WR, Fuks Z, Reuter VE. Altered expression of the retinoblastoma gene product: prognostic indicator in bladder cancer [see comments]. J Natl Cancer Inst 1992; 84: 1251–1256.
132. Cordon-Cardo C, Zhang ZF, Dalbagni G, Drobnjak M, Charytonowicz E, Hu SX, et al. Cooperative effects of p53 and pRB alterations in primary superficial bladder tumors. Cancer Res 1997; 57: 1217–1221.
133. Cote RJ, Dunn MD, Chatterjee SJ, Stein JP, Shi SR, Tran QC, et al. Elevated and absent pRb expression is associated with bladder cancer progression and has cooperative effects with p53. Cancer Res 1998; 58: 1090–1094.
134. Grossman HB, Liebert M, Antelo M, Dinney CP, Hu SX, Palmer JL, Benedict WF. p53 and RB expression predict progression in T1 bladder cancer. Clin Cancer Res 1998; 4: 829–834.
135. Jahnson S, Karlsson MG. Predictive value of p53 and pRb immunostaining in locally advanced bladder cancer treated with cystectomy. J Urol 1998; 160: 1291–1296.
136. Logothetis CJ, Xu HJ, Ro JY, Hu SX, Sahin A, Ordonez N, Benedict WF. Altered expression of retinoblastoma protein and known prognostic variables in locally advanced bladder cancer [see comments]. J Natl Cancer Inst 1992; 84: 1256–1261.
137. Cordon-Cardo C, Sheinfeld J, Dalbagni G. Genetic studies and molecular markers of bladder cancer. Semin Surg Oncol 1997a; 13: 319–327.
138. Fujimoto K, Yamada Y, Okajima E, Kakizoe T, Sasaki H, Sugimura T, Terada M. Frequent association of p53 gene mutation in invasive bladder cancer. Cancer Res 1992; 52: 1393–1398.
139. Soini Y, Turpeenniemi-Hujanen T, Kamel D, Autio-Harmainen H, Risteli J, Risteli L, et al. p53 immunohistochemistry in transitional cell carcinoma and dysplasia of the urinary bladder correlates with disease progression. Br J Cancer 1993; 68: 1029–1035.
140. Matsuyama H, Pan Y, Mahdy EA, Malmstrom PU, Hedrum A, Uhlen M, et al. p53 deletion as a genetic marker in urothelial tumor by fluorescence in situ hybridization. Cancer Res 1994; 54: 6057–6060.
141. Moch H, Sauter G, Moore D, Mihatsch MJ, Gudat F, Waldman F. p53 and erbB-2 protein overexpression are associated with early invasion and metastasis in bladder cancer. Virchows Arch A Pathol Anat Histopathol 1993; 423: 329–334.
142. Sarkis AS, Dalbagni G, Cordon-Cardo C, Zhang ZF, Sheinfeld J, Fair WR, et al. Nuclear overexpression of p53 protein in transitional cell bladder carcinoma: a marker for disease progression. J Natl Cancer Inst 1993; 85: 53–59.
143. Lipponen PK. Over-expression of p53 nuclear oncoprotein in transitional-cell bladder cancer and its prognostic value. Int J Cancer 1993; 53: 365–370.
144. Sarkis AS, Bajorin DF, Reuter VE, Herr HW, Netto G, Zhang ZF, et al. Prognostic value of p53 nuclear overexpression in patients with invasive bladder cancer treated with neoadjuvant MVAC. J Clin Oncol 1995; 13: 1384–1390.
145. Furihata M, Inoue K, Ohtsuki Y, Hashimoto H, Terao N, Fujita Y. High-risk human papillomavirus infections and overexpression of p53 protein as prognostic indicators in transitional cell carcinoma of the urinary bladder. Cancer Res 1993; 53: 4823–4827.
146. Sauter G, Moch H, Gasser TC, Mihatsch MJ, Waldman FM. Heterogeneity of chromosome 17 and erbB-2 gene copy number in primary and metastatic bladder cancer. Cytometry 1995; 21: 40–46.

147. Sardi I, Dal Canto M, Bartoletti R, Guazzelli R, Travaglini F, Montali E. Molecular genetic alterations of c-myc oncogene in superficial and locally advanced bladder cancer. Eur Urol 1998; 33: 424–430.

148. Sardi I, Dal Canto M, Bartoletti R, Montali E. Abnormal c-myc oncogene DNA methylation in human bladder cancer: possible role in tumor progression. Eur Urol 1997; 31: 224–230.

149. Schmitz-Drager BJ, Schulz WA, Jurgens B, Gerharz CD, van Roeyen CR, Bultel H, et al. c-myc in bladder cancer. Clinical findings and analysis of mechanism.Urol Res 1997; 25: S45–S49.

150. Novara R, Coda R, Martone T, Vineis P. Exposure to aromatic amines and ras and c-erbB-2 overexpression in bladder cancer. J Occup Environ Med 1996; 38: 390–393.

151. Ravery V, Grignon D, Angulo J, Pontes E, Montie J, Crissman J, Chopin D. Evaluation of epidermal growth factor receptor, transforming growth factor alpha, epidermal growth factor and c-erbB2 in the progression of invasive bladder cancer. Urol Res 1997; 25: 9–17.

152. Underwood M, Bartlett J, Reeves J, Gardiner DS, Scott R, Cooke T. C-erbB-2 gene amplification: a molecular marker in recurrent bladder tumors? Cancer Res 1995; 55: 2422–2430.

153. Lianes P, Orlow I, Zhang ZF, Oliva MR, Sarkis AS, Reuter VE, Cordon-Cardo C. Altered patterns of MDM2 and TP53 expression in human bladder cancer [see comments]. J Natl Cancer Inst 1994; 86: 1325–1330.

154. Shiina H, Igawa M, Shigeno K, Yamasaki Y, Urakami S, Yoneda T, et al. Clinical significance of mdm2 and p53 expression in bladder cancer. A comparison with cell proliferation and apoptosis. Oncology 1999; 56: 239–247.

155. Schmitz-Drager BJ, Kushima M, Goebell P, Jax TW, Gerharz CD, Bultel H, et al. p53 and MDM2 in the development and progression of bladder cancer. EEur Urol 1997; 32: 487–493.

3 Diagnosis of Bladder Cancer

Ichabod Jung, MD, Edward M. Messing, MD, and Yves Fradet, MD, PHD

CONTENTS

INTRODUCTION

The initial diagnosis of bladder cancer (BC) is suspected by signs and symptoms which are subsequently confirmed by cystoscopy and biopsy. The majority of patients with BC have superficial tumors which are adequately treated by transurethral resection. However, since more than 60% of these patients will experience recurrences, constant monitoring of the bladder is required. The invasive nature of current investigations and the easy access to shed cells or tumor by-products in the urine has stimulated an intensive research effort over the last decade to develop noninvasive diagnostic tests for BC. It has also been recognized that some populations are at higher risk for developing BC and that effective screening methods for early detection could potentially reduce the morbidity and mortality of the disease. This chapter provides an update on the current status of diagnostic methods that are likely to change in the near future the diagnostic algorithm for BC.

From: *Current Clinical Urology: Bladder Cancer: Current Diagnosis and Treatment*
Edited by: M. J. Droller © Humana Press Inc., Totowa, NJ

CLINICAL PRESENTATION AND EVALUATION
Symptoms Suggestive of Bladder Cancer

COMMON SYMPTOMS

The most common presenting symptom of BC is painless gross hematuria, which is often intermittent, leading to occasional delays in consultation. Bladder cancer will be found in approximately 25% of adult patients with gross hematuria. In almost all patients with cystoscopically detected cancer, microhematuria will be found if enough consecutive testings are performed. On the other hand, BC will be detected in only 2% to 4% of all adult patients presenting with microhematuria which represents a dilemma to physicians in recommending invasive investigation for such low yield. The same is true for the second most common presenting symptoms of bladder irritability, urinary frequency, urgency and dysuria. Although this symptom complex will most commonly be associated with diffuse carcinoma *in situ* or invasive BC, depending on the severity of the symptoms, BC will only be found in approximately 5% of these patients. Bladder cancer will more rarely present with flank pain from ureteral obstruction or other symptoms of more advanced disease such as weight loss and abdominal or bone pain.

HEMATURIA INTERMITTENCY

Hematuria arising from BC is often intermittent and appears in only scant amounts *(1,2)*. If one looks often enough at urine, almost all patients with bladder cancer will have hematuria at some time *(1)*. On the average with truly early tumors, not more than one of three or fewer voidings will have blood in it *(3)*. Additionally, once above a threshold level of 2–3 RBC/HPF, the degree of microhematuria is unrelated to the seriousness of its underlying cause *(2)*. Thus, even if there is no subsequent hematuria after a single episode, complete urologic evaluation is warranted since a negative result on one or two specimens has little meaning in ruling out the presence of BC. Additionally, if any screening for BC using hematuria is to be done, a minimum of 7–10 voidings other than those following vigorous physical or sexual activity or prolonged recumbency *(4)* may need to be tested (microscopically or by chemical reagent strip) to assure the potential superior sensitivity *(1,2,5,6)* of this tool.

GLOMERULAR VS COLLECTING SYSTEM HEMATURIA

Hematuria arising from BC or other urothelial sources can be differentiated from that arising from the glomerulus by special examination of urinary sediment *(7)*. Hematuria originating from a glomerular defect is characterized by abnormally shaped ("dysmorphic") erythrocytes, but this usually must be identified by phase constrast microscopy or with Coulter counter analysis (7). Red blood cell casts also indicate a glomerular source, and can be seen by light microscopy. Schramek et al. have suggested no urologic evaluation is necessary for patients with solely dysmorphic erythrocytes in the urinary sediment (8). Similarly, Fracchia et al. have demonstrated that 98% of patients with solely dysmorphic erythrocytes and red blood cell casts, suggesting glomerular bleeding, have no evidence of significant urologic disease after full evaluation (9). In patients with evidence of a glomerular defect only, a 24-h urine protein excretion and creatinine clearance should be obtained (8).

MICROHEMATURIA IN WOMEN

It is unclear whether all women with asymptomatic microhematuria need to undergo a full urologic evaluation given that women are much less likely to have BC than men (1:3 ratio). Bard evaluated 177 women (89 of whom were above age 60) with asymptomatic microhematuria and found a highly significant lesion in only 3.4% (10). None of these lesions were detected by cystoscopy, leaving Bard to conclude that full evaluation need only consist of intravenous urography, urine culture and urine cytology in this group of patients. Benson and Brewer concluded that although most patients with asymptomatic microhematuria deserved a full evaluation, young women with a positive urine culture and signs and symptoms of an uncomplicated cystitis probably did not (11). These patients should be treated with antibiotics and a full hematuria evaluation reserved for those in whom urinalysis remains abnormal despite sterilization of urine. In general, a complete evaluation is appropriate for all women with asymptomatic microhematuria except women under age 40 with an obvious urinary tract infection treatable with antibiotics.

RECURRENT OR PERSISTENT MICROHEMATURIA

In a large number of individuals, asymptomatic microhematuria will persist or recur despite an initially negative complete urologic evaluation. Continued followup of patients with unexplained microhematuria seems warranted since the appearance of hematuria can precede the diagnosis of BC by many years (12). However, data supporting periodic evaluation in individuals with asymptomatic microhematuria appear unconvincing. Golin and Howard initially reported the discovery of five highly significant lesions (2 ureteral calculi, 2 renal lesions, 1 BC) in patients with initially unexplained asymptomatic microscopic hematuria using a followup protocol that involved repeat urinalysis and cytology at 6-month intervals with repeat cystoscopy and IVP alternating biannually *(13)*. In a longer followup study however *(14)*, they reported no discovery of genitourinary malignancies in 155 patients with asymptomatic microhematuria who were followed-up for 10–20 yr after an initial evaluation demonstrated either no lesion or an insignificant lesion. This lead Golin and Howard to abandon routine periodic studies in individuals with persistent microhematuria and advised studies only for patients who became symptomatic. Even patients who remain asymptomatic should probably be evaluated periodically especially individuals who are at high risk (age over 50 yr, tobacco use, occupational exposure) *(15)*. It seems reasonable that periodic (e.g., semiannual) urinary cytology (or some of the tests described below) be used in followup for at least several years, but few studies have addressed this important issue. Certainly, however, the appearance of grossly visible hematuria, flank or abdominal pain, or irritative voiding symptoms in such patients clearly merits an immediate complete re-evaluation.

Clinical Investigation

CONVENTIONAL URINARY CYTOLOGY

Since its first description in 1945 by Papanicolaou and Marshall *(16)*, urinary cytology has gained widespread acceptance as a clinical tool for detection of bladder transitional cell carcinoma (TCC). The malignant transitional cells observed on microscopic examination of urinary sediment have large nuclei with irregular, coarsely textured chromatin. Most studies over the recent years have shown a high specificity, usually over 95%, and high positive predictive value when obvious cancer cells are identified. However, criteria used to determine the presence of malignant cells are prone to subjectivity from cytopathologists, particularly in the interpretation of specimens with atypical or dysplastic cells. The main limitation of microscopic cytology is the low sensitivity for detecting the most common well-differentiated tumors which often shed cytologically normal appearing cells. Therefore, microscopic cytology is more sensitive in patients with high-grade tumors or carcinoma *in situ*. However, even in these patients, urinary cytology may be false negative in up to 10–20% of cases.

False-positive cytology is usually due to urothelial atypia, inflammation or changes caused by radiation therapy or chemotherapy. The overall sensitivity of cytology ranges between 30–50% in most studies. While the sensitivity can be increased to over 70% when "suspicious cells" are considered "positive," this decreases specificity to approximately 70% *(17)*. Bladder washes provide far more cellular specimens than those obtained through voiding and this method has been proposed to increase the sensitivity of cytology. However, it is an invasive method that is almost as uncomfortable as flexible cystoscopy. Moreover, Grégoire et al. recently reported no increase in sensitivity for bladder wash cytology over that of urinary cytology *(17)*. Thus, the main clinical utility of urinary cytology is the identification of cancer which may not be detectable yet by visual cystoscopy, such as the high-risk carcinoma *in situ*. The persistence of unequivocally positive urinary cytology in patients with negative cystoscopy after tumor resection leads inevitably to tumor recurrence and, in the face of a negative upper tract evaluation, should be an indication for prophylactic intravesical therapy. The study of the DNA content of cells obtained by bladder irrigations using flow cytometry analysis has been regarded as a potential new objective tool for bladder cancer detection. However, in comparative studies with urine cytology, DNA flow cytometry adds little information in terms of sensitivity and specificity and thus is of no additional diagnostic value *(17)*.

INTRAVENOUS UROGRAPHY

Excretory urography is indicated for the investigation of all patients with hematuria. Although not a very sensitive means of detecting bladder tumors, large tumors may appear as filling defects on the cystogram phase of the urogram. Urography is particularly useful in examining the upper urinary tract for associated urothelial tumors or for the identification of ureteral obstruction. The latter is usually a sign of muscle-invasive cancer and is frequently associated with presence of metastases in the lymph nodes.

CYSTOSCOPY AND BIOPSY

Cystoscopy remains the gold standard method for diagnosing new or recurrent bladder tumors. Abnormal areas should be biopsied for histologic confirmation. It is important to realize that cystoscopy is not 100% sensitive or specific. For example, it will not recognize carcinoma *in situ* that does not have the typical red velvety appearance. It may also miss some tumors when performed in patients who are actively bleeding or with enlarged prostates and trabeculated bladders. The diagnosis of BC will be confirmed in approximately 90% of biopsies of cystoscopically suspected small tumors. Selected site mucosal biopsies from areas adjacent to the tumor as well as remote from the tumor site have been recommended at the time of resection of visible tumors. While this approach is mandatory if considering partial cystectomy for localized muscle-invasive cancer, it appears unnecessary in the most common condition, that of papillary superficial tumors. Propper sampling of the bladder mucosa can probably be obtained more effectively using bladder washes.

NEW DIAGNOSTIC TESTS

Objectives and Clinical Utility

A substantial body of work over the last decade has brought about a number of diagnostic markers for BC. Five tests are currently commercially available which imply that the assays have been standardized and test kits are produced under quality control for reproducibility. A significant number of clinical studies have been performed with these assays and it is intriguing to see the amount of variability observed between results of different groups which probably reflect in good part the patient population being studied. Other tests are currently at different stages of development by a number of investigators and some will eventually join the group of available tests. Most published studies have reported test results that were better than urinary cytology. This in general meant that sensitivity was higher but in every case, for the commercially available tests, specificity was much lower than that obtained by urinary cytology.

To determine the potential clinical utility of these tests and adopt any one of them in clinical practice, it is important to consider the clinical needs that such tests could fulfill and the clinical conditions under which they would be used. A diagnostic test may be used to screen individuals at risk for BC, to help diagnose new bladder cancer in individuals with microscopic hematuria or irritative voiding symptoms, or to monitor patients following a diagnosis of TCC treated by transurethral surgery. A urine test could be used for one of two possibilities: to rule out BC or to identify cancers not detected by cystoscopy.

The most important characteristic for a test to rule out BC is a high sensitivity which means that few patients with bladder tumors should have a negative test and be undetected. A highly sensitive test will lead to a decreased need for cystoscopy if the clinician is confident that the likelihood of cancer is low. The level of sensitivity required will vary depending on clinical conditions. In high risk cancers, one will not tolerate missing cases. On the other hand, in the monitoring of patients with low grade low stage bladder tumors, a highly sensitive test could lead to decreased frequency of followup cystoscopy. A number of epidemiologic studies have identified simple and reliable criteria, based on the finding at diagnosis and first control cystoscopy, to determine categories of patients at various risks of recurrence *(18)*. In monitoring, the specificity is less of a problem since a positive test would result in a cystoscopy that would have been done in any case if the diagnostic test was not available. Low specificity is far more of an issue for screening individuals without BC histories, since a major driving force in the success of a screening paradigm is its cost, which of course is raised by unnecessary cystoscopies. It is noteworthy however, that PSA is currently used for detection of prostate cancer with a sensitivity of 85% and a specificity as low as 30%. Nam et al. recently compared conventional strategies with strategies using diagnostic tests for followup of superficial bladder cancer using decision analysis *(19)*. The model confirmed the common wisdom of a sensitivity of 90% and above as being a threshold where physicians would feel comfortable and cost savings would be optimized. Above this level, cost savings is dependent on the specificity of the test and the number of cystoscopies saved.

For a test to detect non visible cancer, a high specificity is required. Such test if positive would trigger a thorough investigation and a tight followup to detect the missed cancer. In that regard, urinary cytology, when positivity is limited to the presence of suspicious cancer cells, has a high specificity and is almost diagnostic. Tests that would be better than cytology should have at least similar specificity and higher sensitivity. Thus, the high specificity of urinary cytology finds its value as a complement to cystoscopy to trigger further investigation if the test is clearly positive in absence of visible tumor. On the other hand, high sensitivity is required to rule out bladder cancer and decrease or avoid the need for cystoscopy in select group of patients such as those suspected of cancer because of microhematuria or irritative voiding symptoms, and patients monitored for recurrence who are at low risk of progression.

Commercially Available Tests

The following is a review of the performance characteristics of the tests commercially available according to the type of assay (Table 1). The "point of care" tests are tests that can be performed in the physicians' office in few minutes. This includes the BTA Stat and the Aura Tek FDP test. The biochemical tests, NMP-22 and BTA Trak are quantitative assays performed in clinical laboratories using standard ELISA methodology. The cell-based assay, ImmunoCyt, is designed to complement urinary cytology and to be performed in cytopathology laboratories.

POINT OF CARE TESTS

These tests were developed to be performed in the physician's office as a way to rapidly indicate the probability of tumor. The first available was the BTA test which detected bladder tumor associated analytes in urine using human IgG *(20)*. The antigen recognized was a human complement factor H-related protein and the BTA *Stat* test was later developed using two monoclonal antibodies. The test is performed in 5 min using 5 drops of voided urine placed into a well of a disposable device. The initial report by Sarosdy et al. evaluated the performance of BTA

Table 1
Performance Characteristics of Commercially Available Diagnostic Tests

| Author (year) | Patient number | | % Sensitivity | | % Specifity |
	Tumors	Controls	Overall	Ta	
Office Tests					
BTA stat					
Sarosdy 1997 *(21)*	220	555	58	45	72
Wiener 1998 *(22)*	91	200	57	55	68
Lyeh 1999 *(23)*	107	124	65	53	64
Ramakumar 1999 *(24)*	57	139	74	60	73
Pode 1999 *(25)*	128	122	83	72	69
Aura Tek FDP					
Johnston 1997 *(26)*	60	70	81	74	75
Ramakumar 1999 *(24)*	52	134	52	45	91
Clinical Chemistry Tests					
NMP-22					
Landman 1998 *(28)*	47	30	81	81	77
Wiener 1998 *(22)*	91	200	48	49	70
Del-Nero 1999 *(29)*	105	—	83	66	—
Ramakumar 1999 *(24)*	57	139	53	48	60
Sanchez-Carbayo 1999 *(30)*	111	49	75	62	90
BTA-TRAK					
Ellis 1997 *(31)*	216	—	72	—	97
Thomas 1999 *(32)*	100	120	66	—	69
Cytopathology Test					
ImmunoCyt					
Fradet 1997 *(33)*	198	102	95	96	76
Mian 1999 *(34)*	79	167	90	88	79

Stat in 220 patients with recurrent bladder cancer, 167 healthy volunteers, 107 patients with previous bladder tumors but without evidence of disease at the time of testing and 283 patients with benign GU conditions or cancers other than those of the urothelium *(21)*. The overall sensitivity of the test was 58% compared to a low 23% sensitivity of urinary cytology. Since more than 80% of bladder tumors are stage Ta, Table 1 lists separately the sensitivity of the different tests for this common tumor stage. BTA *Stat* had a sensitivity of 45% for Ta tumors compared to 7% for urinary cytology. The specificity in patients with non-malignant GU conditions was 72% and 95% in healthy volunteers. Wiener et al. found an overall sensitivity of 57% for Ta tumors, but this was not different than the sensitivity of their urinary cytology which was 59% *(22)*. By contrast, the specificity of BTA S*tat* was 68% compared to 100% for cytology. Lyeh et al. found a similar sensitivity of 65% overall and 53% for Ta tumors and a specificity of 64% *(23)*. Ramakumar et al. found a slightly higher sensitivity of 74% overall and 60% for Ta with a specificity of 73% *(24)*. Finally, Pode et al. observed the highest reported sensitivity of 83% overall and 72% for Ta tumors with a specificity of 69% *(25)*. Based on these results, the BTA *Stat* test is expected to detect approximately two-thirds of tumors and slightly more than half of Ta tumors with a specificity of roughly 70%.

The Aura Tek FDP (Fibrin/fibrinogen Degradation Products) is a lateral flow immunoassay device using monoclonal antibodies that was developed to determine qualitatively the presence of urinary FDP. The FDP in urine come from the degradation of the fibrin cloth formed by the blood plasma proteins, fibrinogen and clothing factors released through tumor microvasculature. This release is mediated by angiogenic factors produced by the cancer cells which induce vessel wall permeability. Johnson et al. reported 81% overall sensitivity and 74% sensitivity for detection of Ta tumors with a specificity of 75% in patients with non-malignant genitourinary conditions *(26)*. They also noted a trend for increased intensity of color in relation to the grade of the tumors. On the other hand, Ramakumar et al. found a lower sensitivity of 52% overall and 45% in Ta tumors, but a higher specificity of 91% using the same test kit *(24)*.

Biochemistry Assays

The NMP-22 is an enzyme immunoassay for the quantification of nuclear matrix proteins in voided urine. Nuclear matrix proteins are part of the internal structural framework of the cell nucleus associated with DNA replication and regulation of gene expression. The assay was designed to detect with monoclonal antibodies complexed and fragmented nuclear matrix proteins in urine which have been stabilized by a solution provided by the manufacturer. The initial study reported by Soloway et al. evaluated the ability of the NMP-22 test, performed ten days after transurethral resections of bladder tumors, to predict the subsequent statuses of patients *(27)*. Of patients with NMP-22 less than 10 units (72% of the total), 86% had no malignancy on subsequent cystoscopies while 70% of those with values higher than 10 units had recurrences. These results suggest that the NMP-22 test may be helpful to tailor monitoring and intravesical therapy according to short term risk of recurrence. Landman et al. reported the value of NMP-22 to detect existing bladder tumors *(28)*. They reported a high overall sensitivity of 81% (and a sensitivity of 81% in Ta tumors) with a specificity of 77%

in 30 patients with non bladder cancer conditions. Wiener et al. compared NMP-22 to BTA *Stat* and urinary cytology and found a sensitivity of 48% overall (49% in Ta tumors) with a specificity of 70% *(22)*. Ramakumar et al. also found a low sensitivity of 53% overall and 48% in Ta tumors with a specificity of 60% *(24)*. On the other hand, Del-Nero et al. observed an overall sensitivity of 83% and 66% in Ta *(29)*, while Sanchez-Carbayo et al. had a much higher specificity of 90% with sensitivities of 75% overall and 62% in Ta tumors *(30)*.

The BTA-TRAK assay is a quantitative immunoassay for the detection of the human complement factor H-related protein. Essentially, it is measuring the same analytes as the BTA *Stat* test but the assay is performed in a clinical laboratory. The two studies performed so far by Ellis et al. *(31)* and Thomas et al. *(32)* showed an overall sensitivity of 72% and 66% respectively with a specificity of 75% and 69% in patients with nonBC genitourinary conditions and a 90% specificity in healthy volunteers. These results are quite similar to those obtained with NMP-22. Both assays will detect approximately 70% of tumors with a specificity in the 70% range. Again results have been quite variable between individual laboratories, with sensitivities ranging from as low as 50% to as high as 80%.

CELL-BASED ASSAYS

The ImmunoCyt is a fluorescence-based assay using monoclonal antibodies to a mucin antigen (in green) and a bladder cancer glycoform of the carcinoembryonic antigen (in red) designed to complement voided urinary cytology. The assay is performed in cytopathology laboratories where urine fixed in ethanol at the time of collection is filtered and the cells recovered and applied to slides. Slides are then incubated with a drop of a cocktail of directly labeled antibodies and read with a fluorescence microscope. Cytology can be performed using light microscopy on the same slide after counterstaining with Papanicolau reagents. The test results provide the number of positive cells and different cutoff values can be used to assign the risk of presence of tumors.

Fradet et al. reported the results of a study performed in a central laboratory on 198 patients with cystoscopy proven tumors and 102 controls *(33)*. The overall sensitivity of ImmunoCyt combined with cytology was 95% and was 96% for Ta tumors. The specificity was 76% when a test was considered positive if any green or red cell was seen. However, when a cutoff of 5 positive red cells or one green cell was used, the specificity was 90% with a sensitivity of 89% overall. Mian et al., who evaluated all of the diagnostic tests described above, also evaluated ImmunoCyt in 264 consecutive patients *(34)*. The sensitivity of their cytology overall was 47%, slightly lower than that reported in their previous studies, with a specificity of 98%. The overall sensitivity of ImmunoCyt with cytology was 89.9%. The sensitivity was 88% for pTa tumors and 97% for grade 3 cancers. The specificity in patients undergoing cystoscopy for the followup of previous bladder tumors or for suspicion of new bladder tumor was 79% overall. The authors concluded that when combined with cytology, ImmunoCyt may replace cystoscopy in select patients, especially in followup protocols of low grade tumors. Interestingly, both groups noticed that up to one-third of patients with a negative followup cystoscopy but a positive ImmunoCyt test had recurrences within the next three to six months, suggesting that the assay could detect persistent field defect. Thus, the ImmunoCyt test appears to complement urinary cytology by providing a sensitivity above 90% for tumor detection and above 95% for high grade cancers, while preserving the high specificity of urinary cytology which can be performed on the same slide. Although these results are very promising, independent confirmation in noncentralized cytology laboratories, which are designed to be the primary performers of this assay, should be done before it is recommended for widescale use.

Investigational Tests

A number of tests based on other molecular features of BC are currently under investigation in several laboratories. They provide additional possible means to complement existing tests and should be evaluated with the same criteria for their performance and utility in specific clinical circumstances. Tests to "rule out" BC should have high sensitivity and tests to rule in BC or to identify cancers not visible at cystoscopy should have high specificity.

TELOMERASE ASSAY

Telomeres are specialized structures involved in stabilizing chromosomes. Telomeres shorten with each cellular division in normal somatic cells, and this process has been linked to cell senescence. The enzyme telomerase synthesizes telomeric DNA, which maintains telomere length resulting in cell immortality. Inappropriate telomerase activity has been detected in a variety of tumors with a frequency surpassing 90%. Telomerase activity is measured by the telomeric repeat amplification protocol (TRAP) assay. Cells are collected from 30–50 mL of voided urine, treated with detergents, and the cellular extract incubated with specific primer sequences that are then amplified by PCR. The results of the amplification are then analyzed on gels. This is a rather complex laboratory assay with still subjective interpretation components. Kavaler et

al. reported an overall 85% sensitivity in 104 BC patients *(35)*. This
sensitivity was constant across all grades including grade 1. The specificity was 100% in healthy volunteers but 66% in patients with non-
malignant urologic conditions. However, Dalbagni et al. reported a much
lower sensitivity of 35% in voided urine specimens compared to 71% for
urine cytology *(36)*, and Muller et al. reported only a 7% sensitivity with
the TRAP assay in 30 patients with BC *(37)*. Muller et al. also described
a technique for the detection of human telomerase messenger RNA
using reverse transcriptase-PCR (RT-PCR) which detected 83% of the
tumors. The specificity was 73% in patients with non BC urologic conditions and 85% in healthy controls *(37)*. By contrast, Ramakumar et al.
in a study of 57 patients with bladder tumors showed a sensitivity of 70%
overall and 76% for stage Ta tumors *(24)*. Their specificity was 99% in
138 control patients. Despite the high promise of some of the results
reported, the marked discrepancies between the different studies highlight the importance of having standardized and reproducible test kits
before considering the widespread use of this, or any, new diagnostic
method.

HYALURONIC ACID AND HYALURONIDASE

The glycosaminoglycan hyaluronic acid (HA) promotes tumor metastases. Hyaluronidase (HAase), an endoglycosidase, degrades HA into
small fragments that promote angiogenesis. Lokeshwar et al. developed
two ELISA-like assays that utilize a biotinylated HA binding protein for
detection of HA and HAase levels in urine *(38)*. These levels were normal-
ized to total urinary protein. The HA and HAase tests showed a combined sensitivity of 91.9% in 261 bladder tumors with a specificity in
84% in 243 control patients. Sensitivity for Ta tumors was 87.5%. These
results certainly warrant further development and confirmatory studies.

FLUORESCENCE *IN SITU* HYBRIDIZATION (FISH)

Fluorescence *in situ* hybridization (FISH) techniques may aid in the
detection of BC by using fluorescently labeled DNA probes that bind to
specific chromosome regions. Deletions of chromosome 9, the most common genetic aberration in BCs, are found in >60% of all bladder tumors
across all grades and stages *(39)* and may be detected using FISH analysis.

Chromosome 9 FISH analysis can be performed on epithelial cells
derived from bladder irrigations and can help detect bladder tumors
(40). Reeder et al. were able to combine chromosome 9 FISH assays with
DNA cytometry and detected BC with a sensitivity ranging from 69%
(grade 1) to 92% (grade 3) and a specificity of 92%. Chromosome 9 FISH
analysis has many disadvantages and remains investigational. As with
cytology, sufficient cell numbers are more readily obtained in bladder

barbotage specimens than in voided urine, requiring minimally invasive collection techniques. The cost of reagents and equipment (for quantification) and the labor intensiveness of chromosome 9 FISH analysis makes it prohibitively expensive to use in most clinical settings currently. This limits the test to large laboratory centers where large volumes of specimens and available technical expertise make the cost of performing FISH analyses acceptable. Another disadvantage is that false negatives may arise from lesions not sampled by the bladder washings (e.g., upper tract or prostatic urethral TCC) or that do not readily slough off into the barbotage resulting in insufficient cells for analysis (41). False positives may arise from hybridizations that appear as one fluorescent spot but really represent two distinct hybridizations. The use of an additional reference or control probe however should eliminate this artifact. Despite these disadvantages, chromosome 9 FISH is useful as a means of detecting chromosomal aberrations in patients with BC and may serve as an adjunctive tool to conventional cytology. Additionally, when examined by automated techniques, such as image analysis, it permits development of quantitative thresholds for more objective analysis.

MICROSATELLITE DNA REPEATS

Microsatellite repeats are polymorphic repetitive sequences of DNA that can be used as markers to detect the clonal evolution of neoplastic cells. Microsatellite analysis of exfoliated urinary cells has been used successfully to help diagnose BC with high sensitivity and specificity (42). The test requires a voided urine sample and a blood sample to compare DNA patterns in exfoliated cells with genomic DNA. Mao et al. were able to correctly identify 19 of 20 patients with BC with a combination of PCR based microsatellite analysis and loss of heterozygosity analysis of chromosome 9. Using the same techniques, the same group followed-up patients with BC and were able to correctly identify 10 of 11 patients with recurrent TCC (43). The assay was negative in 10 of 10 patients who had no cystoscopic evidence of BC. Interestingly, they found 2 patients with molecular changes prior to findings seen on cystoscopy supporting the notion that molecular tests can detect disease before imaging or cystoscopy. More recently, Mourah et al. have performed the same techniques and have demonstrated similar results by identifying 10 of 12 patients with BC during followup for recurrence (44).

The basic principals behind this analysis are that genomic instability is a fundamental property of malignantly transformed cells, and that these genetic errors are retained by and added to malignant clones. While some of the defects in DNA repair and mechanisms directing apoptosis are lethal, enough defects affect either noncritical segments of DNA or actually provide growth advantages for these clones and/or encourage tumor progression that they are retained in the tumors' daughter cells. As such microsatellite analysis does not provide information about mutations of specific genes; however it permits the screening of clonally expanded populations without requiring precise information about the functional importance of specific genetic alterations in the primary tumor. This may be particularly useful if cells are truly of clonal origin. However, given the field defect commonly seen in the urothelium, multiple clones may render microsatellite analysis difficult to interpret. In fact, in Mourah's study, the 2 patients in whom they failed to diagnose BC by microsatellite analysis likely involved a different panel of microsatellite markers from those used in the index study. Nevertheless, microsatellite analysis is a molecular method which shows great promise in the surveillance of patients with BC.

EPIDERMAL GROWTH FACTOR AND EGF RECEPTORS

Urinary EGF concentration appears to be reduced in patients with BC compared to controls (45,46). Lower levels of EGF in the urine of BC patients may reflect binding of EGF to abnormally expressed receptors for EGF (EGF-Rs). Reduce urinary EGF levels do not appear to be associated with tumor grade or stage and have little prognostic value (49,50) but they appear to increase after bladder tumor resections, leading to the possibility that measuring urinary EGF in BC patients may be most useful in serially monitoring to predict tumor persistence or recurrence (50).

Immunohistochemical over-expression of EGF-Rs appears to correlate with higher grade and stage and overall poorer prognosis (47). EGF-Rs are normally expressed in the basal layer of urothelial cells (48) but are abnormally distributed throughout all urothelial layers in BCs. This abnormal distribution is also seen in dysplastic and normal appearing urothelium both nearby and remote from TCCs regardless of tumor grade or stage (48). This information supports the concept of a field defect of the urothelium involving premalignant lesions in normal appearing areas, identified by the presence of increased EGF-R expression. In general, EGF-R status appears to be most helpful as a prognostic marker, as an aid to understanding the biology of BC initiation and progression, and as a potential target of TCC therapy (49).

FUTURE APPROACHES

INTRAVESICAL ULTRASOUND

Transurethral intravesical ultrasound can be used to diagnose, stage and aid in treatment of BC. Intravesical ultrasound relies on using an endoscopic probe with up to 3 interchangeable transducers of 60, 90 and

120 degrees, with a frequency of 5.5 MHz to 7.5 MHz. By changing the amount of filling of the bladder, the degree of fixation or muscle infiltration may be studied by ultrasonography. Koraitim and colleagues studied 115 patients *(50)* by intravesical ultrasound either prior to transurethral resection (76) or radical cystectomy (39) and compared their findings to standard pathology. Intravesical ultrasound detected all superficial (Ta, T1) tumors (31 of 31), 95.7% (22 of 23) and 96.8% (30 of 31) of muscle invasive tumors (stage T2 and stage T3 respectively). Intravesical ultrasonography detected BC that could not be visualized by cystoscopy due to hematuria in three patients and bladder diverticuli in two. Moreover, intravesical ultrasonography proved useful in monitoring the extent of tumor resection in 69 of 76 cases (91%). However, in the remaining seven cases, although ultrasonography showed complete resection, pathological examination showed tumor cells in specimens from the base of the resected areas.

There are however several limitations of transurethral intravesical ultrasonography. It cannot distinguish between stage Ta and T1 disease which not only have different prognoses but also require different therapies. Furthermore, intravesical ultrasonography has difficulty in staging tumor invading perivesical fat or adjacent structures (70% accuracy) nor can involvement of pelvic lymph nodes or prostate gland be determined. In a larger prospective study by Schulze et al., 166 patients suspected of having BC underwent transurethral ultrasonography prior to cystoscopy, and less impressive results were obtained. Eight of the 108 patients with histologically confirmed BC were missed by ultrasonography (sensitivity 93%) and 9 patients had false positive results by ultrasonography. More importantly, with respect to staging, their study was less skewed and more accurately reflected the spectrum of disease typically seen by a urologist (No tumor 58; Ta 38; T1 22; T2A 9; T2B 20; T3 12; T4 7). Intravesical ultrasonography accurately detected 73% (44 of 60) of superficial tumors (Ta, T1), 59% (17 of 29) of muscle invasive tumors (T2A, T2B) and 58% (11 of 19) with extravesical disease (T3, T4). This led the authors to conclude that transurethral intravesical ultrasonography could add additional information but was unreliable by itself and should be carried out only after cystoscopy. Despite these deficiencies, transurethral intravesical ultrasonography may serve as a useful guide in determining the extent of resection and as a useful adjunct in the staging of disease that may be easily mastered by urologists.

Virtual Cystoscopy/Ureteroscopy

Virtual cystoscopy or ureteroscopy relies on the use of three-dimensional helical computer tomographic (CT) scan datasets to help delineate the mucosal surface of the bladder or ureter thereby detecting irregularities such as tumors. Contrast medium (delivered intravenously) or air (delivered via foley catheter) is required to create a 'visual gradient' between the mucosal surface and the lumen. By insufflating with air, Hussain et al. were able to detect 26 of 26 masses (mean size 1.7 cm) in six patients with BC by virtual cystoscopy *(51)*.

Perhaps far more promising is the use of this technology for upper tract evaluation, particularly for those in whom complete ureteroscopic and renal calyceal inspection is technically difficult and possibly as an adjunct to upper tract surveillance in patients who previously underwent percutaneous management of upper tract TCC.

There are several disadvantages to virtual cystoscopy. Besides the radiation and potential allergy to contrast medium, virtual cystoscopy cannot detect flat lesions such as carcinoma *in situ* since it cannot appreciate discoloration or subtle urothelial changes. Virtual cystoscopy also has a very difficult time detecting small tumors and characterizing their nature (papillary vs sessile). In a study of 27 patients with known tumors by Narumi et al., only 23 of 30 (77%) tumors less than 10 mm were identified and of these only 9 (39%) were correctly characterized. Information important for preoperative planning such as the location of the ureteric orifices cannot be obtained. In a recent study by Merkel and colleagues, although virtual cystoscopy detected bladder tumors in 11 of 11 patients, all with diameters of at least 5 mm, multiple tumors were often not seen and the ureteric orifices were not visualized *(52)*.

The clinical role of virtual cystoscopy needs to be fully studied in the diagnosis of BC given these limitations. To date, there are no studies documenting clear and convincing evidence that virtual cystoscopy is equal to standard cystoscopy. As it is a "noninvasive" test, virtual cystoscopy does not allow pathological examination of specimens from bladder irrigations or biopsies and hence cannot provide this valuable diagnostic and staging information. Furthermore, the "noninvasiveness" of placing a foley catheter necessary for bladder insufflation prior to virtual cystoscopy should be questioned over the "invasiveness" of flexible cystoscopy. Additionally, few studies have documented the time and cost of performing virtual cystoscopy and compared these to standard cystoscopy. Clearly, prospective studies are necessary and current limitations of virtual cystoscopy need to be addressed (e.g., inability to detect small tumors) before it can be recommended as a modality comparable to standard cystoscopy. Nevertheless, virtual cystoscopy and ureteroscopy represent exciting new modalities whose methods will only improve with more powerful computing algorithms addressing many of these disadvantages.

FLUORESCENCE CYSTOSCOPY

Fluorescent diagnosis of BC was developed and reported by Jocham et al. in the 1980s using systemic photophrin II *(53)*. More recently, Kriegmair et al. used intravesical instillation of 5-aminolevulinic acid (ALA) and a xenon light source to detect BC with high sensitivity *(54)*. ALA is a naturally occurring heme precursor that is selectively taken up by TCC. It's metabolite, photoporphyrin IX and can be readily detected by fluorescence induced with violet light. Biopsies guided by ALA-associated flurescence were found to increase sensitivity for detecting urothelial dysplasia and TCC in BCG treated patients from 61.5% using white light to 96.2% *(54)*. Another potential advantage for ALA fluorescence cystoscopy is the detection of carcinoma in situ that may appear as normal urothelium under white light cystoscopy. D'Hallewin et al. reported a sensitivity of 94% using ALA fluorescence cystoscopy for detecting carcinoma *in situ* compared to only 28% using conventional white light cystoscopy *(55)*.

Some of the disadvantages to fluorescence cystoscopy relate to the potential side effects of the fluorescence inducing drugs as well as its low specificity for detecting BC. The most serious complication from systemic photophrin II usage is a phototoxic skin reaction. However, this has not been seen with intravesical ALA usage *(56)*, so patients no longer need to avoid direct sunlight after cystoscopy. Kriegmair et al. attributed the low specificity (70%) of fluorescence cystoscopy to inflammatory changes especially at the trigone and bladder neck *(54)*. Recently, Filbeck et al. documented the low specificity of fluorescence cystoscopy in detecting BC after TURBT and also attributed this to the inflammatory reaction found in the resected regions *(57)*. The low specificity of fluorescence cystoscopy however does not negate its benefit of offering guided biopsies over random biopsies. Overall, fluorescence cystoscopy is a new exciting method of detecting forms of BC not easily visible by conventional cystoscopy with minimal documented complications.

MICROSCOPIC CHROMOCYSTOSCOPY

Microscopic chromocystoscopy relies on the use of a contact microcystoscope that enables observation of cytological details of the stained urothelium of the bladder. Methylene blue is intravesically delivered prior to cystoscopy and stains the nuclei. Contact microcystoscopy can be performed by increasing magnification up to 150 times by switching the lens optical system. Iguchi et al. performed microscopic chromocystoscopy in 65 patients with superficial BC (Ta, T1) and were able to detect dysplasia and carcinoma *in situ* in 15 of these patients *(58)*. In 12 of the 15 patients, the abnormal biopsies were from stained portions that could not be identified by conventional cystoscopy.

Major disadvantages of microscopic chromocystoscopy include not only the additional time required for methylene blue instillation and micro-cystoscopic viewing but also the high false positive rate. Of the 75 methylene blue stained biopsies obtained by Iguchi and colleagues, only 21 were considered microscopically abnormal and only 10 of these had BC (9 CIS, 1 TCC). Methylene blue staining can be iatrogenically caused by instrument trauma to the urothelium. Inflammatory changes also account for a large number of false-positive stainings but can to a certain extent be differentiated by microscopic cystoscopy. Overall, it appears that microscopic chromocystoscopy may aid in the detection of dysplasia and carcinoma *in situ* but because of poor sensitivity (only 9 of 13 cases of CIS were accurately diagnosed by Iguchi and colleagues) random punch biopsies are also advocated *(58)*.

EARLY DETECTION AND SCREENING

RATIONALE FOR SCREENING/EARLY DIAGNOSIS

Bladder cancer is a common serious condition and because metastases are almost exclusively associated with prior or concomitant muscle invasion *(59,60)*, there should be time between its occurrence on the urothelial surface and deep invasion, in which a diagnosis can be made, and effective treatment associated with relatively little morbidity, instituted. Unfortunately, the vast majority of patients with muscle-invading BCs have muscle invasion at the time of their first BC episode *(61,62)*. Thus, surveillance and treatment strategies for recurrent superficial tumors, although critically important to the patients themselves, are unlikely to significantly reduce BC mortality without being combined with some form of early detection. Even in patients with high-grade TCCs that are highly refractory to conservative therapy, Freeman and colleagues reported roughly an 80% 5-yr disease-specific survival, with the vast majority who died from BC found actually to have had muscle-invasive or more advanced disease at the time of cystectomy *(60)*. This confirms the belief that very few BCs metastasize before detrusor invasion occurs. In those patients with high-grade, frequently recurrent superficial tumors (including T1 lesions) or CIS, by the time cystectomy is contemplated, roughly one-third actually have microscopic evidence of muscularis propria involvement, and roughly half the patients who are upstaged already have extravesical extension or metastases. Thus in upstaged individuals, where survival is worse, if cystectomy had been done earlier, it may have been curative.

Additional characteristics of BC that make it particularly suitable for screening are that:

1. If BC is detected before it is muscle invading, based on standard histologic and cytologic criteria, one can predict with considerable accuracy which superficial tumors probably would have invaded deeply had they not been detected earlier.
2. Death from BC is usually within 18–24 mo of the diagnosis of muscle invasion, so lead time bias poses less of a serious problem in evaluating the efficacy of screening than it does for so many other malignancies *(63)*.
3. Specific target populations at high risk for developing BC (based on age, race, gender, and various environmental and industrial exposures) are well described, and the yield of screening can be increased by focusing on these groups.
4. BC is almost never found incidentally at autopsy *(64)*, indicating that subjects in whom BC is detected by screening are unlikely to suffer the effects of over diagnosis and treatment.

BIASES AND PITFALLS IN SCREENING

Bladder cancer screening would only be of value if it decreases mortality and/or morbidity in individuals who are screened compared to an unscreened population. However, a variety of biases may render screening tests hard to evaluate, including:

1. Lead time bias: a screening program will bring forward the time of diagnosis, appearing to prolong survival even though the time of death from the cancer remains unchanged.
2. Length bias sampling: a screening program will more likely detect slower growing rather than faster growing tumors and hence diagnose more indolent cancers, with apparent improvement in survival.
3. Selection bias: a screening program will tend to recruit individuals who are more health conscious, thus making them more likely to seek earlier medical attention and have fewer comorbid conditions than those who chose not to participate.

For these reasons, only a prospective study that randomizes screened and unscreened individuals and follows subjects for outcome from the disease can truly evaluate the efficacy of screening.

DEFINING INDIVIDUALS AT RISK

The individuals at highest risk for BC are those with previously resected TCCs *(65)*. Indeed, they are currently screened at very frequent intervals with invasive procedures, including cystoscopy and lavage cytology. That no more than 10% of such patients go on to die from their malignancies *(6,66)* pays tribute to the success of early detection and aggressive therapy for superficial TCC. However, asymptomatic individuals without a history of BC would never undergo such invasive modalities without some evidence, based on noninvasive testing, that they were indicated. Subjects at less risk than these, but still increased from the general population, particularly middle-aged and elderly men with histories of cigarette smoking or exposure to BC carcinogens, may be ideal for repeated, less invasive screening studies.

MEANS OF SCREENING

Currently, BC is almost always diagnosed because it produces hematuria which is detected either by microscopic evaluation of urinary sediment or chemical reagent strip testing of voided urine. However, because of intermittency, for hematuria detection to be a successful screening strategy for BC, repetitive testings are needed *(1)*. There are newer promising screening tests that are more sensitive than hematuria testing of a single specimen, and more specific than hematuria detection in multiple specimens, which rely on biologic tumor markers excreted in urine. Candidate tests are discussed earlier in this chapter and others are being investigated. Since these tests are relatively expensive, they may not be suitable for use in general populations without prior histories of BC because of the relatively low proportion of subjects likely to have BC. Furthermore, many of these markers are expressed in normal urothelium and cutoff values can markedly influence the sensitivity and specificity of any detection technique. Despite these limitations and the clear need for further studies to define the performance of each test in various settings, the possibility of combining a variety of marker tests either by themselves or in individuals who have microhematuria to determine who should go on to cystoscopy, holds a great deal of promise for screening.

OUTCOMES OF SCREENING STUDIES

In four separate screening studies, Messing et al. in Wisconsin, USA *(5,6,67)* and Britton et al. in Leeds, England *(68,69)* asked men age 50 or 60 and older who were believed to be healthy and free of histories of hematuria-producing diseases, current hematuria (microscopic or macroscopic), or histories of genitourinary tract tumors, to take part in repetitive home testing with chemical reagent strips for hematuria. Although protocols varied slightly between the studies and only the Wisconsin study had repeated testing periods after the initial screening, the findings of the studies were remarkably similar. In each, 14–21% of participants had hematuria at entry, as defined by at least one positive test in the first 10–14 testings, and each was asked to undergo a work-up that included a physical examination, medical history, microscopic urine analysis, serum creatinine, prothrombin time, complete blood count, upper tract evaluation with ultrasound or intravenous urography, cystoscopy, and urine or bladder wash cytology. In each study, 6–8% of those evaluated were found to have genitourinary malignancies, of which over two-thirds were BCs. Each of these studies confirmed that the quantity of hematuria was unrelated to the seriousness of the underlying cause and demonstrated that hematuria often was intermittent.

To determine if hematuria screening effected earlier diagnoses and reduced BC mortality, Messing et al. *(6)* compared tumor types, grades, stages, and outcomes in the men with BCs detected by hematuria screening with those of men with BC diagnosed through standard clinical presentation in a comparable unscreened population. The unscreened population consisted of all Wisconsin men age 50 and over with newly diagnosed BCs reported to the state tumor registry in 1988 (the year between the two Wisconsin hematuria screening studies). Additionally, to determine if self-selection played a role in the findings, the 55% of men who were solicited but decided not to take part in hematuria screening were followed for a diagnosis of BC (as reported to the tumor registry) within 12 mo of the last home testing date scheduled (had they take part in screening) and for disease-related mortality within two years of diagnosis. The pathology materials from all newly diagnosed BCs in unscreened and screened populations were reviewed by a single pathologist unaware of the clinical diagnosis or whether subjects were screening participants or not.

A total of 21 BCs were detected in the 1575 men (1.3%) who participated in the screening programs. Twenty-three BCs were detected and reported to the state tumor registry in the 1940 men (1.2%) who chose not to be screened within 12 mo of what would have been their final testing date had they taken part in screening.

The proportions of low-grade (grade 1 and 2) superficial (stage Ta and T1) vs high-grade (grade 3) or invasive (stage $\geq$ T2) cancers in the screened and unscreened populations were not significantly different (52.4% vs 47.7% in 21 screened and 56.8% vs 43.3% in 511 unscreened cases [P = 0.20 between screened and unscreened cases]). However, only 4.8% of screening detected cancers actually invaded the muscularis propria, whereas 23.9% of all unscreened cancers were not diagnosed until they were muscle invading or more advanced (P = .007 between screened and unscreened cancers).

At 24 mo after diagnosis of the primary tumor, a total of 84 of the 511 men in the unscreened population had died from BC (16.4%). At 3–8 yr after diagnosis of the index tumor, 2 of the men in the screened population had died. However, both died from causes other than BC (esophageal and lung cancer), and neither had experienced BC recurrence at the time of death. The remaining 19 screened men with BC are alive 3 to 8 yr after the initial diagnosis and have been disease free for at least 2 yr (at last followup). From this study, the estimated efficacy of screening in preventing BC death is between 0.47 and 1.00, indicating that unscreened men who develop BC are much more likely to die from this malignancy than screened men.

Thus, hematuria screening appeared to reduce BC mortality, by detecting high-grade TCCs before they became muscle invading. However, this study, because it was not randomized, can be criticized because of possible biases. Although the populations were similar in terms of several known risk factors (e.g., age, gender, history of smoking), they may have differed in other ways causing a sampling bias. Additionally, although the followup in the screened population was far longer than in the unscreened one (3–8 yr vs 2 yr) —thus limiting the influence of lead-time bias, it may still have played a role in the more favorable outcomes in screened cases. Similarly, length bias sampling, which would favor finding indolent tumors in the screened group may have occurred, although a higher proportion of screened cancers were high-grade malignancies than unscreened cases. It is also possible that intentional self-selection had a significant impact on the screened population, although this is inconsistent with the finding that men who were solicited but declined to take part in screening had the same prevalence and incidence of BC as the screened group. Finally, it is possible that unscreened men with BC received less than optimal therapy. Such a bias is unlikely, however, because the 2-yr BC mortality rates of 16.4% for all unscreened BC cases and nearly 36% for high-grade or invasive unscreened BC are similar to what one would expect using available treatment regimens or what occurs in the country as a whole. Clearly, a randomized prospective trial of BC screening with unscreened controls is needed to clarify these matters and to determine whether screening is as promising as it appears to be from these data.

Screening Populations
Exposed to Putative Environmental Carcinogens

In 1986, the Drake Health Registry Study initiated bladder cancer screening for 366 persons at high risk because of occupational exposure to B-naphthylamine *(70)*. The screening protocol consisted of urinalysis, cytology and quantitative fluorescence image analysis (QFIA). Of the 26 positive results, most have been based on abnormal cytology *(3)* or abnormal image analysis *(13)* or both *(8)*. Bladder abnormalities were found among the 18 participants who went on to a complete diagnostic evaluation (cystoscopy). Given the relative youth of the cohort (60% had less than 20 yr exposure history), it is not surprising that no tumors were visible at cystoscopy as it is likely to take several years for symptomatic disease to occur. Nevertheless, screening by QFIA did prove effective in detecting various bladder pathologic conditions.

Mason and Vogler screened workers in a 3-yr case-control study at the Dupont Chamber Works for BC *(71)*. Those workers who were exposed to B-naphthylamine, benzidine, and 4,4-methlenebis (2-chloroaniline) were followed quarterly by urinalysis. Participants tested their urine for microhematuria using chemical reagent strips for 14 consecutive days every other quarter. Through the first 7 periods of screening, two new cases and one recurrence of TCC of the bladder were detected *(72)*.

Therialult et al. screened aluminum workers exposed to benzene-soluble coal tar pitch volatiles in Quebec *(73)*. They had reported that annual urinary cytology examinations have effected a shift of tumors to pre-muscle-invasive stages when compared with historical controls from the 1970s (39% non-muscle-invasive in the 1970s versus 63% non-muscle-invasive in 1980s) without any alteration in tumor grade (roughly 40-45% in both the 1970s and the 1980s groups had high grade tumors). However, potential biases exist that may account for this observed stage shift. Because of a heightened awareness about BC, workers in the 1980s may have been more sensitive to the need for aggressive evaluation of hematuria than workers in the 1970s were. Also, because of lead time issues, and because the unscreened control group had been followed longer, that mortality in the screened group (1980s) was significantly less is not surprising. Nevertheless, this study indicates that such workers may be appropriate subjects for screening programs.

SUMMARY

The current standard for diagnosing and monitoring BC relies upon cystoscopy, urinary or bladder wash cytology, and ultimately biopsy. A variety of already commercially available tests may aid in the diagnosis of BC, none that have yet been tested on large populations have sufficient sensitivity to replace the need for cystoscopy in the adult patient with micro- or macroscopic hematuria. However, these tests, perhaps used in patients with prior histories of low grade superficial BCs may reduce the frequency with which they require surveillance cystoscopies. Studies are needed to evaluate their use in this specific scenario. Additionally, tests detecting and/or measuring molecular tumor markers in urine or exfoliated cells are being evaluated, and several hold promise as surveillance and even diagnostic aids, particularly because of their increased sensitivity for low grade TCCs. However, without large trials, it is premature to advocate their use as a replacement for current modalities and practice standards.

Because of its biological and clinical behavior, BC is a potentially excellent disease for screening endeavors, although this has yet to be demonstrated in a prospective randomized trial following participants for outcome from this disease. Because of expense, methodological and performance factors, it is unlikely that these molecular tests can be satisfactory screening tools on their own but are likely to be useful, either alone or in combination, to determine which screening subject with hematuria should proceed to cystoscopy.

REFERENCES

1. Messing EM, Valencourt A. Hematuria screening for bladder cancer. J Occup Med 1990; 32: 838–845.
2. Messing EM. Early stage bladder cancer. Wis Med J 1987; 86: 14–17.
3. Messing EM, Young TB, Hunt VE, et al. Hematuria home screening: repeat testing results. J Urology 1995; 154 : 57–61.
4. Addis T. The number of formed elements in the urinary sediment of normal individuals. J Clin Invest 1926; 2: 409–415.
5. Messing EM, Young TB, Hunt VE, et al. Home screening for hematuria: results of a multiclinic study. J Urol 1992; 148: 289.
6. Messing EM, Young TB, Hunt VB, et al. Comparison of bladder cancer outcome in men undergoing hematuria home screening versus those with standard clinical presentations. Urology 1995; 45: 387.
7. Birch DF, Fairley FK. Hematuria: glomerular or non-glomerular? Lancet 1979; 2: 845.
8. Schramek P, Schuster FX, Georgopoulos M, et al. Value of urinary erythrocyte morphology in assessment of symptomless microhematuria. Lancet 1989; 2: 1316.
9. Fracchia JA, Motta J, Miller LS, et al. Evaluation of asymptomatic microhematuria. Urology 1995; 46: 484.
10. Bard RH. The significance of asymptomatic microhematuria in women and its economic implications: A ten-year study. Arch Intern Med 1988;148: 2629.
11. Benson GS, Brewer ED. Hematuria: algorithms for diagnosis. II. Hematuria in the adult and hematuria secondary to trauma. JAMA 1981; 246: 993.
12. Hiatt RA, Ordonez JD. Dipstick urinalysis screening, asymptomatic microhematuria, and subsequent urological cancers in a population-based sample. Cancer Epidemiol Biomarker Prev 1994; 3: 439.
13. Howard RS, Golin AL. Long-term followup of asymptomatic microhematuria. J Urol 1991; 145: 335.
14. Golin AL, Howard RS. Asymptomatic microscopic hematuria. J Urol 1980; 124: 389.
15. Sutton JM. Evaluation of hematuria in adults. JAMA 1990; 263: 2475.
16. Papanicolaou GN, Marshall VF. Urine sediment smears as a diagnostic procedure in cancers of the urinary tract. Science 1945; 101: 519.
17. Grégoire M, Fradet Y, Meyer F, Têtu B, Bois R, Bédard G, et al. Diagnostic accuracy of urinary cytology and DNA flow cytometry and cytology on bladder washings during follow-up for bladder tumors. J Urol 1997; 157: 1660–1664.
18. Allard P, Bernard P, Fradet Y, Têtu B. The early clinical course of primary Ta and T1 bladder cancer: a prognostic index. Brit J Urol 1998; 81: 692–698.
19. Nam RK, Redelmeier DA, Spiess PE, Sampson HA, Fradet Y, Jewett MAS. Comparison of molecular and conventional strategies for followup of superficial bladder cancer using decision analysis. J Urol 2000; 163: 752–757.

20. Sarosdy MF, deVere White RW, Soloway MS, Sheinfeld J, Hudson MA, Schell-hammer PF, et al. Results of a multicenter trial using the BTA test to monitor for and diagnose recurrent bladder cancer. J Urol 1995; 154: 379–393.

21. Sarosdy MF, Hudson MA, Ellis WJ, Soloway MS, deVere White R, Sheinfeld J, et al. Improved detection of recurrent bladder cancer using the Bard BTA stat test. Urology 1997; 50: 349–353.

22. Wiener HG, Mian C, Haitel A, Pycha A, Schatzl G, Marberger M. Can urine bound diagnostic tests replace cystoscopy in the management of bladder cancer? J Urol 1998; 159: 1876.

23. Leyh H, Marberger M, Conort P, Sternberg C, Pansadoro V, Pagano F, et al. Comparison of the BTA stat test with voided urine cytology and bladder wash cytology in the diagnosis and monitoring of bladder cancer. Eur Urol 1999; 35: 52–56.

24. Ramakumar S, Bhuiyan J, Besse JA, Roberts SG, Wollan PC, Blute ML, O'Kane DJ. Comparison of screening methods in the detection of bladder cancer. J Urol 1999; 161: 388–394.

25. Pode D, Shapiro A, Wald M, Nativ O, Laufer M, Kaver I. Noninvasive detection of bladder cancer with the BTA stat test. J Urol 1999; 161: 443–446.

26. Johnston B, Morales A, Emerson L, Lundie M. Rapid detection of bladder cancer: a comparative study of point of care tests. J Urol 1997; 158: 2098–2101.

27. Soloway MS, Briggman V, Carpinito GA, Chodak GW, Church PA, Lamm DL, et al. Use of a new tumor marker urinary NMP22, in the detection of occult or rapidly recurring transitional cell carcinoma of the urinary tract following surgical treatment. J Urol 1996; 156: 363–367.

28. Landman J, Chang Y, Kavaler E, Droller MJ, Liu BC-S. Sensitivity and specificity of NMP-22, telomerase, and BTA in the detection of human bladder cancer. Urology 1998; 52: 398–402.

29. Del Nero A, Esposito N, Curro A, Biasoni D, Montanari E, Mangiarotti B, et al. Evaluation of urinary level of NMP22 as a diagnostic marker for stage pTa-pT1 bladder cancer: comparison with urinary cytology and BTA test. Eur Urol 1999; 35: 93–97.

30. Sanchez-Carbayo M, Herrero E, Megias J, Mira A, Soria F. Comparative sensitivity of urinary CYFRA 21-1, urinary bladder cancer antigen, tissue polypeptide antigen and NMP22 to detect bladder cancer. J Urol 1999; 162: 1951–1956.

31. Ellis WJ, Blumenstein BA, Ishak LM, Enfield DL. Clinical evaluation of the BTA TRAK assay and comparison to voided urine cytology and the BARD BTA test in patients with recurrent bladder tumors. The Multi Center Study Group. Urology 1997; 50: 882–887.

32. Thomas L, Leyh H, Marberger M, Bombardieri E, Bassi P, Pagano F, et al. Multicenter trial of the quantitative BTA TRAK assay in the detection of bladder cancer. Clin Chem 1999; 45: 472–477.

33. Fradet Y, Lockhart C, and the ImmunoCyt™ Trialists. Performance characteristics of a new monoclonal antibody test for bladder cancer: ImmunoCyt™. Can J Urol 1997; 4: 400–405.

34. Mian C, Pycha A, Wiener H, Haitel A, Lodde M, Marberger M. ImmunoCyt: a new tool for detecting transitional cell cancer of the urinary tract. J Urol 1999; 1612: 1486–1489.

35. Kavaler E, Landman J, Chang Y, Droller MJ, Liu BC. Detecting human bladder carcinoma cells in voided urine samples by assaying for the presence of telomerase activity. Cancer 1998; 82: 708–714.

36. Dalbagni G, Han W, Zhang ZF, Cordon-Cardo C, Saigo P, Fair WR, et al. Evaluation of the telomeric repeat amplification protocol (TRAP) assay for telomerase as a diagnostic modality in recurrent bladder cancer. Clin Cancer Res 1997; 3: 1593–1598.

37. Muller M, Krause H, Heicappell R, Tischendorf J, Shay JW, Miller K. Comparison of human telomerase RNA and telomerase activity in urine for diagnosis of bladder cancer. Clin Cancer Res 1998; 4: 1949–1954.
38. Lokeshwar VB, Obek C, Pham HT, Wei D, Young MJ, Duncan RC, et al. Urinary hyaluronic acid and hyaluronidase: markers for bladder cancer detection and evaluation of grade. J Urol 2000; 163: 348–356.
39. Knowles MA, Elder PA, Williamson M, Cairns JP, Shaw ME, Law MG. Allelotype of human bladder cancer. Cancer Res 1994; 54: 531–538.
40. Reeder JE, O'Connell MJ, Yang Z, Morreale JF, Collins L, Frank IN, et al. DNA cytometry and chromosome 9 aberrations by fluorescence in situ hybridization of irrigation specimens from bladder cancer patients. Urology 1998; 51(Suppl 5A): 58–61.
41. Zhang FF, Arber DA, Wilson TG, Kawachi MH, Slovak ML. Toward the validation of aneusomy detection by fluorescence in situ hybridization in bladder cancer: comparative analysis with cytology, cytogenetics, and clinical features predicts recurrence and defines clinical testing limitations. Clin Cancer Res 1997; 3: 2317–2328.
42. Mao L, Schoenberg MP, Sciccitano M, Erozan YS, Merlo A, Schwab D, Sidransky D. Molecular detection of primary bladder cancer by microsatellite analysis. Science 1996; 271: 659–662.
43. Steiner G, Schoenberg MP, Linn JF, Mao L, Sidransky D. Detection of bladder cancer recurrence by microsatellite analysis of urine. Nat Med 1997; 3(6): 621–624.
44. Mourah S, Cussenot O, Vimont V, Desgrandchamps F, Teillac P, Cochant-Priollet B, et al. Assessment of microsatellite instability in urine in the detection of transitional-cell carcinoma of the bladder. Int J Cancer 1998; 79: 629–633.
45. Messing EM, Murphy-Brooks N. Recovery of epidermal growth factor in voided urine of patients with BC. Urology 1994; 44: 502–506.
46. Fuse H, Mizuno I, Sakamoto M, Katayama T. Epidermal growth factor in urine from the patients with urothelial tumors. Urol Int 1992; 48: 261.
47. Messing EM, Hanson P, Ulrich P, Erturk E. Epidermal growth factor-interactions with normal and malignant urothelium: in vivo and in situ studies. J Urol 1987; 138: 1329.
48. Messing EM. Clinical implications of the expression of epidermal growth factor receptors in human transitional cell carcinoma. Cancer Res 1990; 50: 2530.
49. Goldberg MR, Heimbrook DC, Russo P, Sarosdy MF, Greenberg RE, Giatonio BJ, et al. Phase I clinical study of the recombinant oncotoxin TP40 in superficial bladder cancer. Clinical Cancer Res 1995; 1: 57–61.
50. Koraitim M, Kamal B, Metwalli N, Zaky Y. Transurethral ultrasonographic assessment of bladder carcinoma: its value and limitation. J Urol. 1995; 154: 375– 378.
51. Hussain S, Loeffler JA, Babayan RK, Fenlon HM. Thin-section helical computed tomography of the bladder: initial clinical experience with virtual reality imaging. Urology 1997; 50(5): 685–689.
52. Merkle EM, Wunderlich A, Aschoff AJ, Rilinger N, Gorich J, Bachor R, et al. Virtual cystoscopy based on helical CT scan datasets: perspectives and limitations. Brit J Radiol 1998: 71: 262–267.
53. Jocham D, Baumgartner R, Fuchs N, et al. Die Fluoreszenzdiagnose Prophyrin-markierter urothelialer tumoren. Urologe(a) 1989; 28: 59–64.
54. Kriegmair M, Baumgartner R, Knuechel R, et al. Detection of early bladder cancer by 5 aminolevulinic acid induced fluorescence. J Urol 1996; 155: 105–109.
55. D'Hallewin MA, Vanherzeele H, Baert L. Fluorescence detection of flat transitional cell carcinoma after intravesical instillation of aminolevulinic acid. Am J Clin Oncol 1998; 21(3): 223–225.

56. Filbeck T, Wimmershoff M, Pichlmeier, et al. Skin phototoxicity after intravesical instillation of 5-aminolevulinic acid for fluorescence diagnosis of bladder cancer. J Urol 1999; 161(4)Suppl Abstract 580.

57. Filbeck T, Roessler W, Knuechel R, Straub M, Kiel HJ, Wieland WF. 5-Amino-levulinic acid-induced fluorescence endoscopy applied at secondary transurethral resection after conventional resection of primary superficial bladder tumors. Urology 1999; 53(1): 77–81.

58. Iguchi A, Kinoshita N, Masaki Z. In vivo detection by microscopic chromocysto-scopy of concurrent urothelial atypia in superficial bladder cancer. Brit J Urol 1992; 70 : 152–155.

59. Jewett HJ, Strong GH. Infiltrating carcinoma of the bladder: relation of depth of penetration of the bladder wall to incidence of local extension and metastases. J Urol 1946; 55: 366.

60. Freeman JA, Esrig DE, Stein JP, et al. Radical cystectomy for high risk patients with superficial bladder cancer in the era of orthotopic urinary reconstruction. Cancer 1995; 76: 833.

61. Kaye KW, Lange PH. Mode of presentation of invasive bladder cancer: reassess-ment of the problem. J Urol 1982; 128: 31.

62. Hopkins SC, Ford KS, Soloway MS. Invasive bladder cancer: support for screen-ing. J Urol 1983; 130: 61.

63. Prout GR, Barton BA, Griffin P, Friedell G. Treated history of noninvasive grade 1 transitional cell carcinoma. J Urol 1992; 148: 1413–1419.

64. Kishi K, Hirota T, Matsumoto K, et al. Carcinoma of the bladder: a clinical and pathological analysis of 87 autopsy cases. J Urol 1981; 125: 36–39.

65. Lamm DL. Long-term results of intravesical therapy for superficial bladder cancer. Urol Clin North Am 1992; 19: 573–580.

66. Cookson MS, Sarosdy MF. Management of stage T1 superficial bladder cancer with intravesical bacillus Calmette-Guerin therapy. J Urol 1992; 148: 797–801.

67. Messing EM, Young TB, Hunt VB, Wehbie JM, Rust P. Urinary tract cancers found by home screening with hematuria dip stick in health men over 50 years of age. Cancer 1989; 64: 2361–2367.

68. Britton JP, Dowell AC, Whelan P. Dipstick hematuria and bladder cancer in men over 60: results of a community study. Br Med J 1989; 299: 1010–1012.

69. Britton JP, Dowell AC, Whelan P, Harris CM. A community study of bladder cancer screening by the detection of occult urinary bleeding. J Urol 1992; 148: 788–790.

70. Marsh GM, Callahan C, Pavlock D, Leviton LC, Talbott EO, Hemstreet G. A protocol for bladder cancer screening and medical surveillance among high-risk groups: the Drake health registry experience. J Occup Med 1990; 32: 881.

71. Mason TJ, Vogler WJ. Bladder cancer screening at the Dupont Chamber Works: a new initiative. J Occup Med 1990; 32: 874.

72. Masib TJ, Walsh WP, Lee K, Vogler W. New opportunities for screening and early detection of bladder cancer. J Cell Biochem Suppl 1992; 16l: 13–22.

73. Theriault GP, Tremblay CG, Armstrong BG. Bladder cancer screening among pri-mary aluminum production workers in Quebec. J Occup Med 1990; 32: 869.

4 Diagnostic Imaging in Urothelial Cancer

Lynn Ladetsky, MD, Harold Mitty, MD, and Rosaleen B. Parsons, MD

CONTENTS

INTRODUCTION
CONVENTIONAL UROGRAPHY
CONCLUSION
REFERENCES

INTRODUCTION

Radiology's role in the detection of bladder cancer is limited. However, imaging plays an important role in staging bladder tumors. This chapter discusses the different imaging modalities used to stage bladder cancer and the advantages and disadvantages of each. Urography is often the initial study performed for evaluation of urothelial tumors. CT and MRI are conventionally used for staging bladder cancer, with the highest accuracy seen for staging more invasive tumors. Investigational techniques such as CT cystoscopy and advanced MRI post-processing methods will undoubtedly improve radiographic detection and staging of bladder cancer. The use of traditional ultrasound is of limited value for staging bladder tumors but transurethral ultrasound and ultrasound contrast agents should improve its accuracy .The role of nuclear medicine, and in particular positron emission tomography (PET) for detection and staging continues to emerge *(1)*. Tumor targeting potential of radionuclides has shown some promise in animal models *(2)*.

From: *Current Clinical Urology: Bladder Cancer: Current Diagnosis and Treatment*
Edited by: M. J. Droller © Humana Press Inc., Totowa, NJ

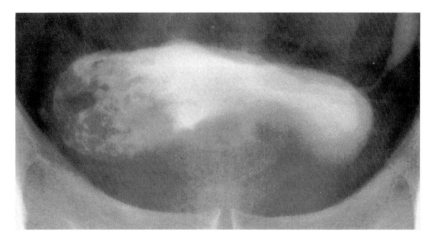

Fig. 1. Papillary transitional carcinoma. Note the contrast material between the fronds of tissue giving a stippled appearance.

CONVENTIONAL UROGRAPHY

Intravenous urography provides a method for the demonstration of bladder masses as well as the general status of the kidneys, ureters, and surrounding structures. Since small urothelial neoplasms of the collecting system and ureter may occur synchronously with a bladder tumor, it is important to demonstrate these structures. Urography remains a sensitive method for detection small upper tract lesions that are often clinically occult. Since urography provides visualization of the lumen of the bladder it is not as effective as CT, ultrasound, and MRI for showing the extent of disease. Urographic findings such as hydronephrosis and ureteral displacement are generally associated with more advanced disease.

Papillary tumors produce intraluminial filling defects that have an irregular surface which has been described as stippled. This appearance is due to the presence of contrast material between the fronds of tissue (Fig. 1). Because of the large volume of the filled bladder small papillary lesions may be missed by urography. In fact, an attempt to demonstrate small bladder lesions urographically is rarely made since they are usually directly visualized at cystoscopy.

Transitional cell tumors that are more infiltrative tend to produce a contour defect in the bladder wall which is manifested as a flattening at the site of tumor growth (Fig. 2). This appearance is not specific as it may be produced by adjacent inflammatory disease (Fig. 3), hematoma, previous treatments, or rare conditions such as amyloidosis involving the bladder. In addition, this type of flattening may be due to direct invasion by other neoplasms.

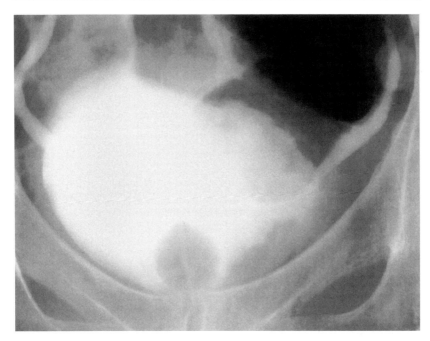

Fig. 2. Infiltrating transitional cell carcinoma. The irregular tumor has produced a contour defect at the left bladder base as it infiltrates the wall.

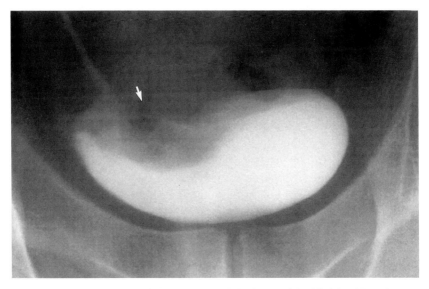

Fig. 3. Crohn's disease with fistula to the right dome of the bladder. Note the gas in the mid superior aspect of the bladder defect (*arrow*), and nodular contour, mimicking tumor infiltration.

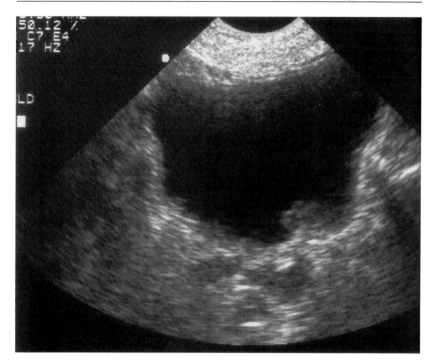

Fig. 4. Transabdominal ultrasound in the transverse plane showing a peduncu-lated tumor the left at bladder base.

Ultrasound

Ultrasound evaluation of the bladder can be performed quickly and is readily available. When the bladder is distended the wall is thin and smooth measuring up to 3 mm in thickness *(3)*. Transitional cell carcinoma typically appears as a single or multifocal mass which is slightly more echogenic than bladder mucosa and submucosa (Fig. 4). However, the differential diagnosis for a thick walled bladder is extensive and includes tumor invading from contiguous organs, cystitis, trabeculation and thickening from long-standing outlet obstruction, adherent blood clot or debris, and postoperative changes *(4)*.

Transabdominal ultrasound is limited in its ability to detect and stage bladder tumors. One study reported a false-negative rate of 24% of cystoscopically detected tumors *(3)*. Technical difficulties such as patient obesity, postoperative changes, and tumor location contribute to this unacceptably high false-negative rate. Tumors located in the bladder trigone and near the dome are missed in 40% of the cases *(3)*. Tumors located in the lateral walls are easier to visualize. Larger size tumors, above 2 cm, are more easily detected than those measuring less than 5 mm.

Because of the limitations of transabdominal ultrasound, transurethral ultrasound was introduced *(5)*. A transducer is introduced through a 24F sheath, under anesthesia. Smaller transducers of higher frequency may also be introduced through a standard cystoscope. Visualization of the tumor is accomplished by the acoustic differences between the fluid surrounding the transducer, the bladder wall and the tumor. Transducers with ability to scan at multiple angles are used to allow complete visualization of the entire bladder wall. Because of scattering, the transition between bladder wall and perivesical fat may not be clearly visualized. High frequency transducers produce high-resolution images of structures near the transducer. However, the high frequency ultrasound beam is limited in its ability to penetrate and therefore poorly visualizes structures outside the bladder.

There has been limited experience with transurethral ultrasound. In several studies it has been found to be most accurate for local staging and for tumor confined to the bladder wall. The accuracy decreases for tumors with extravesical extension *(6)*. Distensibility of the bladder wall is assessed during filling of the bladder with irrigation fluid. Superficial tumors do not cause fixation or distortion of the wall. Muscle invasive tumors, limit the distensibility of the bladder wall and cause fixation and distortion of the bladder wall. Superficial tumors appear as masses projecting into the bladder lumen and are nonmobile as opposed to stones and clots. Invasion of muscle layers appears as interruption of the smooth and curved echo pattern of the bladder wall. One particular advantage of transurethral ultrasound is the detection of tumor within diverticuli, which might not be seen with cystoscopy.

An investigational technique is the introduction of ultrasound contrast agents. Carbon dioxide microbubbles, are injected into the blood vessels to improve the tissue contrast. In a recent study this technique was used to follow patients with muscle invasive bladder cancer who were being treated with low dose cisplatin and radiotherapy. The investigators found this method improved visualization of the tumor when compared to conventional ultrasound *(7)*. This technique holds more promise than color doppler alone which has not been found to be useful for staging *(8)*.

Computed Tomography

There is currently no role for diagnostic imaging in screening for bladder carcinoma or staging superficial disease. Cystoscopy, transurethral resection and bimanual examination are more accurate than imaging for staging T1 and T2 lesions. However once invasive bladder carcinoma is detected there is a role for imaging. Traditionally this has been performed

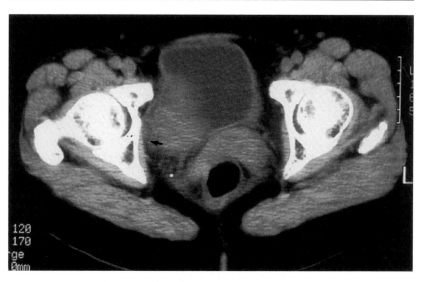

Fig. 5. Noncontrast CT scan shows a lobulated carcinoma along the right poste-rolateral aspect of the bladder with an intraluminal component as wall as extravesical extension (*arrow*) into the perivesical fat.

with CT. Both CT and Magnetic resonance imaging overstage tumor when imaging occurs after intervention. CT is usually more accessible and cost effective than MRI. A major drawback of CT is its inability to depict the extent of intramural invasion due to the similar attenuation of the bladder wall and carcinoma.

The morphology of the intraluminal component of bladder tumors appears similar on CT and MRI. Bladder neoplasms may present as either a sessile or pedunculated soft tissue mass or diffuse bladder wall thickening (Fig. 5, 6A,B). On non-contrast scans the attenuation characteristics of bladder tumors are similar to the bladder wall. However on dynamic scanning after the intravenous injection of iodinated contract, bladder tumors appear denser than the bladder wall. Tumor extension beyond the bladder wall causes blurring of the perivesical fat planes (Fig. 7). With invasive disease the tumor may be seen directly extending into adjacent organs such as rectum, vagina, prostate and seminal vesicles or muscles. Obliteration of the normal seminal vesicle angle with the posterior wall of the bladder is not a reliable sign of tumor extension as overdistension of the rectum may cause the angle to be distorted in some normal patients. False positive results may occur when a distinct fat plane between contiguous organs is not visualized and early invasion is suspected. Perivesical inflammation and fibrosis is indistinguishable from tumor and a frequent cause of overstaging. The overall staging accuracy

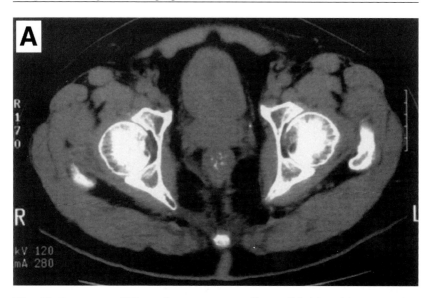

Fig. 6A. Precontrast CT scan demonstrates a collapsed bladder with a suggestion of polypoid intraluminal masses.

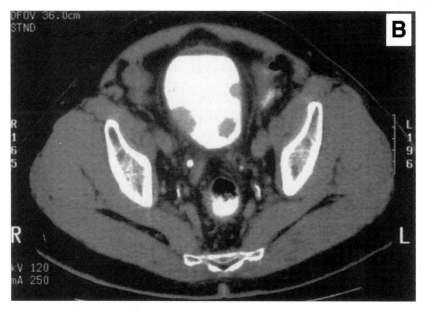

Fig. 6B. Delayed postcontrast image. The polypoid intraluminal masses are shown to better advantage.

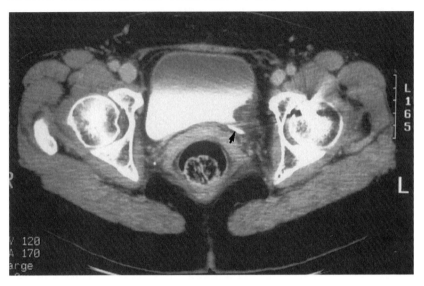

Fig. 7. Postcontrast CT scan shows a bladder tumor adjacent to the left ure-terovesical junction (*arrow*) projecting into the bladder lumen.

for primary tumors with CT ranges from 40–92% (mean 74%). The over-all accuracy of MR staging is higher ranging from 73–96% (mean 85%).

Spiral CT scanning technology has produced great advancements in CT scanning. Coverage of the entire abdomen and pelvis can occur dur-ing a single breath hold, which enables better contrast utilization and lessens respiratory misregistration. Partial volume effects are reduced and overlapping slice reconstruction as well as three-dimensional recon-struction has become practical. All of these advances have improved the quality of multiplanar reformatted images.

Bladder pseudolesion artifacts are unique to spiral CT and are produced by the opacified urine entering the bladder during contrast enhanced dynamic scanning. By obtaining delayed images through the bladder, pseudolesions can be distinguished form true lesions *(11)*.

With the advent of helical CT scanning technology and postprocess-ing software, helical CT data sets can be used to produce three-dimen-sional shaded surface display images of the bladder as well as virtual cystoscopy. Narumi et al. *(12)* imaged patients with suspected bladder cancer prior to cystoscopy and then used the helical CT data to produce a 3D display of the bladder. In order to obtain the maximum density difference between the wall of the bladder and the bladder lumen, air was injected into the bladder through a urethral catheter. The data acquired was reconstructed to produce a 3D shaded-surface display. In Narumi's study, 52 (85%) of 61 tumors seen on cystoscopy were identified by 3D shaded-surface display.

These 3D techniques have advantages over cystoscopy in that they offer a wider field of view and can visualize the anterior wall near the bladder base. They can more objectively measure the tumor and provide preoperative mapping prior to transurethral resection as well as follow up after chemotherapy. The 3D shaded-surface display technique is limited in the identification of lesions smaller than 10 mm and those which are flat in morphology.

Vining et al. *(13)* used helically acquired data sets of the bladder to perform virtual cystoscopy. This requires several manipulations of the data utilizing computer technology, which was originally developed for special effects in the movie industry. The steps after acquiring the data include data transfer, volume formation, image segmentation, 3D rendering and video recording. The images are transferred to a Silicon Graphics (SGI, Mountainview, CA) work station computer via an Ethernet network. Explorer (SGI) software program generates 3D surface rendered images of the bladder. These images can be viewed from any projection within the bladder lumen thus simulating a cystoscopic exam. The Explorer software and the real time rendering capabilities of the SGI computer allows the user to navigate through video images of the bladder with a computer cursor directed by a mouse.

Subsequent investigations of the efficacy of detecting bladder cancer by CT virtual cystoscopy have drawn conflicting conclusions. Merkle et al. *(14)* studied 11 patients with both virtual and real cystoscopy. All of the bladder tumors identified at fibreoptic cystoscopy were seen with virtual cystoscopy. The latter was however, not reliable for detection of the ureteral orrifices. The authors concluded that virtual cystoscopy had not reached the quality of the fibreoptic examination and recommended its use in specific cases such as patients with urethral strictures.

Hussain et al. *(15)* found virtual cystoscopy accurate in detecting bladder masses, which were discovered on conventional cystoscopy. They concluded that it may represent a radiological adjunct to conventional cystoscopy for initial evaluation of patients with hematuria and for surveillance of patients after bladder tumor resection. Clearly CT cystoscopy is in its infancy and additional studies will be needed to determine the future role of this new technique in staging bladder cancer.

Finally, CT plays an important role in surveillance. Lymphadenopathy is readily seen with CT. Diagnosing lymph node metastases depends on size criteria. Lymphatic spread usually occurs first in the medial or obturator followed by the middle group of external iliac nodes. Then the internal iliac and common iliac node chains become involved. Lymph nodes measuring less than 1 cm are considered normal, nodes measuring between 1.0 and 1.5 cm are indeterminate and nodes greater than 1.5 cm are abnormal. If an enlarged node is detected, CT guided biopsy, which is widely available, may be performed to assess for tumor involvement.

MRI

MRI has unique strengths, including multiplanar capabilities and superior tissue contrast. Because the bladder wall and the perivesical fat are well defined and have characteristic signals on different sequences, bladder wall invasion of tumor and extension into perivesical fat can be well visualized. Multiplanar capabilities allow three dimensional lymph node measurements as well as better visualization of tumor involving the bladder dome or base.

MRI examination of the bladder does not require any special patient preparation. The exam can be performed using standard commercially available units and coils. Depending on the size of the patient either a body or torso coil is adequate. In some instances where tumor extension into the prostate is questioned there may be a benefit to performing endorectal MRI. The imaging parameters can be adjusted depending on the tumor location. T1 weighted spin echo sequences are obtained in the axial plane with 5mm slice thickness and a gap of 2 mm and a 300–700 msec TR and 10–20 msec TE. Matrix size of 256×192 with 2 NEX and field of view of 32–40 cm. A corresponding axial FSE sequence is also obtained 4000–5000 TR and 102 (effective) TE. This is then followed with either a coronal or sagittal FSE. There may be an advantage to performing additional imaging following the intravenous injection of gadopentatate dimeglumine, as will be described later in the chapter.

T1 weighted images are used to determine tumor extension into perivesical fat and to visualize the endoluminal component of the tumor. On T1 weighted sequences carcinoma is similar in intensity to skeletal muscle, urine is low in signal and perivesical fat is high in signal. The endoluminal component of tumor can be easily demonstrated on T1 (Fig. 8). The depth of intramural invasion cannot be distinguished on T1 because of the similar signal intensity of tumor and muscle. Extravesical disease may be conspicuous against the high signal perivesical fat. Lymph node and bone metastases are best seen with T1 weighted sequences.

FSE weighted images help to determine depth of tumor infiltration into bladder wall. The signal of the bladder wall is lower than that of the tumor. Urine is higher in signal intensity compared with tumor. Therefore the endoluminal component can be visualized (Figs. 9 and 10). The zonal anatomy of prostate and uterus is seen on FSE weighted images allowing assessment of invasion into surrounding organs. Seminal vesical

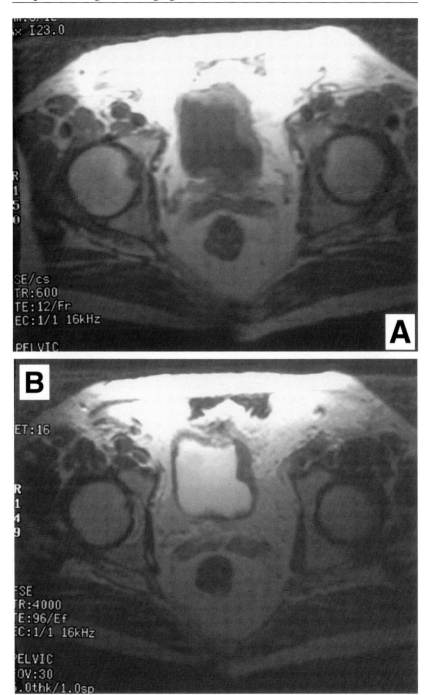

Fig. 8A,B. Axial T1 and FSE (**B**) weighted MRI shows dark signal urine outlining an infiltrating transitional cell carcinoma.

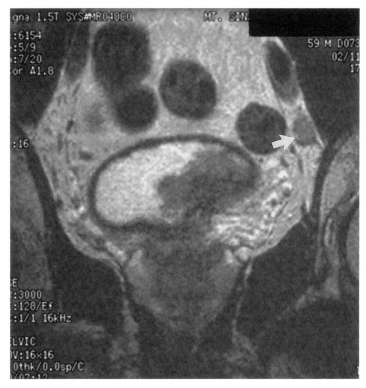

Fig. 9. Coronal FSE weighted MRI demonstrates a polypoid carcinoma project-ing into the bladder lumen. High signal urine outlines the bladder mass. A patho-logically enlarged left iliac chain lymph node is identified (*arrow*).

invasion can also be assessed because of the contrast difference between high signal intensity of the seminal vesicals and relative hypointensity of tumor (Fig. 11).

MRI has been limited in its ability to stage superficial tumors and to dis-tinguish post-biopsy changes and inflammation from superficial tumor. It has also been shown that MRI may overestimate tumor stage when there is perivesical inflammation or inflammatory changes in adjacent organs and the pelvic side wall. Therefore staging becomes more diffi-cult after diagnostic and therapeutic procedures. Other limitations of MRI include high cost and limited access

Recent studies have shown that dynamic contrast enhanced sequences improved the accuracy of MRI in staging both superficial and invasive tumors as well as staging tumors after transurethral biopsy *(17,18)*. When fast MRI sequences such as single section turbo fast low-angle shot (FLASH) are used during the first pass of the contrast bolus with images acquired every 2 s, the timing of urinary bladder cancer enhance-

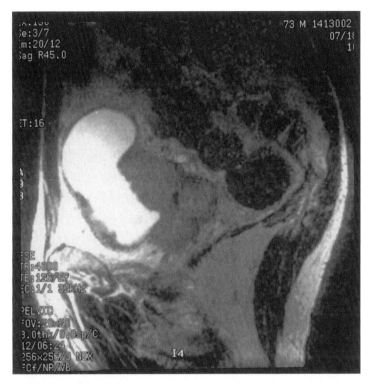

Fig. 10. Sagittal FSE weighted images demonstrates an irregular bulky exophytic tumor along the inferior half of the bladder.

ment can be assessed. Barentsz *(18)* showed that bladder cancer starts to enhance 6.5 sec ± 3 sec(SD) after the beginning of arterial enhancement. Postbiopsy tissue enhanced later, 13.6 sec ± 4.2 sec (SD) after arterial enhancement. Postprocessing color-coded time and slope images are generated to further analyze the timing of enhancement. Using unenhanced as well as fast dynamic first-pass enhanced imaging with time analysis the overall accuracy of staging improved from 67–84% (Fig. 12). Once excreted contrast is demonstrated in the bladder the tumor becomes inconspicuous.

This first pass technique is also helpful for evaluating lymph node metastases which show enhancement characteristics similar to bladder cancer.

Other MRI sequences besides conventional two-dimensional spin echo sequences are of value in staging bladder cancer. Barentsz *(19)* describes the use of magnetization prepared-rapid gradient-echo (MP-RAGE) as a three dimensional T1 weighted MR imaging sequence for staging. A-3 dimensional acquisition can be used to reformat the image in a plane,

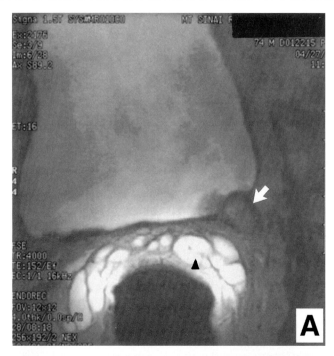

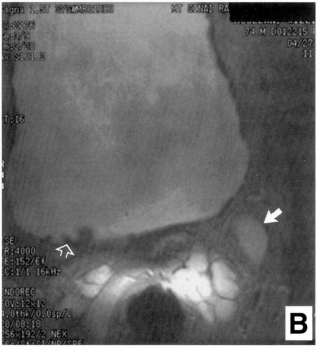

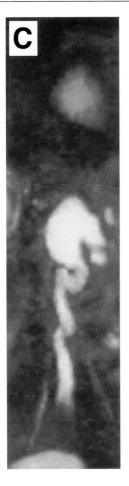

Fig. 11A,B. (*opposite page*). Axial FSE weighted MRI using an endorectal coil demonstrates the small polypoid bladder tumor at the left ureterovesical junction causing obstruction (*arrow*). The bright serpiginous structures posterior to the bladder are the seminal vesicles (*black arrowhead*). Note the multiple tiny polypoid intraluminal bladder masses (*open arrow*) along right posterolateral aspect of bladder in same patient. (**C**) MR urogram showing left hydroureteronephrosis secondary to the obstructing bladder tumor.

which better characterizes tumor extent and involvement of lymph nodes. With MP-RAGE sequences, there were fewer motion artifacts as compared with conventional T1-weighted spin echo sequences. Spatial resolution and fluid-tumor contrast improved. An application of this technique allows oblique imaging that can be used for directed biopsy a suspicious node that would be inaccessible to CT.

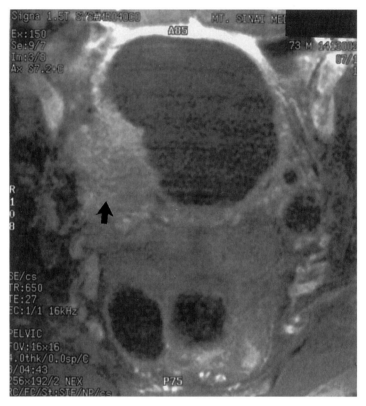

Fig. 12. Early dynamic post contrast enhanced axial T1 weighted MRI showing a bulky enhancing tumor with gross extravesical extension.

CT shares some of MRI's limitations of overstaging tumor especially when imaging occurs after interventions. CT is usually more accessible and cost effective than MRI. Because the density of bladder tumor is similar to normal bladder wall on CT scanning, a major drawback of CT is its inability to depict extent of intramural invasion (stage T1 from T2). MRI is more promising for evaluating deep muscle invasion by tumor because of the higher signal intensity of tumor and lower signal of bladder wall on FSE weighted sequences. CT is limited to axial plane imaging whereas MRI images in the coronal and sagittal planes. This multiplanar capability enables better depiction of tumor involving the base and dome of the bladder, which would be imaged tangentially in the axial plane. Determining size of lymph nodes may also be more accurate on MRI given that the lymph node may be visualized in a third plane. However both MRI and CT are limited in the diagnosis of tumor in a normal sized lymph node. Size continues to be the main criteria for diagnosing lymph node involvement. Advantages of CT over MRI include lack of specific MRI artifacts such as chemical shift and breathing artifacts, which degrade the images. Reduced spatial resolution and signal to noise ratio occur in FSE weighted sequences. The study by Kim in Radiology 1994 *(16)* found that CT and MRI performed comparably well in the detection of tumors. MRI was more accurate in staging than CT. Dynamic contrast enhanced MR imaging with gadopentetate dimeglumine appears promising for staging superficial disease and for detection of tumor in normal sized nodes.

CONCLUSION

With investigational techniques of CT generated virtual cystoscopy and newer MRI pulse sequences and post-processing methods, radiology is making inroads into the detection of bladder cancer as well as continuing to improve the accuracy of staging bladder cancer.

There is currently no role for diagnostic imaging in screening for bladder carcinoma or staging superficial disease. Cystoscopy, transurethral resection and bimanual examination are more accurate than imaging for staging T1 and T2 lesions. However once invasive bladder carcinoma is detected there is a role for imaging. Traditionally this has been performed with CT. Both CT and Magnetic resonance imaging overstage tumor when imaging occurs after intervention. CT is usually more accessible and cost effective than MRI. A major drawback of CT is its inability to depict the extent of intramural invasion because the density of the bladder wall is similar to carcinoma. MRI is more promising for evaluating deep muscle invasion by tumor because of the higher signal intensity of tumor and lower signal of the bladder wall on FSE weighted sequences.

The role of MRI and in particular dynamic enhanced MRI for staging bladder cancer continues to evolve and in the future it is likely to become the imaging modality of choice for staging.

REFERENCES

1. Ahlstrom H, Malmstrom PU, Letocha H, et al. Position emission tomography in the diagnosis and staging of urinary bladder cancer. Acta Radiol 1996; 37(2): 180–185.
2. Van-Den-Abbelle AD, Tutrone RF, Berman RM, et al. Tumor-targeting potential of radioiodinated iododeoxyurdine in bladder cancer. J Nucl Med 1996; 37(2): 315–320.
3. Djavan B, Roehrborn CG. Bladder ultrasonography. Semin Urol 1994; 12(4): 306–319.
4. Rumak UM, Wilson SR, Charboneau JW. Diagnostic ultrasound. Mosby, St. Louis, MO, 1991; (1): 247–248.

5. Holm HH, Northered A. A transurethral ultrasonic scanner. J Urol 1984; 111: 238–241.
6. Korartim M, Kamal B, Metwalli N, et al. Transurethral ultrasonographic assessment of bladder carcinoma: its value and limitation. J Urol 1995; 154: 375–378.
7. Akimoto T, Matsumoto M, Mitsuhashi N, et al. Evaluation of effect of treatment for invasive bladder cancer by ultrasonography with intra-arterial infusion of carbon dioxide microbubbles. Invest Radiol 1997; 32(7): 396–400.
8. Horstman WG, McFarland RM, Gorman JD. Color doppler sonogarphic findings in patients with transitional cell carcinoma of the bladder and renal pelvis. J Ultrasound Med 1995; 14: 129–133.
9. Barentsz JO, Witjes JA, Ruijs JHJ. What is new in bladder cancer imaging. Urol Clin A 1997; 24(3): 583–602.
10. Lee JKT, Sagel SS, Stanley RJ, Heiken JP. Computed body tomography with MRI correlation. Lippincott Williams and Williams, PA, 1998, pp. 1218–1225.
11. Olcott EW, Nino-Murcia M, Rhee JS. Urinary bladder pseudolesions on contrast-enhanced helical CT: Frequency and clinical implications. AJR 1998; 171: 1349–1354.
12. Narumi Y, Kumatani T, Sawai Y, et al. The bladder and bladder tumors: imaging with three-demensional display of helical CT data. AJR 1996; 167: 1134 –1135.
13. Vining DJ, Zagoria RJ, Liu K, et al. CT cystoscopy: an innovation in bladder imaging. AJR 1996; 166: 409–410.
14. Merkle EM, Wunderlich A, Aschoff AJ, et al. Virtual cystoscopy based on helical CT scan datasets: perspectives and limitations. Br J Radiol 1998; 71(843): 262–267.
15. Hussain S. Loeffler JA, Babayan RK, et al. Thin-section helical computed tomography of the bladder: initial clinical experience with virtual reality imaging. Urology 1997; 50(5): 685–688.
16. Kim B, Semelka RC, Ascher S, et al. Bladder tumor staging: comparison of contrast-enhanced CT, T1 and T2-weighted MR imaging, dynamic gadolinium-enhanced imaging, and late gadolinium-enhanced imaging. Radiology 1994; 193: 239–245.
17. Scattoni V. DaPozzo LF, Colombo R, et al. Dynamic gadolinium-enhanced magnetic resonance imaging in staging of superficial bladder cancer. J Urol 1996; 155: 1594 –1599.
18. Barentsz JO, Jager GJ, vanVierzen PBJ, et al. Staging urinary bladder cancer after transurethral biopsy: value of fast dynamic contrast-enhanced MR imaging. Radiology 1996; 201: 185–193.
19. Barentsz JO, Jager G, Mugler JP, et al. Staging urinary bladder cancer: value of T1-weighted three-dimensional magnetization prepared-rapid gradient echo and two-dimensional spin-echo sequences. AJR 1995; 164: 109–115.

5

Urinary Cytology and its Role in Diagnosis and Monitoring of Urothelial Carcinoma

Hans Wijkström, MD, PHD,
William C. Baker, MD, Arline D. Deitch, PHD,
and Ralph W. deVere White, MD

CONTENTS

INTRODUCTION
COLLECTION TECHNIQUES
CYTOLOGIC FINDINGS OF URINARY SEDIMENTS
INTERPRETATION OF CYTOLOGIC SEDIMENTS
THE CYTOLOGY REPORT AND DIAGNOSTIC NOMENCLATURE
REVIEW AND QUALITY ASSURANCE
CLINICAL ROUTINES AT DETECTION AND FOLLOWUP
SUMMARY AND SUGGESTED GUIDELINES
    IN CLINICAL PRACTICE
ACKNOWLEDGMENT
REFERENCES

INTRODUCTION

From the time of Hippocrates until the present, the examination of urine has been shown to be useful in the diagnosis of patients with urinary disorders. Lambl (1856), Beale (1864) and Sanders (1864) were among the first to report extensively on identifying cancer cells in the urine *(1)*. The widespread acceptance of the use of urinary cytology awaited Papanicolaou and Marshall's 1945 development of criteria for interpretation of transitional cell carcinoma (TCC) cells in voided urine.

From: *Current Clinical Urology: Bladder Cancer: Current Diagnosis and Treatment*
Edited by: M. J. Droller © Humana Press Inc., Totowa, NJ

Table 1
Pertinent Clinical Information
that Should Accompany a Requisition for Cytologic Evaluation

Collection

Type of specimen: Urine, bladder washings.

Location of obtained specimen: Urethra, urinary bladder, bladder substitute, reservoirs or conduits, ureters or renal pelves (origin left/right).

Way of obtaining specimens: Voiding, catheter (permanent or not), cystoscopy, selective ureteral catheterization, brushings.

Synchronous surgical procedures: Biopsies, transurethral resections.

Medical history

Previous health and earlier medication (alkylating agents), current medication and symptoms (irritative, hematuria, infection, urinary lithiasis).

History of bladder cancer and treatment: Resection only, intravesical chemo- or immunotherapy, radical surgery, irradiation.

Endoscopy findings

Exophytic tumor or not. Size, number, location and configuration of tumor. Indication of invasion, bimanual palpation.

Enthusiasm for this technique increased in the late 1950s after Solomon developed a membrane filter that improved the cellular yield and accuracy of diagnosis. The development of a semi-automatic method of specimen processing as reported by Bales in 1981 greatly enhanced the reliability of specimen processing *(2)*.

Following this report, a flurry of research in the 1980s defined the pathologic and clinical usefulness of this technique, which has remained the standard for evaluating transitional cell carcinoma. Urinary cytology plays a major role in the diagnosis and monitoring of carcinoma *in situ*. Recent research efforts have been directed toward exploring the use of different tumor antigens in noninvasive analysis of transitional cell carcinoma. Cytology remains the standard against which these new tests will be compared and evaluated for their clinical usefulness.

COLLECTION TECHNIQUES

To minimize diagnostic errors, cytologic evaluation should be done in close collaboration with the clinician. The latter should provide the cytopathologist with pertinent clinical information that might influence cytologic interpretation. This should include reference to previously submitted specimens (Table 1). Ideally, especially when examining for field change disease, concurrently obtained tissue samples should also be examined. Review of earlier cytologies and histopathologies is highly desirable. Many of the pitfalls encountered in urinary cytology occur because of inappropriate sampling techniques. The type of specimen and variations in sampling affect the accurate interpretation of cytologic results. Careful methods of cell preservation and preparation are mandatory for correct microscopic interpretation.

Urine Sampling

Fresh samples of voided urine are the most practical routine form of urine collection. Three successive daily collections have been found to increase diagnostic accuracy. Since this is not clinically practical, most centers prefer to obtain the first or second voided specimen of the day for analysis. The first morning void produces the richest yield of cells for evaluation. However, the first morning urine often contains many degenerating cells and is therefore not always recommended. Recent papers suggest that the patient should ingest one 1000-mg Vitamin C tablet the night prior to urine collection *(3)*. This reduces the caustic effects of overnight urine, and helps to preserve the cells well enough to get satisfactory cytological preparations.

Freshness is the key to obtaining samples sufficient for a definite diagnosis *(4)*. The specimen should be processed as soon as possible but fresh samples of voided or catheterized urine, not infected or mingled with blood, can be refrigerated overnight, without preservatives or additives and still offer adequate cell preservation. We have found that either the first morning specimen enhanced by Vitamin C or the second morning void yields the most clinically practical samples giving high cellular yields that help insure accurate cytologic diagnosis.

Urine from ileal conduits or the increasing number of bladder substitutions has to be managed appropriately because of abundant mucus production from the intestinal component of the graft. The composition of these sediments has been thoroughly studied. The mucosal fragments are often degenerated and render the search for tumor cells difficult. However, if the specimen is adequately prepared with good staining, detecting tumor cells is not too difficult *(4)*.

Voided urine is less reliable in the diagnosis of tumors of the ureter and renal pelvis. The poor cellular yield and preservation of cells from the upper tracts needs special attention. When the suspicion of tumor is strong, a ureteral catheterization should be performed. In some centers the use of a shallowly inserted ureteral catheter, with or without lavage has been shown to double the sensitivity of cytology.

Bladder Washings (Barbotage)

The use of bladder washings circumvents some of the problems of studying voided urine. Bladder washings can yield the largest and most diverse population of cells, and this technique is therefore considered by many to be the best way to obtain samples for cytopathology *(5–7)*. Bladder irrigation using isotonic saline done in conjunction with cystoscopy should be obtained after the bladder has been emptied of urine without undue manipulation, and before any surgery or bimanual palpation. When washings are obtained without cystoscoping the patient, an 18F catheter should be used. It is important that the bladder is fairly vigorously irrigated or the number of cells obtained will be inadequate *(8)*. However, voided urine samples should always be preferred unless instrumentation is clinically justified. Unlike urine, bladder washing specimens have to be brought to the laboratory as soon as possible for further processing.

Brushings

The use of brush cytology for the upper tract is mostly of historical interest. Brushing causes a significant disruption and abnormal exfoliation of epithelial cells, making diagnostic evaluation especially difficult. Brushings can contribute to diagnostic errors and because of that should not be considered the preferred method of sampling for cytologic evaluation *(9)*. Because upper tract endoscopy with biopsy is available, the use of blind brushings of the upper urinary tract is likely to be used less and less in modern urology.

Cell Preservation and Processing

Cell preparation from urinary sediments is very demanding *(10)* requiring dedication and skill, together with the experience of evaluating specimens in sufficient numbers on a regular basis. The different types of specimen require different processing and the clinician should identify the type of specimens before sending it to the laboratory. The prevention of cell loss and satisfactory preservation of morphologic details are the main goals of the various technical procedures *(10)*. Regardless of the technique used, it should be standardized and cell loss and optimal staining controlled carefully *(4)*. Without standardized cell preparation, accurate cytologic interpretation is seriously hampered.

CYTOLOGIC FINDINGS OF URINARY SEDIMENTS

The Normal Urinary Sediment

Transitional epithelium which lines all but the terminal squamous portion of the adult urinary tract exhibits more variability in size and shape than found in most other types of epithelium. Microscopic evaluation of desquamated urothelium involves the recognition of two normal cell types: large, so-called umbrella cells from the superficial layers and smaller, tightly packed cells from the deeper epithelial layers.

SUPERFICIAL CELLS AND DEEP CELLS

The superficial cells are called umbrella cells because they each have the ability to cover several smaller deep cells when the uncontracted urothelium is examined histologically in cross section. Since these cells are in direct contact with urine, they desquamate more readily than the deeper layers. The latter are usually seen only in disease states, especially in lithiasis but arc also sccn sccondary to instrumcntation or after palpation of the bladder prior to obtaining samples for cytologic analysis. The superficial umbrella cells are usually very large and can be multinucleated and are usually larger than their counterparts having single nuclei. Multinucleated cells are also commonly found in cancers (11).

Superficial umbrella cells are the most common component of the urinary sediment regardless of whether the cells are obtained from voided urine or from bladder washings. They can be distinguished from deeper cells by their size and their elongated, often flattened appearance. These cells are usually larger than other cells in the sediment but they have a low nuclear to cytoplasmic ratio indicative of benign cells. The cells from the deeper epithelial layer are often found in clusters. They are more commonly seen in disease processes that have eroded the superficial cell compartment. They are also frequently observed after instrumentation. In the absence of inflammation they usually desquamate in clusters, so much so that they can assume an almost papillary type of appearance. Cells from the deeper layers are usually tightly bound to one another. In this cell type, cytoplasmic extensions can be observed that are derived from cytoplasmic interconnections of the adherent type. The cytoplasm of cells from the deeper layers is more basophilic than that of the superficial layers, especially when observed in sediment from voided urine.

SQUAMOUS CELLS

Squamous cells are also commonly seen in the voided urinary sediment. In females, these cells may originate from the vagina, the vulva and the cervix. The amount of squamous epithelium present in female urine varies according to estrogen status and will change during menstruation, menopause and if the patient is on estrogen replacement therapy. In males, squamous cells originate from the fossa navicularis and, as in females, can show variability in appearance and frequency, especially if the patient is undergoing concomitant therapy for prostate cancer.

RENAL TUBULAR CELLS

Renal tubular cells may be seen occasionally as a normal component of voided urine. These cells are usually small and are most often accompanied by poorly preserved renal casts, whether hyaline, granular or cellular in nature. Usually the presence of renal casts reflects an underlying problem which should be evaluated separately. Other cells seen are derived from the peripheral circulation and consist of erythrocytes, leukocytes, macrophages and occasionally eosinophils.

Noncancerous Conditions Causing Cellular Changes

Stones can cause cells to exfoliate abnormally and are a major cause of incorrect diagnosis of low-grade papillary TCC. However, one must always be aware that these conditions can appear concurrently. Inflammation of the urinary tract can also present difficulties in interpretation. A variety of conditions not only can cause cells to desquamate, they induce changes in nuclear morphology. These include cystitis, senile prostatitis, calculus, chemotherapy and radiotherapy effects, all of which can cause cellular atypia *(12)*. Calculus, postsurgical trauma, ulceration and other inflammatory processes can also lead to shedding these fragments. Such fragments can present troubling features to the cytologist including multinucleation, increased nuclear size, chromatin coarseness, prominent nucleoli, and mitotic activity *(12)*. Furthermore prostatic massage may expel seminal vesicle cells into the voided cell mass. These can have enlarged, hyperchromatic polypoid nuclei and exhibit brown cytoplasmic pigment *(13)*.

VIRUSES

While many changes caused by viruses are well known to the experienced cytologist, certain viral infections such as polyoma cause significant nuclear changes that are reminiscent of cancer. The human polyoma virus (HPV) in particular causes changes in the nuclear to cytoplasmic ratio that mimic cancer *(14)*. Furthermore, HPV infection results in the formation of large basophilic nuclear inclusions that might cause them to be mistaken for cancer cells *(9)*. The difficulty in interpretation of urine sediments is to distinguish transitional cells with unusually active nuclear structures from differentiated carcinoma cells. To increase diagnostic accuracy, the cytopathologist should be notified at the time of sample submission of the existence of conditions listed in Table 1.

Urothelial Tumors

The underlying concept in the study of cancer cells in urine is that, as cells become more abnormal, they lose the character of cellular adhe-

Table 2
Table on Abnormalities

Cell of origin	Papillary hyperplasia	Dysplasia and carcinoma in situ
DNA ploidy	Predominately diploid	Predominately anueploid
Chromosomal abnormalities	Absent	Loss and translocation
Cell adhesion abnormalities	Uncommon	Present
Invasive capability	Low	High
Recurrence rate	Low to moderate	High
Cytological recognition	Poor	Good

siveness. Moreover, abnormal urothelial cells have aberrant nuclear and cytoplasmic characteristics. Recent investigations have shown that loss of adhesion is related to the grade and aggressiveness of the tumor (15,16).

Diverse systems of transmembrane proteins mediate cell-to-cell adhesion. These molecules include the integrins, cadherins and selectins. Cadherins have been the most investigated of these proteins. Loss of these molecules not only allows for these cells to be exfoliated into the urine, it helps to mediate tumor aggressiveness by increasing cellular motility and invasion.

Like cytologic diagnosis in other systems, the grade of the abnormality is directly dependent upon the severity and frequency of these abnormalities (Table 2). Furthermore the rate at which cells are exfoliated into the urine is characteristic of the underlying pathology. There is a normal low rate of cell shedding into urine, which becomes increased under pathological conditions such as inflammation or tumor formation. Studies using DNA flow cytometry have shown that exfoliated cells are more likely to be more aneuploid than are those that do not shed. A prime example is carcinoma in situ. CIS cells are more likely to be aneuploid than are cells from low-grade papillary carcinoma.

Most frequently papillary TCCs are low-grade tumors composed of morphologically normal cells supported by an organized fibrovascular stalk. High-grade papillary TCC consist of morphologically abnormal cells that may surround a fibrovascular core in papillary formation, but they will often arise as a flatter (or nodular) type of lesion.

Our ability to detect bladder cancer by cytology is directly dependent upon which type of cancer is present. Low-grade carcinomas are difficult to detect using cytology, while high grade TCC and carcinoma in situ are more readily detectable. In low-grade papillary carcinoma, the cellular characteristics are more closely similar to those of normal cells. These cells are predominantly diploid. While shedding of papillary clusters of cells is diagnostic of papillary TCC, it can be confused with the

Table 3
Cellular Features of Urothelial Neoplasia[a]

	Low grade	High grade
Cells		
Arrangement	Papillary and loose clusters	Isolated and loose clusters
Size	Increased, uniform	Increased, pleomorphic
Number	Often numerous	Variable
Cytoplasm	Homogeneous	Variable
Nuclear/Cytoplasmic ratio	Increased	Increased
Nuclei		
Position	Eccentric	Eccentric
Size	Enlarged	Variable
Morphology	Variable within aggregates	Variable
Borders	Irregular (notches, creases)	Irregular
Chromatin	Fine, even	Coarse, uneven
Nucleoli	Small/absent	Variable

[a]Murphy WM (1990) with permission (21).

effects of instrumentation. The difficulty in interpretation of urinary sediments lies in distinguishing transitional cells with unusually active nuclear structure from well differentiated carcinoma cells. Since transitional cells frequently exhibit a wide range of normal morphology, as noted above, this requires that marked nuclear aberrations be identified before diagnosing cancer on the basis of urinary cytology.

INTERPRETATION OF CYTOLOGIC SEDIMENTS

Description of the cellular features of the normal and abnormal urinary sediment are extensively discussed in the literature (10,17,18), taught in cytologic tutorials (International Academy of Cytology, IAC) (4) and found in generally accessible audiovisual teaching aids (19).

The cellular yield from urine and bladder washings is poor in the normal urinary bladder, but the shed cells have distinctive features that are recognizable by the experienced cytologist. Usually the cellularity is sufficient to make a cytological diagnosis of a benign sample (20). There is, however, always a risk that overinterpreted normal or reactive constituents of the urinary sediments may be taken as being malignant.

By strictly adhering to defined criteria characterizing neoplasia (Table 3), it has been stated by Murphy that "almost all true transitional cell carcinomas (WHO grade II and III) and carcinoma in situ of the urinary bladder can be detected using urinary cytology" (21). However, disagreements in interobserver concurrence, and the differing quality and experience of cytologists will affect the quality of diagnosis from center to center, and low grade TCC may be missed unless other parameters such as immunohistochemistry of tumor antigens are added.

Squamous cell carcinoma can often be readily identified and primary adenocarcinomas, although rare, will be recognized by the mere presence of these cells, however, they are often not identified as neoplastic *(21)*.

Cytologic accuracy can be evaluated by comparison to the histology of the tissue in question. The comparison between neoplastic cells in smears and the various degrees of histopathologic differentiation cannot be performed for all tissue types. Some of the features used to identify low grade tumors in tissue sections cannot be identified as easily in cytological specimens, or not at all, as some of the cells are almost identical to those of the normal mucosa. Low grade tumors also exfoliate less than more aggressive tumors and, in addition, the changes characteristic of low grade malignancy require considerable training for accurate identification *(21)*. In Figs. 1–4 cytological samples with concurrently obtained tissue specimens, grade I, IIA, IIB and III, are shown.

Cytological Grading of Urothelial Neoplasias

From a clinical standpoint the identification of low grade tumors in cytologic smears plays a minor role, while identification of tumors of higher grades is crucial. Comparison of cytology and histopathology findings in the clinical context is therefore of great value. A comparison can be performed if the criteria for both methods are clearly defined.

As long ago as 1972 Esposti, using analysis of exfoliated cells in smears from over 300 patients showed that it was possible to assess the cytological grade of malignancy, separating transitional cell tumors of low-grade, moderate and high-grade atypia. The histological basis for this cytologic grading was solely the grade of cellular atypia in tissue specimens *(23)*. The 1965 histological classification by Bergkvist suggests grading of transitional cell tumors into 5 grades from 0–IV according to the severity of cellular deviation from transitional epithelium with the borderline between benign and malignant types being drawn between grades I and II. This classification has been widely utilized in Scandinavia with a later modification, dividing grade II tumors into two entities "a" and "b", thereby further separating tumors of low malignancy from those of high malignancy. This separation was an attempt to better define the histological parameters for the large and heterogeneous group of moderately differentiated tumors (corresponding to grade II WHO) (Figs. 2, 3) *(24,25)*.

The separation into grades IIa and IIb has proven to be reproducible and of great clinical value as reflected in survival figures. In a followup

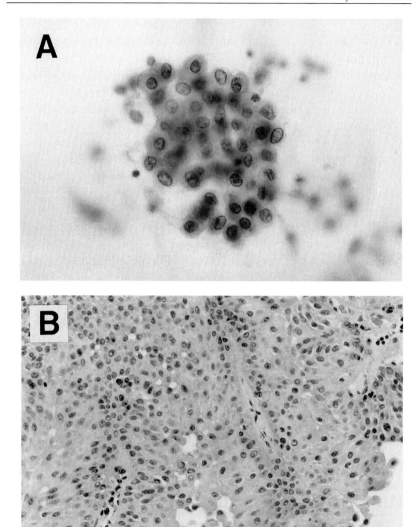

Fig. 1. (A). Cytology: A loose cluster of cells with slightly enlarged nuclei and some hyperchromasia. This pattern is diagnostic for a urothelial carcinoma grade I (Pap, × HP). **(B)** Histology: A grade I carcinoma, same case as Fig. 1A, with somewhat irregular cells which appear in more layers than in the normal bladder urothelium (H&E, × HP).

study from Stockholm, the 5-yr survival rate for patients with grade IIa tumors was 92% while it was 43% for those with grade IIb tumors *(26)*. These results are further supported by studies using flow cytometry that separate grade II tumors into diploid and aneuploid tumors *(27)*.

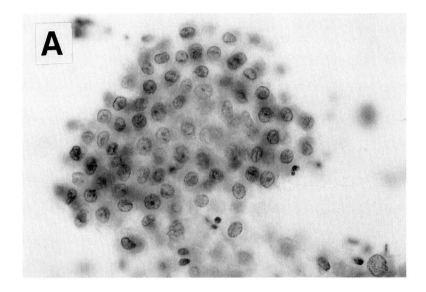

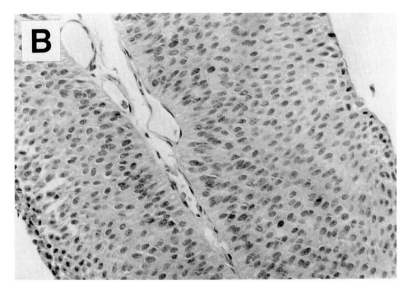

Fig. 2. (A). Cytology: A cluster from a grade II A carcinoma. The cells have enlarged nuclei that are hyperchromatic but without pleomorphism (Pap, ×HP). **(B)** Histology: Section from the case depicted in Fig. 2A. There are many more layers of cells than in the normal urothelium. The cells still show some polarity. The pattern of Grade II A tumors is also characterized by: *"Slight to moderate variation in nuclear size with clearly less than a 2-fold variation in each diameter as the same axis among adjacent cells at the same level, moderately prominent but a smooth nuclear membrane and an even very fine chromatin pattern, and few mitoses" (25).* (H&E, × HP).

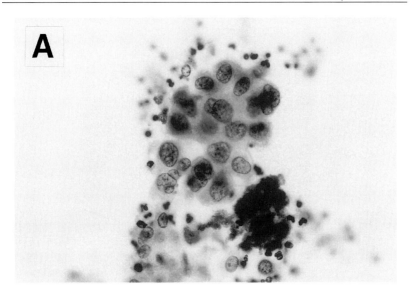

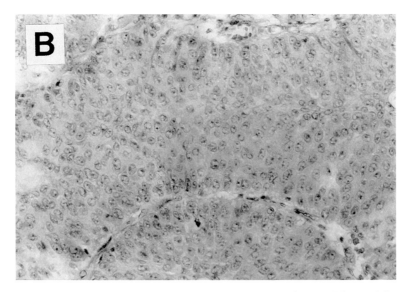

Fig. 3. (A). Cytology: A cluster from a Grade II B carcinoma. The nuclei are irregular, hyperchromatic and vary markedly in size (Pap, × HP). (**B**) Histology: Same case as in Fig. 3A. The Grade II B is characterized by the following features. *"Moderate to strong variation in nuclear size with at least a 2-fold variation in each diameter at the same axis among adjacent cells at the same level, prominent nuclear membrane and a fine hyperchromatic chromatin pattern, increased nuclear-to-cytoplasmic ratio and mitoses easily found" (25)*. (H&E, × HP).

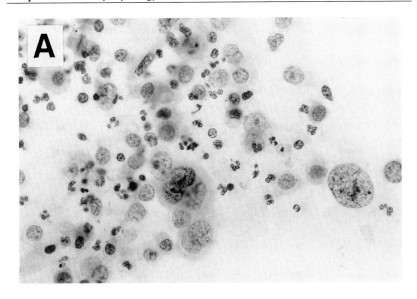

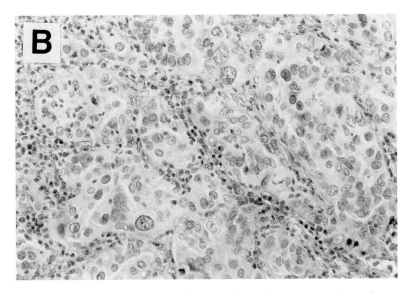

Fig. 4. (A). Cytology: The tumor cells from a Grade III carcinoma have pleomorphic nuclei with distinctly abnormal chromatin. Naked nuclei are common and there is a low tendency to form clusters (Pap, × HP). **(B)** Histology: Grade III carcinoma (same case as in Fig. 4A). The distinctly pleomorphic tumors cells have lost their polarity and are invasive (H&E, × HP).

Although the classification originally was adapted to categorization of tissue specimens, the later modification *(25)* was formulated to adapt these parameters to cytology samples. This enables comparison of the two diagnostic modalities and gives added information. The modified classification is currently used in routine clinical practice. This type of subdivision, discriminating between low and high grade malignancy, has been proposed by others in equivalent systems *(28,29)* and has now been proposed in the latest issue of the WHO histological typing of urinary bladder tumors *(30)*. A comparison between different grading systems is outlined in Table 4.

THE CYTOLOGY REPORT
AND DIAGNOSTIC NOMENCLATURE

The cytology report should be descriptive and predictive of histologic findings *(32)* and should also be in conformity with the needs of the clinician. There is, however, a lack of universal consensus on the diagnostic criteria and terminology to be used in cytology. Using standardized terminology would facilitate the dialogue between pathologists, urologists and oncologists. This would permit reporting clinical findings in a reproducible way to facilitate interinstitutional exchanges of information. Proposals (Table 5) *(33)* have also been made to correlate cytology to current histologic classification systems, in order to make cytology an integrated part of therapeutic decisions.

Negative Cytology
(Including Reactive Cells)

A designation should be given as to whether the samples are representative and/or adequate for evaluation. In the event that the specimen is inadequate, a subsequent specimen should be requested. A statement recommending further investigation should follow sediments read out as low-grade atypia or suspicious for malignancy.

Atypical/Dysplastic Cells

There is some disagreement on how to report these findings. The lack of consensus on cytologic criteria for dysplasia makes consistent reporting of dysplasia difficult. One suggestion is to divide atypical cells into two categories: atypia with uncertain significance, and atypia suspicious for malignancy *(33)*. Such a categorization may be disputable between expert cytologists, but it would make it more understandable for urologists managing the disease clinically.

Table 4
Comparison Between Different Histological Grading Systems and Urinary Cytology for TCC Cancers

Histology			Cytology			
WHO 1973 (31)	Malmström (24) Carbin (25) 1991	WHO/ISUP (29) 1998	Esposti (22) 1972	Ooms (33) "WHO" 1993	Carbin (25) 1991	Murphy (21) 1990
Grade I	I	Pap. neopl. low malign. potential	Low grade atypia	I	(I)	Negative (low grade TCC)
Grade I, II	IIa	Papillary ca low grade	Moderate atypia	II	IIa	Low grade TCC
Grade II	IIb	Papillary ca high grade	Moderate atypia	II	IIb	High grade TCC
Grade III	III	Papillary ca high grade	High grade atypia	III	III	High grade TCC
Not defined	IV	Marked anaplasia	Not defined	Undiff carcinoma	IV	Undiff; neoplasm

[a] From Ooms (1993) (33), who proposes a terminology corresponding to WHO, 1973.
[b] From Murphy (1990) (21), whose terminology is equivalent to WHO, 1998.
[c] TCC: transitional cell carcinoma. WHO: World Health Organization. ISUP: International Society of Urologic Pathologists.
[d] In parentheses: neoplasia not readily identified.

Table 5
Proposed Terminology for Urinary Cytology[a]

Negative cytology
Atypical cells, significance uncertain
Atypical cells, suspicious for malignancy
Neoplastic cells present:
  grade I carcinoma
  grade II carcinoma
  grade III carcinoma
  carcinoma *in situ* (CIS)
  squamous cell carcinoma
  adenocarcinoma
  small cell undifferentiated carcinoma
  others

[a]The terminology corresponds to the international classification of the World Health Organization for tumours of the bladder.
[b]Ooms ECM (1993) by permission *(33)*.

Transitional Cell Carcinoma

When malignant cells are identified, they should if possible be graded (from I–III, WHO), a basic description of the cellular features of the sediment should be documented, and a conclusion drawn. There have been earnest efforts to come to a consensus that would be morphologically accurate, understandable and meet the clinical needs of the physician (Table 5) *(33)*.

In a report comparing different grading systems, the 1973 WHO system although more descriptive, was regarded as being less logical than other systems that differentiate only between high and low grade neoplasms *(21)*. The latest edition from WHO *(30)* on histological typing, however, proposes dividing transitional cell carcinoma solely into low- and high-grade lesions. This grading system corresponds well with these efforts and makes possible a compromise that would further consensus on cytological matters for clinical purposes.

REVIEW AND QUALITY ASSURANCE

Central Review Cytopathology

There is a lack of consistency and interobsever reproducibility in histologic and cytologic grading of bladder tumors at different institutions, raising the question of whether we need reference panel review, especially in clinical trials. These are important in the development of new pathologic assessments *(34)*, but they may not have an influence on treatment results *(35,36)*. Even when there is significant disagreement on eligibility criteria between local and regional pathologists, it is essential that data integrity be maintained in multicenter studies. Clinical trials should therefore always include detailed information on the histopathologic standards used in the study plan. The need to audit variations in pathologic diagnoses has been pointed out, and the statistical methodology needed for such a study is available *(37)*. This type of study, addressing key questions on diagnostic criteria in cytology, may have a major impact on the future use of cytology in the diagnosis and monitoring of bladder cancer.

However, a recent alarming report that questions the ability of local pathology under routine clinical conditions showed that both histopathology and cytology may have low sensitivity and specificity *(36)*.

Quality Assurance

There are many ways of improving the routine use of cytology in the management of bladder cancer. Standardization of clinical routines and terminology will have an immediate impact on diagnostic accuracy. Regular conferences where clinicians and cytopathologists interact and review newly detected tumors, before therapy, especially in controversial cases, will also contribute to establishing clinical standards. Most misinterpretations of adequate samples are done by inexperienced cytologists. Supervision by a senior cytologist should be maintained for an adequate length of time, and regular consultations among colleagues should be part of the routine. For example tutorials covering all aspects of the field of cytology are held twice annually by the IAC (International Academy of Cytology). Tutorials such as this represent another example of a modern approach to improve the skill and diagnostic ability of the cytopathologist. The differing results in cytologic interpretation at various institutions also call for specially designed quality assurance programs and such programs for the cytopathology laboratory have been outlined and adopted *(38)*.

CLINICAL ROUTINES
AT DETECTION AND FOLLOWUP

Clinical Utility of Urinary Sediments at Detection

It was stated in the report from the WHO Bladder Consensus Conference Committee 1998 that "pathological consultations based on urinary samples should be recommended as an integral part of any program monitoring patients with neoplasms of the lower urinary tract," provided limitations are observed and common pitfalls avoided *(29)*. This statement has, however, already been challenged by an increasing number of new noninvasive techniques that promise both immediate results (point-of-care), improved sensitivity and specificity, as well as an improved indication of the degree of tumor differentiation *(39)*.

However, sensitivity has remained controversial. It often appears to be very operator-dependent. This has led to extensive evaluation of image analysis and flow cytometric studies. Recent research efforts have been directed towards exploring the use of different tumor antigens or molecular probes as ways of improving the sensitivity of cytology, while other urine tests based on cytology are being explored. In the future, highly sensitive and specific tests may largely replace conventional cytology and permit the number of cystoscopies and imaging studies to be reduced. This will decrease the immense workload of checkup cystoscopies for both low and high-risk patients. However, at the present time the available markers do not offer an acceptable alternative to cytology *(40)*.

In an effort to overcome subjective grading and poor standardization, quantitative image analysis by various techniques have been utilized concurrently with cytology or histology *(41–43)*. This kind of technique has been reported to be superior to standard analysis of cytology specimens. New marker assays (as for any innovative technique) still have to be tested in large-scale studies to validate their accuracy and should at present only be used as an adjunct to conventional diagnostic modalities *(40)*. A request for cytology should, however, be considered as a medical consultation rather than merely a laboratory test *(44)*.

A complete work up of a patient with symptoms indicative of a bladder tumor usually include cystoscopy and cytology and the WHO committee has emphasized that "cytologic evaluation is of significant assistance as an adjunct to cystoscopy in the classification of newly detected bladder neoplasms" *(29)*. However, the use of cytology in this setting is controversial and one of the authors of this chapter (deVere White) feels that cytology seldom is required in the primary work up because of the poor sensitivity and specificity of this test in recent point-of-service studies (Table 6). Regrettably the WHO report lacks a detailed definition of diagnostic criteria for the interpretation of smears.

In the preliminary evaluation of patients, cytology plays a minor role since the majority of tumors found consist of low-grade, mostly non-aggressive papillary lesions making them less sensitive for detection. However, given adequate samples almost all potentially aggressive bladder neoplasms can be detected with urinary cytology *(21)* and cytology should therefore be performed initially in order to rule out high grade tumors. Although most centers agree on the high specificity of bladder tumor cytology, the diagnostic accuracy varies among reporting centers,

Table 6
Reported Diagnostic Accuracy of Cytology
(Percentage Malignant Specimens)
in Histologically Confirmed TCC Bladder Tumors with Regards to Grade

First author	N tum.	Grade I	Grade II	Grade III	Grade IV
Esposti (22) (1972) BW	326	3% (3/87)	68% (67/99)	89% (125/140)[*]	
Kern (45) (1988) U	699	29% (44/152)	42% (105/248)	70% (209/299)[**]	
Maier (46) (1995) BW	361	29%	77%	92%	
Farrow (47) (1997) U	634	22% (22/98)	62% (180/291)	84% (181/215)	83% (25/30)
Sarosdy (48) (1997) U	126	8% (3/40)	18% (6/33)	38% (2053)	
Wiener (49) (1998)U	91	17% (4/23)	61% (23/38)	90% (27/30)	
V. d Poel (50) (1998) BW	54	29% (2/7)	30% (8/27)	75% (15/20)	
Leyh (51) (1999) U	107	4% (1/26)	20% (9/45)	69% (25/36)	

[a]In the last 4 studies, cytology was compared with new urine-based diagnostic tests.
[b]In parentheses proportion of cytologically detected tumors.
[c]TCC: transitional cell carcinoma; BW: bladder washings; U: urine.
*Grade 3 + 4.
**Grade 3 + 4 including 65 carcinoma *in situ* tumors.

(Grade I: 3–29%; Grade II: 18–77% and Grade III: 38–92%), (Table 6). This table includes both older studies, only evaluating cytological accuracy in urine or bladder washings, and more recent ones with the view of comparing the sensitivity of cytology to the new diagnostic markers. Discrepancies are most pronounced in grade I and grade II tumors and may be caused in part by differing definitions among institutions. The newly proposed separation of papillary cancers into low and high grade tumors, if accepted by clinicians, may improve reporting in the future.

Positive Cystoscopy: Positive Cytology (Table 7)

Cytology is complementary to resected tissue samples in examination of the lower urinary tract and both samples should be evaluated concurrently. When a tumor is found and cytology is positive whether due to TCC or other lesions, there may or may not be agreement between histology and cytology. Concordance will confirm the diagnosis while discrepancy calls for an extended evaluation. Synchronous lesions out-

Table 7
Possible Combinations of Endoscopic, Cytologic and Histopathological
Findings at Initial Work Up for Suspected Bladder Tumor[a]

Cystoscopy	Cytology	Histopathology	Comments
Positive	**Pos/mal**		
Visible lesion	LG TCC	G1, 2a/Ta-1	High specificity, low sensitivity for LG tumors
	HG TCC	G2b, 3/Ta-1+, Tis,	High specificity and sensitivity for HG tumors
	Susp TCC	Cancer (any)	Discrepancy cytol/histol: may be conc. *CIS*, upper tract tumor or unrepresentative biopsy
	Non TCC	Non TCC	Non-TCC (Adeno/Squamous) may be primary, metastatic or overgrowth
Positive	**Negative**		
Visible lesion	Benign	Any Ca, NNC	Unusual with false negative cytological findings in HG tumors
	Insufficient	Any Ca, NNC	Common with false negative findings in LG tumors
Negative	**Pos/mal**		
Normal	LG TCC	NA	May be due to missed exophytic tumor, *CIS* or upper tract tumor
	HG TCC	NA or *CIS*	Further investigation warranted
Endoscopy	Susp TCC	NA	
Negative	**Negative**		
Normal			
endoscopy	Benign	NA	May be false-negative cytology or endoscopy
	Insufficient	NA	Repeat study if symptomatic

[a]Ca: cancer; G: Grade; LG: Low-grade; HG: High grade; Susp: Suspicious, but not indicative of TCC; TCC: Transitional Cell Carcinoma; NA: Not available; Conc *CIS*: Concomitant carcinoma *in situ*; NNC: Non-neoplastic condition.

side the area of visible tumor always have to be kept in mind *(31)*. If the bladder biopsy shows a low-grade lesion and cytology reveals a higher-grade lesion, this is indicative of either a missed high-grade lesion or concomitant carcinoma *in situ*. It may also mean that a coexistent high-grade upper tract lesion is present. The positive cytology may also represent a focus of high-grade cancer not recognized in the biopsy.

Random biopsies are considered by many to be an integral part of initial workup. However, the value of biopsies routinely taken at the time of detection has been questioned *(52)*. A good alternative is to collect urinary specimens about two weeks after resection. It has been reported that voided urine has a better predictive value than random biopsies *(53)*. A primarily positive urinary cytology from voided urine has been shown to be an independent negative prognostic factor in long time followup of bladder cancer patients *(54)*.

Positive Cystoscopy: Negative (Normal) Cytology (Table 7)

When a tumor is seen at cystoscopy and cytology is negative, the lesion is probably low grade. Accordingly, there should be no coexistent high grade lesion in other parts of the urinary tract. In conditions mimicking malignancy, such as enterovesical fistulas, cystitis glandularis or in patients with chemical or radiation cystitis, cytologic examination is highly valuable to rule out malignancy in cases having negative biopsies. In such difficult cases, repeated cytologic evaluations will eventually disclose most high grade lesions.

Negative Cystoscopy: Positive Cytology (Table 7)

The most evident diagnostic advantage of cytology is its ability to sample areas not seen cystoscopically (e.g., distal ureters, prostatic urethra, Brunn's nests) or that is uncharacteristic in appearance (carcinoma *in situ*). Diagnosing carcinoma *in situ* is the most important reason for examining of urinary sediments. This has become increasingly appreciated with the growing awareness that *CIS* is not always recognizable through the cystoscope. While the diagnostic sensitivity of cytology is less in upper tract tumors than in the bladder, the specificity is the same. A tumor of the upper tract must be ruled out when a positive cytology cannot otherwise be explained.

In an excellent review, the sinister significance of clinically unconfirmed positive urinary cytology has been pointed out *(55)*. Specific guidelines have been outlined for these cases and an aggressive evaluation of extravesical sites has been recommended for previously untreated patients having positive cytologies as well as for those with a complete response to intravesical chemotherapy who are without evidence of disease for one year. Biopsy of the prostatic urethra has been recommended to rule out TCC in all case of high grade positive cytologies, even if other bladder foci have been identified. Another explanation for positive cytology may be a missed tumor at first cystoscopy. This possibility emphasizes an additional value of cytology. Atypical specimens in patients having known conditions like urinary stones should also be checked after treatment since a simultaneous neoplasm can be present.

Negative Cystoscopy: Negative Cytology (Table 7)

A distinction must always be made between the normal sample, the inadequate sample, or the urinary sediment of unknown significance (i.e., "dysplasia, low grade neoplasm cannot be excluded"). It is always a clinical dilemma to balance between an extended followup and terminating the investigation. In cases having indeterminate cytology ("not clearly indicative of malignancy" or "not clearly negative"), those patients who are nonsmokers and do not have hematuria or a prior history of urothelial cancer are at low risk for harboring malignancy (56). There is, of course, always the risk of false negative examinations by both the urologist and the cytologist.

Careful evaluation of each case that has serious symptoms and negative findings should be performed since negative examinations do not definitively rule out tumors. If clinically indicated, these examinations should be repeated in order to avoid lulling the urologist into false security. The much-criticized limitation of urine cytology in missing low grade tumors is of far less clinical importance, since most of these tumors will be detected by cystoscopy in connection with symptoms like hematuria. Small low grade tumors missed at first cystoscopy will eventually cause further symptoms, necessitating a new endoscopic approach, usually without a change in prognosis. The risk of missing low grade tumors because of insensitive cytology is minor compared to that caused by a delay in evaluating patients who have serious symptoms and negative cystoscopies.

Followup of Bladder Tumors

Urinary cytology is used as an adjunct to cystoscopy in monitoring patients treated for bladder cancer with a view toward improved detection of residual or recurrent disease. Cytologic evaluation may be used as an extra safety measure between cystoscopies with the frequency of the request being tailored to the clinical evaluation of the individual patient. Cytology is also valuable after resection of large or multiple tumors in locations that are not readily accessible.

If cytology at the two week checkup after resection is still positive, it is a strong indication that residual tumor is present. If, however, the cytological grade is higher than that for the resected tumor, this requires extensive further evaluation. Alternatively, if the cytology has returned to normal, the resection can be deemed to be complete.

Positive or suspicious cytology may also precede tumor recurrence for a considerable length of time. Intravesically-given chemo- or immunotherapy may cause misinterpretation of the sediment as being malignant despite complete response to treatment. However, as a rule the changes caused by topical agents can be recognized and are distinguishable from malignancy (21).

Monitoring Carcinoma **In Situ** *(CIS)*

The single most valuable indication for using urinary cytology is the detection and monitoring of CIS. Awareness of its occurrence, its role in preceding muscle-invasive disease, as well as the success of intravesical therapy using BCG, have all increased the use of cytology. There are 3 types of carcinoma *in situ*: primary, concomitant, and secondary, with the common agreement that all these lesions should be classified as grade III (high-grade intraurothelial neoplasia including "severe dysplasia" in the latest WHO classification) *(29)*. Although attempts to grade carcinoma *in situ* have been made, most laboratories only classify lesions as carcinoma *in situ* if the sample is cytologically highly positive with severe nuclear atypia corresponding to grade 3 WHO and contain many isolated cancer cells indicating a low cohesivity. In many reports, the sensitivity of cytology to detect CIS is almost complete *(10)*, thus establishing the importance of cytology in this context and making it a useful tool for monitoring this type of bladder cancer. Although intravesical treatment with BCG has revolutionized the outcome for patients with CIS at least in the short term, maintenance treatment is recommended for prolonged periods of time and close surveillance of these high-risk patients is mandatory.

The great advantage of cytology is that when visible lesions are not present, cytology can reliably detect residual or recurrent tumor, since the changes secondary to BCG are easily recognizable. Furthermore, positive cytology can herald the onset of recurrence well before a visible lesion is identified. Because of this, repeated and numerous biopsies can be circumvented, especially when negative cytologies are reported. A change in the status of cytology can be relied upon to be a good indicator of treatment efficacy. However, failure primarily or in the form of recurrent carcinoma *in situ* with or without exophytic tumor necessitates a confirming tissue diagnosis before radical treatment is instituted.

Monitoring Low Grade *(GI-GIIA)*
Ta-T1 Tumors With or Without Instillation Therapy

Urinary cytology has a lower sensitivity for detecting low grade tumors. Detection of recurrences or residual disease after resection is therefore not as useful in the followup of these patients, especially when the initial cytology was negative. These primary tumors have a low prospect of recurrence and progression. The most important prognostic information comes from their initial designation as invasive (T1) or noninvasive (Ta). Their further subdivision into single and/or multiple tumors, including the result from the first checkup cystoscopy, has led to a proposal, that includes an initial, single instillation of chemotherapy *(57)*, that could substantially decrease the number of followup cystoscopies *(58)*. Based on these prognostic factors, the need for lifelong surveillance has been challenged, at least in noninvasive low grade tumors without recurrence at the first checkup cystoscopy. This implies that some of these patients may be discharged after an appropriate followup interval while others need to be followed more closely *(58)*, as recent longterm reports in high risk patients have shown *(59)*. Well organized, prospective controlled studies are required to scrutinize traditional strategies in the followup of superficial bladder cancers including the role of routine use of cytology *(60)*.

Monitoring High Grade (GIIB-GIII)
Ta-T1 Tumors With or Without Instillation Therapy

These highly unpredictable tumors have to be followed with the utmost caution. They can progress to muscle invasion and have a high frequency of concomitant CIS. Grade II tumors with the characteristics described as grade IIb carry almost the same risks as grade III tumors *(35)*. When a conservative approach is chosen instead of immediate cystectomy, this usually requires intravesical chemotherapy with BCG and a followup protocol similar to that for primary carcinoma *in situ*. Needless to say, the initial resection should include sufficient muscle tissue for evaluation, with early reconfirmation to exclude undetected muscle invasion. A renewed requisition for cytology on voided urine after roughly 2 weeks is also valuable to rule out TCC or concomitant CIS.

In a report from the first Consensus Conference on Bladder Cancer, cystoscopy and cytology are recommended for high-risk patients twice during the first 6 mo. After that, if the bladder is clear, cystoscopy is recommended at 6-mo intervals and cytology at 3-month intervals. In this declaration there is a detailed description of the cytologic technique to be used *(61)*.

Muscle Invasive Tumors (T2+) All Grades

CONSERVATIVE APPROACH

Although cystectomy is the standard treatment worldwide for muscle invasive bladder cancer, bladder saving protocols, including chemoradiotherapy *(62)* or extensive transurethral resections and adjuvant chemotherapy *(63)*, have given what some consider to be acceptable results in carefully selected cases. In a combined chemotherapy-radiation protocol instituted by the Massachusetts General Hospital, with a view toward bladder sparing, all controls include cytology for classification. A complete response is defined as negative biopsies accompanied by cytologically negative bladder washings *(62)*. Cytology specimens may be difficult to evaluate after irradiation *(21)*. Positive cytology directly after irradiation may represent residual disease and/or concomitant carcinoma *in situ* that has not responded to irradiation. Positive cytology may also precede an exophytic recurrence by a long interval or it may represent a secondary carcinoma *in situ*.

It is also important to decide whether we are dealing with a curative or palliative situation. In the curative setting, cytology may prove to be extremely valuable in detecting minor residual or early recurrent disease. Positive cytologies may lead the clinician to initiate prompt salvage cystectomy as part of a bladder sparing protocol.

The majority of patients with high grade muscle-invasive cancer will have invasive disease at first presentation *(64)*. It has, however, been reported that home screening for hematuria can detect high-grade cancers before they become invasive of muscle muscle *(65)*. Urinary cytology could be used during this brief preclinical period to verify these findings.

AFTER RADICAL TREATMENT

Periodic cytological examination of urine from patients who have had a cystectomy should be included in the followup *(32)*. The purpose of such studies is to monitor upper tract and urethral recurrences. If malignant cells are found in urine after cystectomy, the ureters are difficult to catheterize through a conduit or a bladder substitute, making retrograde sampling almost impossible. In these cases, one has to rely on radiological techniques to localize the lesion. Urethral cytology after cystectomy is an absolute indication, and the prognosis of positive urethral cytology is ominous.

MONITORING THE UPPER TRACT

Surveillance of the upper tracts after treatment is important especially for all high grade tumors. Patients with high grade tumors are more disposed to develop new tumors in these locations which are known for their insidious symptoms. The poor cell yield from the upper tracts renders diagnosis difficult, but when malignant cells are found the specificity is high. However, patients who have positive urinary cytology immediately after a complete transurethral resection of bladder tumors or after receiving intravesical therapy, will almost always have recurrent transitional cell carcinoma of the bladder and initially do not require aggressive extravesical evaluation *(55)*. In high grade exophytic tumors and carcinoma *in situ*, sensitivities of 90–100% are not uncommon using ureteral catheterization. This procedure is an excellent, yet minimally invasive technique for monitoring high grade TCC of the upper tract.

Guidelines for screening extravesical sites in high-risk patients are given in a recent report. Whenever cytology is positive without evidence for bladder cancer recurrence, the recommendation is for intravenous pyelograms and urethral biopsy to be performed yearly *(66)*.

SUMMARY AND SUGGESTED GUIDELINES IN CLINICAL PRACTICE

Collection of Cytologic Samples

Careful sampling in a standardized manner is carried out with the goal of ensuring fresh specimens for swift processing. Samples should be accompanied by complete clinical information for the cytopathologist. Cytological and histological samples obtained concurrently should be examined together. Review of earlier cytologies and histologies is desirable.

If the pitfalls and limitations of these tests are familiar to both the urologist and the cytopathologist, their close collaboration and the use of standardized terminology in the cytology report should ensure optimal patient management.

Interpretation of Cytologic Samples

The cytologist should have the experience of evaluating specimens in sufficient numbers on a regular basis. The diagnostic accuracy, as well as laboratory techniques, has to be carefully monitored using accepted quality assurance programs.

Clinical Utility of Urinary Cytology

AT THE DIAGNOSIS OF BLADDER CANCER

Analysis of cytologic specimens may be useful in conjunction with cystoscopy as part of the primary work up for newly diagnosed bladder tumors, but the clinical value for all tumors is controversial. Cytology has a high specificity with extremely few false positive findings. It has a low sensitivity for low-grade tumors, but on the other hand its sensitivity is high for high-grade tumors with relatively few false negative findings.

IN THE INTERVALS BETWEEN CYSTOSCOPIES

While cytologic evaluation can never replace cystoscopy, if it is performed shortly after resection, it may prove predictive of residual disease or prove valuable in the detection of unrecognized tumors or carcinoma *in situ*. Cytology, which may become positive prior to the detection of exophytic tumors, may be used to prolong the intervals between endoscopic examinations or be used as an extra safety measure in surveillance of bladder tumors without causing discomfort to the patient. Cytology is, however, not nearly sensitive enough to be used in place of regular cystoscopic examinations in high-risk patients.

IN MONITORING BLADDER CANCER AS AN ADJUNCT TO CYSTOSCOPIES

1. Cytology is valuable at checkup cystoscopies of low grade tumors to rule out a concurrent higher grade tumor, either CIS or upper tract tumor.
2. To monitor conservatively-managed high grade tumors, T1/GIII or higher both in the bladder and upper tract.
3. To monitor carcinoma *in situ* during or after instillation therapy.
4. To monitor upper tracts and urethra after cystectomy.
5. To monitor patients after irradiation therapy.

The value of new point-of-care tests should be confirmed in large scale studies before being used in the clinical context.

ACKNOWLEDGMENT

All cytologic and tissue samples (Figs. 1–4) were prepared and photographed by Professor Lambert Skoog, Department of Pathology, Karolinska Hospital, Stockholm, Sweden.

REFERENCES

1. Koss LG. The cellular and acellular components of the urinary sediment. In: *Diagnostic Cytology of the Urinary Tract with Histopathologic and Clinical Correlations* (Koss LG, ed.). Lippincott-Raven, Philadelphia, PA, 1996, p. 28.
2. Bales CE. A semiautomated method for preparation of urine sediment for cytologic evaluation. Acta Cytol 1981; 25: 323.
3. Pearson JC, Kromhout CT, King EB. Evaluation of collection and preservation techniques for urinary cytology. Acta Cytol 1981; 25: 327.
4. Rosenthal DL, Mandell DB. Cytologic detection of urothelial lesions. In: *Compendium on Diagnostic Cytology* (Wied GL, Marluce B, Keebler CM, Koss LG, Patten SF, Rosenthal DL, eds.), Eighth Edition. Tutorials of Cytology, Chicago, Illinois, 1997, p. 268.
5. Matzkin H, Moinuddin SM, Soloway MS. Value of urine cytology versus bladder washing in bladder cancer. Urology 1992; 34: 201.
6. Wijkström H, Lundh B, Tribukait B. Urine or bladder washings in the cytologic evaluation of transitional cell carcinoma of the urinary tract. A comparison made under routine conditions supplemented by flow cytometric DNA anlysis. Scand J Urol Nephrol 1987; 21: 119.
7. Tawfik Z, Wajsman Z, Englander LS, Gamarra M, Huben RP, Pontes JE. Evaluation of bladder washings and urine cytology in the diagnosis of bladder cancer and its correlation with selected biopsies of the bladder mucosa. J Urol 1984; 132: 670.

8. Aamodt RL, Coon JS, Deitch AD, deVere White RW, Koss LG, Melamed MR, et al. Flow cytometric evaluation of bladder cancer: recommendations of the NCI flow cytometry network for bladder cancer. World J Urol 1992; 10: 63.

9. Koss LG. The role of cytology in the diagnosis, detection and followup of bladder cancer. In: *Developments in Bladder Cancer* (Denis L, et al., eds.). Alan R. Liss, New York, 1986, p. 97.

10. Koss LG. Tumors of the urothelium (transitional epithelium) of the bladder. In: *Diagnostic Cytology and its Histopathologic Bases,* Fourth Edition. JB Lippincott, Philadelphia, PA, 1992, p. 934.

11. El-Bolkainy MN. Cytology of bladder carcinoma. J Urol 1980; 124: 20.

12. Ro JY, Staerkel GA, Ayala AG. Cytologic and histologic features of superficial bladder cancer. Urol Clin North Am 1992; 19: 435.

13. Melamed MR. Introduction to cytology of the urinary tract. In: *Compendium of Diagnostic Cytology* (Weid GL, Keebler CM, Koss LG, et al., eds.), Sixth Edition. Chicago, International Academy of Cytology, 1998, p. 401.

14. Coleman DV. The cytodiagnosis of human polyoma virus infection. Acta Cytol 1975; 19: 93.

15. Ross JS, del Rosario AD, Figge HL, Sheehan C, Fisher HA, Bui HX. E-Cadherin expression in papillary transitional cell carcinoma of the urinary bladder. Human Pathol 1995; 26: 940.

16. Imao T, Koshida K, Endo Y, Uchibayashi T, Sasaki T, Namiki M. Dominant role of E-Cadherin expression in the progression of bladder cancer. J Urol 1999; 161: 629.

17. Murphy WM. Diseases of the urinary bladder, urethra, ureters and renal pelvis. In: *Urological Pathology.* WB Saunders Company, 1989, p. 34.

18. Atkinson BF. Urinary cytology. In: *Atlas of Diagnostic Cytopathology Urinary Cytology* (Atkinson BF, ed.). WB Saunders Company, 1992, p. 351.

19. Koss LG. Cytology of the urinary tract and its histological bases. 105 illustrations and text. Second edition, revised. Tutorials of Cytology, 1640 East 50th St, Chicago, IL, 1981.

20. Esposti P-L. Urinary cytology for diagnosis, grading and monitoring response to treatment. In: *Bladder cancer. Principles of combination therapy* (Oliver RTD, Hendry WF, Bloom HJG, eds). Butterworths, 1981, p. 9.

21. Murphy WM. Current status of urinary cytology in the evaluation of bladder neoplasms. Hum Pathol 1990; 21: 886.

22. Esposti P-L, Zajicek J. Grading of transitional cell neoplasms of the urinary bladder from smears of bladder washings. A critical review of 326 tumors. Acta Cytol 1972; 16: 529.

23. Bergkvist A, Ljungqvist A, Moberger G. Classification of bladder tumours based on the cellular pattern. Preliminary report of a clinical-pathological study of 300 cases with a minimum follow-up of eight years. Acta Chir Scand 1965; 130: 371.

24. Malmström P-U, Busch C, Norlén BJ. Recurrence, progression and survival in bladder cancer. A retrospective analysis of 232 patients with 5-year follow-up. Scand J Urol Nephrol 1987; 21: 185.

25. Carbin B-E, Ekman P, Gustafson H, Christensen NJ, Sandstedt B, Silverswärd C. Grading of human urothelial carcinoma based on nuclear atypia and mitotic frequency. I. Histological description. J Urol 1991; 145: 968.

26. Carbin, B-E, Ekman P, Gustafson H, Christensen NJ, Silverswärd C, Sandstedt B. Grading of human urothelial carcinoma based on nuclear atypia and mitotic frequency. II. Prognostic importance. J Urol 1991; 145: 968.

27. Tribukait, B. Flow cytometry in surgical pathology and cytology of tumors of the genito-urinary tract. In: *Advances in Clinical Cytology* (Koss LG, Coleman DV, eds.), Second volume. Masson Publishing, New York, NY, 1984, p. 165.

28. Murphy WM, Soloway MS, Jukkola AF, Crabtree WN, Ford KS. Urinary cytology and bladder cancer. Cancer 1984; 53: 1555.
29. Epstein JL, Amin MB, Reuter VR, Mostoffi FK, the Bladder consensus Conference Committee. The World Health Organization/International Society of urological pathology consensus classification of urothelial (transitional cell) neoplasms of the urinary bladder. Am J Surg Pathol 1998; 22: 1435.
30. Mostofi FK, Davis CJ, Sesterhenn IA. Histological typing of urinary bladder tumours. International histological classifications of tumours. World Health Organization, Geneva, Springer-Verlag, Berlin, Heidelberg, 1999.
31. Mostofi FK, Sobin LH, Torloni H. Histological typing of urinary bladder tumours. International histological classifications of tumours 19. World Health Organization, Geneva, 1973.
32. Yazdi HM. Genitourinary cytology. Clin Lab Med 1991; 11: 369.
33. Ooms ECM, Veldhuizen RW. Cytological criteria and diagnostic terminology in urinary cytology. Cytopathology 1993; 4: 51.
34. Freedman LS, Machin D. Pathology review in cancer research. Br J Cancer 1993; 68: 827.
35. Witjes JA, Kiemeney LALM, Schaafsma HE, Debruyne FMJ, the members of the Dutch South East Cooperative Urological Group. The influence of review pathology on study outcome of a randomized multicentre superficial bladder cancer trial. Br J Urol 1994; 73: 172.
36. Sharkey FE, Sarosdy MF. The significance of central pathology review in clinical studies of transitional cell carcinoma in situ. J Urol 1997; 157: 68.
37. Machin D, Parmar MKB. Pathology review and diagnosis of cancer (letter). Lancet 1994; 343: 55.
38. Keebler CM. A quality assurance program for the cytopathology laboratory. In: *Compendium on Diagnostic Cytology* (Wied GL, Marluce B, Keebler CM. Koss LG, Patten SF, Rosenthal DL, eds.), Eighth Edition. Tutorials of Cytology, Chicago, Illinois, 1997, p. 409.
39. Johnston B, Morales A, Emerson L. Lundie M. Rapid detection of bladder cancer: A comparative study of point of care tests. J Urol 1997; 158: 2098.
40. Halachmi S, Linn JF, Amiel GE. Moskowitz B, Nativ O. Urinary cytology, tumour markers and bladder cancer. Br J Urol 1998; 82: 647.
41. Choi, H-K, Vasko J, Bentsson E, Jarkrans T, Malmström P-U, Wester K, Busch C. Grading of transitional cell bladder carcinoma bytexture analysis of histological sections. Analyt Cell Pathol 1994; 6: 327.
42. Ooms ECM, Blok APR, Veldhuitzen RW. The reproducibility of a quantitative grading system of bladder tumors. Histopathology 1985; 9: 501.
43. van der Poel HG, Boon ME, van Stratum P, Ooms ECM, Wiener H, Debruyne FMJ, et al. Conventional bladder wash cytology performed by four experts versus quantitative image analysis. Modern Pathol 1997; 10: 976.
44. Murphy WM, Rivera-Ramirez I, Medina CA, Wright NJ, Waijsman Z. The bladder tumor antigen (BTA) test compared to voided urine cytology in the detection of bladder neoplasms. J Urol 1997; 158: 2102.
45. Kern W. The diagnostic accuracy of sputum and urine cytology. Acta Cytol 1988; 32: 651.
46. Maier U, Simak R, Neuhold N. The clinical value of urinary cyolog: 12 years of experience with 615 patient. J Clin Pathol 1995; 48: 314.
47. Farrow GM. Urine cytology of transitional cell carcinoma. In: *Compendium on Diagnostic Cytology* (Wied GI, Marluce B, Keeble CM, Koss LG, Patten SF, Rosenthal DL, eds.), Eighth Edition. Tutorials of Cytology, Chicago, Illinois, 1997, p. 280.

48. Sarosdy MF, Hudson MA, Ellis WJ, Soloway MS, et al. Improved detection of recurrent bladder cancer using the bard BTA stat test. Urology 1997; 50: 349.
49. Wiener HG, Mian C, Haitel A, Pycha A, Schatzl G, Marberger M. Can urine bound diagnostic tests replace cystoscopy in the management of bladder cancer? J Urol 1998; 159: 1876.
50. Van der Poel HG, Van Balken MR, Schamhart DHJ, Peelen P, et al. Bladder wash cytology, quantitative cytology, and qualitative BTA test in patients with superficial bladder cancer. Urology 1998; 51: 44.
51. Leyh H, Marberger M, Conort P, Sternberg C, et al. Comparison of the BTA stat test with voided urine cytology and bladder wash cytology in the diagnosis and monitoring of bladder cancer. Eur Urol 1999; 35: 52.
52. Richards B, Parmar MKB, Anderson CK, Ansell ID, et al. Interpretation of biopsies of "normal" urothelium in patients with superficial bladder cancer. Br J Urol 1991; 67: 369.
53. Harving N, Wolf H, Melsen F. Positive urinary cytology after tumor resection: an indicator of concommitant carcinoma in situ. J Urol 1988; 140: 495.
54. Zieger K, Wolf H, Olsen PR, Hojgaard K. Long-term survival of patients with bladder tumours: the significance of risk factors. Br J Urol 1998; 82: 667.
55. Schwalb DM, Herr HW, Fair WR. The management of clinically unconfirmed positive urinary cytology. J Urol 1993; 150: 1751.
56. Novicki DE, Stern JA, Nemec R, Lidner TK. Cost-effective evaluation of indeterminate urinary cytology. J Urol 1998; 160: 734.
57. Oosterlink W, Kurth KH, Schröder FH, Bultinck J, Hammond B, Sylvester R. A prospective European Organisation for Research and Treatment of Cancer Genitourinary Group randomised trial comparing transurethral resection followed by a single intravesical instillation of epirubicin or water in single stage Ta, T1 papillary carcinoma of the bladder. J Urol 1993; 149: 749.
58. Hall RR, Parmar MKB, Richards AB, Smith PH. Proposal for changes in cystoscopic follow up of patients with bladder cancer and adjuvant intravesical chemotherapy. BMJ 1994; 308: 257.
59. Cookson MS, Herr HW, Zang ZF, Soloway S, et al. The treated natural history of high risk superficial bladder cancer: 15-year outcome. J Urol 1997; 158: 62.
60. Abel PD. Follow-up of patients with superficial transitional-cell carcinoma of the bladder. In: *Superficial Bladder Cancer* (Pagano F, Fair WR, eds.). Isis Medical Media, Oxford Ltd, 1997, p. 203.
61. Soloway MS, Murphy WM, Johnson DE, Farrow GM, Paulson DF, Garnick MB. Initial evaluation and response criteria for patients with superficial bladder cancer. Report of a workshop. Br J Urol 1990; 66: 380.
62. Shipley WM, Prout GR, Kaufman DS. Advances in laboratory innovations and clinical management, with emphasis on innovations allowing bladder sparing approaches for patients with invasive tumors. Cancer 1990; 65: 675.
63. Thomas DJ, Roberts JT, Hall RR, Reading J. Radical transurethral resection and chemotherapy in the treatment of muscle-invasive bladder cancer: a long-term follow-up. Br J Urol 1999; 83: 432.
64. Kaye KW, Lange PH. Mode of presentation of invasive bladder cancer: reassessment of the problem. J Urol 1982; 128: 33.
65. Messing EM, Young TB, Hunt VB, Newton MA, et al. Hematuria home screening: repeat testing results. J Urol 1995; 154: 57.
66. Herr HW. Extravesical tumour repalse in patients with superficial bladder tumours. J Clin Oncol 1998; 16: 1099.

6

The Use of Tumor Markers in Bladder Cancer and Current Concepts on Clinical Applicability

H. Barton Grossman, MD

CONTENTS

INTRODUCTION
DIAGNOSTIC MARKERS
PROGNOSTIC MARKERS
INTEGRATING MARKERS INTO CLINICAL PRACTICE
REFERENCES

INTRODUCTION

In its broadest sense, a biomarker is anything that can be used to indicate the presence or nature of a disease. This definition includes techniques ranging from molecular analysis to image analysis and can utilize all of the research tools of modern medicine. Biomarkers can be used for either diagnosis or prognosis.

While this categorization is intuitively simple, the distinction between diagnosis (detection) and prognosis (outcome) is often complex. For example, a marker such as urine cytology can detect the presence of bladder cancer cells in the urine when the standard test, cystoscopy, indicates that the bladder is normal. In this common clinical situation, a bladder cancer will eventually grow large enough to be detected by cystoscopy. While it appears that in this case the cytology predicted the development of bladder cancer, it actually was more sensitive in detecting disease that was already present but was below the limits of detection of the standard assay.

From: *Current Clinical Urology: Bladder Cancer: Current Diagnosis and Treatment*
Edited by: M. J. Droller © Humana Press Inc., Totowa, NJ

In contrast to diagnostic markers that may presage the development of a clinical lesion, prognostic markers provide an insight into the biology of bladder cancer that enables prediction of long-term events such as progression in stage or the risk of death from bladder cancer. Biomarkers that are used for chemoprevention further blur the distinction between diagnostic and prognostic markers and share characteristics of both.

When biomarkers are evaluated, the fundamental concepts of sensitivity, specificity, and other derived measures of utility must be kept in mind. Sensitivity is a measure of the ability of a test to detect the presence of disease. Specificity measures the ability of a test to determine the absence of disease. In evaluating sensitivity and specificity, it is important to determine whether the population being tested is representative of the patient population in which the tests will be used. If the test population is considerably different, then the expected results may differ significantly from those actually achieved. The formulas that measure sensitivity, specificity, positive predictive value, negative predictive value, and accuracy are listed below.

$$\text{Sensitivity} = \frac{\text{true positive}}{\text{disease present (true positive + false negative)}}$$

$$\text{Specificity} = \frac{\text{true negative}}{\text{disease absent (false positive + true negative)}}$$

$$\text{Positive predictive value} = \frac{\text{true positive}}{\text{test positive (true positive + false positive)}}$$

$$\text{Negative predictive value} = \frac{\text{true negative}}{\text{test negative (true negative + false negative)}}$$

$$\text{Accuracy} = \frac{\text{true positive + true negative}}{\text{all patients}}$$

Adding additional tests increases the bother and expense of medical care. The goal in adding biomarkers to the treatment of patients with bladder cancer is to obtain information that will enable individualized care based on the information gained from the biomarkers. Nevertheless, accomplishing this task is difficult. While biomarkers can have excellent performance characteristics in a patient population, the performance in specific individuals in that group will either be better or worse than the group as a whole. It is virtually impossible to obtain correct information on all of our patients all of the time because of both variations in laboratory results and undefined individual differences. Nevertheless, the intelligent use of biomarkers may bring us closer to this goal.

DIAGNOSTIC MARKERS

The new diagnostic markers that are now in clinical use can be divided into three categories: (1) qualitative markers that are point-of-care assays —the Accu-Dx and BTA *stat* tests; (2) quantitative makers that must be performed in a clinical laboratory—the BTA TRAK and NMP22 assays; and (3) markers that are used in combination with urine cytology—the DD23 and ImmunoCyt assays. Numerous other markers for diagnosis are under development. Some of the promising ones are the hyaluronic acid/hyaluronidase assays, microsatellite analysis, and telomerase assays.

Cytology/DNA Ploidy

Cytologic evaluation of urine specimens and bladder washings is the standard to which the newer biomarkers must be compared. A bladder biopsy displays the interaction between a tumor and its host and provides information regarding both grade and stage. While cytology cannot reveal differences in stage, it offers the advantage that it can sample the entire urothelial surface. However, cytologic assays are subjective and dependent not only on the expertise of the cytopathologist but also on the variable preservation of cells in a toxic environment. Some quantification can be gained by adding flow cytometry or, more recently, image analysis to conventional cytology.

Cytologic analysis does not reliably detect well-differentiated bladder cancers and has a sensitivity for low-grade tumors reported as low as 20% *(1–3)*. However, this test very efficiently detects high-grade tumors with a reported sensitivity as high as 95%. The overall sensitivity of cytology in experienced hands is approximately 60–85%. However, recent comparisons of newer biomarkers to cytology in multi-institutional studies have demonstrated the overall sensitivity for cytology to be in the 20–30% range *(4,5)*. These reports contrast with other recent data demonstrating the effectiveness of urine cytology *(6)*. Therefore, the diagnostic advantage of the newer biomarkers may be less than anticipated particularly when a good cytopathologist is assessing specimens from a patient with a high grade tumor.

Bladder washing or barbotage can be more efficient than voided urine in providing exfoliated cells of high quality for cytologic analysis. A comparison of urine cytology with bladder barbotage found that a single bladder barbotage was equivalent in sensitivity to three voided urine specimens *(7)*. Although urine cytology has a low sensitivity, especially for low-grade tumors, the specificity of this test is very high when cancer cells are identified. Therefore, a positive cytology is an excellent indicator of occult bladder cancer and indicates the need for an aggressive diagnostic evaluation of the urinary tract including biopsies (8).

The sensitivity or rate of detection of cytology can be improved by adding flow cytometry or image analysis (9). Image analysis requires fewer cells than flow cytometry and is more sensitive to rare events. It has therefore largely replaced flow cytometry for DNA ploidy analysis of urinary cytologic specimens. When image analysis is combined with cytology, the diagnostic sensitivity is improved but the specificity is decreased (10,11). Image analysis of ploidy has a high correlation with cytology when the cytological analysis is either normal or malignant. In these situations, adding DNA ploidy to cytology is confirmatory but does not provide additional clinical information. However, DNA ploidy analysis is useful for those specimens that are cytologically atypical or dysplastic (11). Patients whose specimens exhibit atypical cytology and abnormal ploidy have a higher risk of tumor recurrence than those with diploid cells with rates of recurrence of 20% and 5%, respectively ($p < 0.0001$). Similarly, in patients with dysplastic specimens, the rates of tumor recurrence for patients with specimens with abnormal and normal ploidy were 39% and 16%, respectively ($p = 0.033$).

Accu-Dx

The qualitative, point-of-care Accu-Dx assay detects fibrin/fibrinogen degradation products in the urine. This test is more sensitive than cytology or Hemostix for the detection of recurrent bladder cancer in patients undergoing cystoscopic follow-up (5). The sensitivities of Accu-Dx for Tis, Ta, and T1 bladder cancers were 67%, 62%, and 62%, respectively; the corresponding sensitivities for cytologic analysis were 50%, 0%, and 38%. The largest difference in sensitivity was seen for grade 1 tumors. The sensitivities of Accu-Dx and cytology for these low-grade bladder cancers were 62% and 8%, respectively. In this study, the specificities of Accu-Dx were 86% for patients with urologic disease and 80% for patients undergoing follow-up for a history of bladder cancer. Another study compared the Accu-Dx assay with the original BTA assay, cytology, and Hemostix for the detection of bladder cancer (12). In this report, the sensitivities of the four assays were 81%, 28%, 35%, and 69%, respectively. The specificities of these tests were 75%, 87%, 90%, and 68%, respectively.

BTA

The original Bladder Tumor Antigen (BTA) test was a qualitative point-of-care assay for the detection of a basement membrane complex

in urine specimens. Different clinical studies found it to be either more
(4) or less *(13)* sensitive than cytology in detecting bladder cancer.

Second generation monoclonal antibodies were produced that resulted
in the BTA *stat* and TRAK tests *(14,15)*. Both of these newer tests detect
a human complement factor H-related protein. The qualitative, point-of-
care BTA *stat* assay and the quantitative BTA TRAK assay have similar
performance characteristics. The BTA *stat* assay has been shown to have
better sensitivity than cytology (58% and 23%, respectively) *(14)*. In
patients with benign genitourinary disease, the specificity of the BTA
stat assay was 72%. The BTA *stat* assay was better than cytology in detecting superficial papillary bladder cancer (stages Ta and T1), but these two
tests were equivalent for the detection of carcinoma *in situ*.

Another study evaluated the BTA *stat* test and cytology for the detection of bladder cancer in 162 people with a history of bladder cancer and
in 88 patients with hematuria or voiding symptoms and no prior history
of bladder cancer *(16)*. Of these latter 88 patients, 71 were found to have
bladder cancer. The overall sensitivity and specificity of the BTA *stat*
test were 83% and 69%, respectively. Cytology exhibited a sensitivity
of 40% and a specificity of 95% overall. Interestingly, both the sensitivity and specificity of the BTA *stat* assay was better for primary tumors
(90% and 76%, respectively) than for recurrent tumors (74% and 68%,
respectively). The BTA TRAK assay had a reported sensitivity of 68%
and a specificity of 75% when a value of 14 U/mL was used as the upper
limit of normal *(15)*.

The BTA TRAK and NMP22 assays were compared in a study of 47
healthy subjects and 109 patients with a histologic diagnosis of bladder
cancer *(17)*. With the specificity fixed at 95%, the BTA TRAK and NMP
22 assays were evaluated at cutoffs of 12 and 23 U/mL, respectively.
Despite the fact that a high concordance between the two assays was
observed (73%), the BTA TRAK had better sensitivity in 42 patients
with superficial bladder cancer (36% and 14%, respectively).

While it is intuitive that a quantitative assay should provide more useful information than a qualitative assay, the demonstration of this phenomenon and the determination of how best to use this added information
are critical. Increased levels in the BTA TRAK assay are associated with
an increased risk of tumor recurrence *(18)*. Nevertheless, the effective
use of this information requires considerably more clinical data.

NMP22

The NMP22 assay provides a quantitative measurement of a nuclear
matrix protein in urine specimens. The median NMP22 levels in healthy
individuals and in persons with benign urinary tract conditions are 2.9

and 3.3 U/mL, respectively *(19)*. Limited data demonstrate that urinary tract infections, calculi, and other benign conditions can result in higher levels of the analyte. This phenomenon is not unique to NMP22 and is seen with other markers. In addition, urine NMP22 levels appear to be elevated in people with intestinal urinary diversions *(20)*.

Initially, the NMP22 assay was intended for use after endoscopic removal of a bladder tumor. When this test was performed a median of 22 d after transurethral resection, a cutoff of 10 U/mL provided a sensitivity of 70% and a specificity of 79% for the detection of recurrent bladder cancer *(21)*. More recently, this assay has been evaluated for the detection of bladder cancer prior to cystoscopy. In this setting, a lower cutoff of 6.4 U/mL has been reported to provide a sensitivity of 68% and a specificity of 80% *(22)*. Patients with grade 1 tumors had lower NMP22 levels. The sensitivities for grade 1, 2, and 3 tumors were 31%, 74%, and 81%, respectively. Another group used a cutoff of 10 U/ml in this setting and found a sensitivity of 72% and a specificity of 61% *(23)*.

To determine its role in screening, NMP22 was evaluated in patients with hematuria or other indications suggesting the possibility of bladder malignancy *(24)*. Of 330 screened patients, all 18 patients with bladder cancer were detected by the NMP22 assay using a cutoff of 10 U/mL. Cytology detected 6 tumors. The sensitivity, specificity, positive predictive value, and negative predictive value for NMP22 were 100%, 85%, 29%, and 100%, respectively. The sensitivity, specificity, positive predictive value, and negative predictive value for cytology were 33%, 100%, 100%, and 96%, respectively.

DD23

The monoclonal antibody DD23 binds to a protein dimer expressed on bladder cancer cells *(25)*. By quantitative fluorescence image analysis (QFIA) DD23 had a sensitivity of 85% and a specificity of 95% *(26)*. DD23 is currently being marketed as a diagnostic test to be used in conjunction with cytology. When used in this manner, it has a reported sensitivity of 94% (data from UroCor, Inc., Oklahoma City, OK). In asymptomatic and symptomatic control groups, the specificities were 84% and 87%, respectively.

ImmunoCyt

The ImmunoCyt test utilizes three monoclonal antibodies in combination, two that are directed at different mucins and one that binds to a high-molecular-weight form of carcinoembryonic antigen *(27)*. This immunohistochemical assay is intended to be used with cytologic evaluation. With a cutoff of 1 abnormal cell by immunohistochemistry, Immuno-

Cyt plus cytology yielded sensitivities for Ta, T1, and T2/T3 bladder cancers of 96%, 100%, and 90%, respectively. For the entire group, the sensitivity was 95%. The specificity of this combined analysis in an asymptomatic control group was 76%.

Hyaluronic Acid/Hyaluronidase

Hyaluronic acid is a glycosaminoglycan involved in tumor adhesion and migration. Urinary hyaluronic acid is present in higher concentration in patients with bladder cancer. At a cutoff of 100 ng/mg of protein, the use of urinary hyaluronic acid as a biomarker for detecting bladder cancer had a sensitivity of 92% and a specificity of 93% *(28)*. The concentration of hyaluronic acid did not correlate with tumor grade. The same authors also evaluated urinary hyaluronidase activity. Hyaluronidase activity varied with the grade of the bladder cancer and was elevated in patients with grade 2 and grade 3 bladder cancers *(29)*. Urinary hyaluronidase activity was ≥10 mU/mg in all patients with grade 2 or 3 bladder cancers, while only 9% (2/22) of patients with grade 1 tumors and 12% (6/48) of normal controls had values at this level.

Microsatellite Analyses

Microsatellites are polymorphic, short, tandem segments that are dispersed throughout the genome. Microsatellites are stably inherited and can be assessed from small numbers of cells by polymerase chain reaction (PCR) and gel electrophoresis. Comparing extracted DNA from a specimen (tumor or urine) with DNA from leukocytes will enable the detection of alterations in the patterns of the microsatellites. Because it is impossible to predict which microsatellites may be altered, a panel of microsatellite markers is often used. This analysis is labor intensive and is currently not suited for routine clinical application. However, newer methods of automated, rapid throughput analysis are being developed that may make this type of assay commercially feasible in the future.

Microsatellite instability is frequently seen in cancer cells. Measurement of this instability is being explored as a new method for enhancing the detection of bladder cancer. Urine sediments from 25 patients suspected of having bladder cancer were assayed for changes in 13 microsatellite markers *(30)*. In 20 patients with bladder cancer, matching microsatellite changes were seen in the urine and tumors of 19 patients (95%). This result was better than the cytologic detection rate of 50%.

A second study from this same group examined 20 microsatellite markers in 21 patients with a prior history of bladder cancer *(31)*. At 4–6 mo intervals, patients underwent cystoscopy and microsatellite analysis. Eleven patients had tumor recurrences and 10 of them (91%) were diagnosed by microsatellite analysis of the urine. In two patients, microsatellite detection of recurrence preceded cystoscopic documentation by 4 and 5 mo.

Telomerase

Telomerase is a ribonucleoprotein that enables the synthesis of telomere ends. Telomerase activity is usually assayed by the telomeric repeat amplification protocol (TRAP) and is not specific for malignancy *(32)*. Both telomerase activity and telomerase RNA have been assayed in clinical specimens. The measurement of telomerase activity on bladder barbotage specimens appears to provide better sensitivity for the detection of bladder cancer than voided urine specimens *(33,34)*.

Telomerase activity is frequently detected in low to moderate grade (grades 1 and 2) neoplasms *(33,35,36)*. The TRAP assay exhibited a sensitivity of 62% and a specificity of 96% in a study of 26 patients with bladder cancer and 83 patients without malignant disease *(37)*. In a study comparing TRAP, NMP22, the original BTA, and cytology, telomerase activity and NMP22 yielded the best results *(38)*. The sensitivities of TRAP, NMP22, the original BTA, and cytology were 80%, 81%, 40%, and 40%, respectively with specificities of 80%, 77%, 73%, and 94%, respectively. Another study compared the TRAP assay with cytology, BTA *stat*, NMP22, Accu-Dx, chemiluminescent hemoglobin, and Hemastix using urine specimens from 57 people with bladder cancer and 139 people without evidence of bladder cancer by cystoscopy *(39)*. In this report, the NMP22 cutoff was 3.6 U/mL as determined by receiver operator characteristic analysis of their data. The TRAP assay had the best combination of sensitivity and specificity. The sensitivities of the TRAP assay, cytology, BTA *stat*, NMP22, Accu-Dx, chemiluminescent hemoglobin, and Hemastix were 70%, 44%, 74%, 53%, 52%, 67%, and 47%, respectively; specificities were 99%, 95%, 73%, 60%, 91%, 63%, and 84%, respectively. An *in situ* TRAP assay appears to provide higher sensitivity than a fluorescence based TRAP assay *(40)*. Comparison of telomerase activity determined by TRAP and telomerase RNA detected by the reverse transcriptase polymerase chain reaction (RT-PCR) in urine specimens demonstrated that the RT-PCR assay is more sensitive but less specific than the TRAP assay *(41)*. Additional assays that will directly measure the catalytic component of telomerase are being developed.

PROGNOSTIC MARKERS

A variety of prognostic markers for bladder cancer have been evaluated, but at this point none has been sufficiently validated to warrant a recommendation for routine clinical use. However, enough preliminary data are available so that two markers, the protein products of the tumor suppressor genes TP53 and retinoblastoma (p53 and pRB, respectively), are currently being assessed in ongoing clinical trials. In these studies, both proteins are being measured by immunohistochemical staining. Using this technique, p53 is not detectable in normal urothelial cells and nuclear staining in bladder cancer cells is abnormal. In bladder cancer, unlike some other neoplasms, immunohistochemical staining for p53 has shown a good correlation with mutations in the TP53 gene (42,43). Overexpression of the p53 protein has been reported to be correlated with poor prognosis, tumor progression, and/or increased risk of death from bladder cancer in patients with either superficial or locally advanced disease (44,51). Cellular regulation by TP53 is complex, and therefore, it should not be a surprise that downstream genes such as p21 (WAF1/CIP1) can modulate the prognosis of patients whose tumors exhibit altered p53 expression (52). The clinical evaluation of p53 expression has primarily been performed on tissue specimens. The role of p53 assessment on exfoliated cells in urine and/or bladder barbotage specimens is being explored.

The RB protein is detectable in a weak, heterogeneous nuclear staining pattern in normal cells, and loss of pRB as shown by immunohistochemical analysis is abnormal and correlates with an increased risk of progression of bladder cancer (53,54). More recently, overexpression of pRB has also been demonstrated to be an indicator of a poor prognosis (55,56). The abnormal overexpression of pRB is caused by the loss of p16 (MTS-1/INK4a) function (57). Several studies have also demonstrated that the combined use of p53 and pRB provides better prognostic information in both superficial and locally advanced bladder cancer (55,56,58).

Although the above data indicate that both p53 and pRB are powerful indicators of prognosis in bladder cancer, other investigators have not been able to document this association (59–62). This may reflect differences in study design, antibodies used, and staining techniques. For example, in superficial bladder cancer, progression and recurrence are very different endpoints. A study from The University of Texas M. D. Anderson Cancer Center documented that p53 and pRB were statistically and clinically significant indicators of progression in patients with T1 bladder cancer (56). However, neither marker was an indicator of tumor recurrence. This inability to predict local recurrence of superficial bladder cancer has also been reported by others (63). As discussed above, prediction of recurrence is often a matter of increased sensitivity in detection while prediction of progression is a measure of tumor aggressiveness.

The differences in the literature regarding the utility of p53 and pRB prohibit a recommendation that these markers be used in the routine management of patients with bladder cancer. However, sufficient data now exist to warrant the prospective testing of these markers in controlled clinical trials. Such studies are now ongoing at Memorial Sloan-Kettering Cancer, at The University of Texas M. D. Anderson Cancer Center, and in an international multi-institutional effort organized through the University of Southern California. Issues regarding the challenges of incorporating biomarkers in patient care are discussed in Chapter 15 of this volume.

INTEGRATING MARKERS INTO CLINICAL PRACTICE

The number of biomarkers touted to manage bladder cancer that are either in current use or are likely to be incorporated in the clinical diagnostic armamentarium in the near future is rapidly increasing. Because these novel indicators of bladder cancer fall far from the ideal goal of 100% sensitivity and specificity, the challenge to both the clinician and patient is how to best use these biomarkers effectively in improving individual patient care. To use these markers in a rational fashion, it is incumbent upon the physician ordering these tests to follow several general rules: (1) know the performance characteristics of the marker; (2) know the information expected to be gained from the marker; and (3) be prepared to act on the result of the assay. If any one of these three links is broken, the use of a biomarker in that clinical circumstance can be challenged. It is worthwhile to consider these individual steps in more detail. If the performance characteristics of an assay are not known at least in general, there is no way to gauge the reliability of the result.

After the performance characteristics are understood, consideration must be given to the individual clinical situation to which it is applied. For example, tests for detection differ in sensitivity and specificity. If a diagnostic marker is being used to delay cystoscopy, then a test that maximizes sensitivity should be selected. On the other hand, if cystoscopy is to be performed and the test is being used to detect occult disease, i.e., indicate the need for a biopsy, then a test that has high specificity should be selected. Finally, if the results of a test will not be used in patient management, there is little reason to order the test. Doing so results in expenditure of time and money with no reward.

At the present time, the biomarkers in clinical use are focused on diagnosis. These markers are usually used by urologists for the followup of patients with a history of bladder cancer. Nevertheless, markers can potentially be applied in other ways to the management of patients with bladder cancer if sufficient data are generated to support these new uses.

Markers with high sensitivity, particularly point-of-care assays, could be used for initial screening by primary care physicians and by patients themselves if they experience hematuria. In this circumstance, a positive test, while not necessarily proving the existence of bladder cancer, would indicate the need for a referral to an urologist for a more complete evaluation. Primary care physicians could potentially also assist urologists in the followup of patients with a history of bladder cancer employing sensitive tests to determine when cystoscopy should be used. The obvious risk of these approaches to superficial bladder cancer management is that some tumors will not be recognized at a time when they are still of low stage and that increased morbidity and mortality will result from the delayed detection of invasive tumors. It can not be emphasized too strongly that relevant data in an appropriate patient population are required before new methods of using biomarkers are incorporated into routine clinical practice.

Biomarkers for prognosis have the potential to enable individualized therapy based on tumor phenotype. While the initial observations with the p53 and pRB proteins are promising, the ongoing prospective assessment of these markers in clinical trials will determine whether they should be added to the clinical evaluation of patients with bladder cancer.

Considerable uncertainty remains regarding the optimal use of biomarkers for the management of patients with bladder cancer. Controlled clinical trials in a relevant patient population will provide the means for resolving this dilemma. Fortunately, physicians are accustomed to making decisions with less than complete information and can effectively incorporate biomarkers into their treatment decisions by following the guidelines listed above.

REFERENCES

1. Ro JY, Staerkel GA, Ayala AG. Cytologic and histologic features of superficial bladder cancer. Urol Clin North Am 1992; 19: 435.
2. Murphy WM. Current status of urinary cytology in the evaluation of bladder neoplasms. Hum Pathol 1990; 21: 886.
3. Shenoy UA, Colby TV, Schumann GB. Reliability of urinary cytodiagnosis in urothelial neoplasms. Cancer 1985; 56: 2041.
4. Sarosdy MF, deVere White RW, Soloway MS, Sheinfeld J, Hudson MA, Schellhammer PF, et al. Results of a multicenter trial using the BTA test to monitor for and diagnose recurrent bladder cancer. J Urol 1995; 154: 379.
5. Schmetter BS, Habicht KK, Lamm DL, Morales A, Bander NH, Grossman HB, et al. A multicenter trial evaluation of the fibrin/fibrinogen degradation products test for detection and monitoring of bladder cancer. J Urol 1997; 158: 801.
6. Bastacky S, Ibrahim S, Wilczynski SP, Murphy WM. The accuracy of urinary cytology in daily practice. Cancer 1999; 87: 118.

7. Badalament RA, Hermansen DK, Kimmel M, Gay H, Herr HW, Fair WR, et al. The sensitivity of bladder wash flow cytometry, bladder wash cytology, and voided cytology in the detection of bladder carcinoma. Cancer 1987; 60: 1423.

8. Schwalb DM, Herr HW, Fair WR. The management of clinically unconfirmed positive urinary cytology. J Urol 1993; 150: 1751.

9. Melamed MR. Flow cytometry for detection and evaluation of urinary bladder carcinoma. Semin Surg Oncol 1992; 8: 300.

10. de la Roza GL, Hopkovitz A, Caraway NP, Kidd L, Dinney CP, Johnston D, Katz RL. DNA image analysis of urinary cytology: prediction of recurrent transitional cell carcinoma. Mod Pathol 1996; 9: 571.

11. Slaton JW, Dinney CPN, Veltri RW, Miller MC, Liebert M, O'Dowd GJ, Grossman HB. Deoxyribonucleic acid ploidy enhances the cytological prediction of recurrent transitional cell carcinoma of the bladder. J Urol 1997; 158: 806.

12. Johnston B, Morales A, Emerson L, Lundie M. Rapid detection of bladder cancer: a comparative study of point of care tests. J Urol 1997; 158: 2098.

13. Murphy WM, Rivera-Martinez I, Medina CA, Wright NJ, Wajsman Z. The bladder tumor antigen (BTA) test compared to voided urine cytology in the detection of bladder neoplasms. J Urol 1997; 158: 2102.

14. Sarosdy MF, Hudson MA, Ellis WJ, Soloway MS, deVere White RW, Sheinfeld J, et al. Detection of recurrent bladder cancer using a new one-step test for bladder tumor antigen. J Urol 1997; 157(Suppl): 337.

15. Ellis WJ, Blumenstein BA, Ishak LM, Enfield DL. Clinical evaluation of the BTA TRAK assay and comparison to voided urine cytology and the Bard BTA test in patients with recurrent bladder tumors. The Multi Center Study Group. Urology 1997; 50: 882.

16. Pode D, Shapiro A, Wald M, Nativ O, Laufer M, Kaver I. Noninvasive detection of bladder cancer with the BTA stat test. J Urol 1999; 161: 443.

17. Abbate I, D'Introno A, Cardo G, Marano A, Addabbo L, Musci MD, et al. Comparison of nuclear matrix protein 22 and bladder tumor antigen in urine of patients with bladder cancer. Anticancer Res 1998; 18: 3803.

18. Blumenstein BA, Ellis WJ, Ishak LM. The relationship between serial measurements of the level of a bladder tumor associated antigen and the potential for recurrence. J Urol 1999; 161: 57.

19. Carpinito GA, Stadler WM, Briggman JV, Chodak GW, Church PA, Lamm DL, et al. Urinary nuclear matrix protein as a marker for transitional cell carcinoma of the urinary tract. J Urol 1996; 156: 1280.

20. Miyanaga N, Akaza H, Ishikawa S, Ohtani M, Noguchi R, Kawai K, et al. Clinical evaluation of nuclear matrix protein 22 (NMP22) in urine as a novel marker for urothelial cancer. Eur Urol 1997; 31: 163.

21. Soloway MS, Briggman JV, Carpinito GA, Chodak GW, Church PA, Lamm DL, et al. Use of a new tumor marker, urinary NMP22, in the detection of occult or rapidly recurring transitional cell carcinoma of the urinary tract following surgical treatment. J Urol 1996; 156: 363.

22. Stampfer DS, Carpinito GA, Rodriguez Villanueva J, Willsey LW, Dinney CP, Grossman HB, et al. Evaluation of NMP22 in the detection of transitional cell carcinoma of the bladder. J Urol 1998; 159: 394.

23. Serretta V, Lo Presti D, Vasile P, Gange E, Esposito E, Menozzi I. Urinary NMP22 for the detection of recurrence after transurethral resection of transitional cell carcinoma of the bladder: experience on 137 patients. Urology 1998; 52: 793.

24. Zippe C, Pandrangi L, Agarwal A. NMP22 is a sensitive, cost-effective test in patients at risk for bladder cancer. J Urol 1999; 161: 62.

25. Grossman HB, Washington RW Jr, Carey TE, Liebert M. Alterations in antigen expression in superficial bladder cancer. J Cell Biochem 1992; 161: 63.

26. Bonner RB, Liebert M, Hurst RE, Grossman HB, Bane BL, Hemstreet GP 3rd. Characterization of the DD23 tumor-associated antigen for bladder cancer detection and recurrence monitoring. Cancer Epidemiol Biomarkers Prev 1996; 5: 971.

27. Fradet Y, Lockhart C. Performance characteristics of a new monoclonal antibody test for bladder cancer: ImmunoCyt. Can J Urol 1997; 4: 400.

28. Lokeshwar VB, Obek C, Soloway MS, Block NL. Tumor-associated hyaluronic acid: a new sensitive and specific urine marker for bladder cancer. Cancer Res 1997; 57: 773.

29. Pham HT, Block NL, Lokeshwar VB. Tumor-derived hyaluronidase: a diagnostic urine marker for high grade bladder cancer. Cancer Res 1997; 57: 778.

30. Mao L, Schoenberg MP, Scicchitano M, Erozan YS, Merlo A, Schwab D, Sidransky D. Molecular detection of primary bladder cancer by microsatellite analysis. Science 1996; 271: 659.

31. Steiner G, Schoenberg MP, Linn JF, Mao L, Sidransky D. Detection of bladder cancer recurrence by microsatellite analysis of urine. Nat Med 1997; 3: 621.

32. Belair CD, Yeager TR, Lopez PM, Reznikoff CA. Telomerase activity: a biomarker of cell proliferation, not malignant transformation. Proc Natl Acad Sci USA 1997; 94: 13,677.

33. Kinoshita H, Ogawa O, Kakehi Y, Mishina M, Mitsumori K, Itoh N, et al. Detection of telomerase activity in exfoliated cells in urine from patients with bladder cancer. J Natl Cancer Inst 1997; 89: 724.

34. Muller M, Heine B, Heicappell R, Emrich T, Hummel M, Stein H, Miller K. Telomerase activity in bladder cancer, bladder washings and in urine. Int J Oncol 1996; 9: 1169.

35. Kavaler E, Landman J, Chang YL, Droller MJ, Liu BCS. Detecting human bladder carcinoma cells in voided urine samples by assaying for the presence of telomerase activity. Cancer 1998; 82: 708.

36. Yokota K, Kanda K, Inoue Y, Kanayama H, Kagawa S. Semi-quantitative analysis of telomerase activity in exfoliated human urothelial cells and bladder transitional cell carcinoma. Br J Urol 1998; 82: 727.

37. Yoshida K, Sugino T, Tahara H, Woodman A, Bolodeoku J, Nargund V, et al. Telomerase activity in bladder carcinoma and its implication for noninvasive diagnosis by detection of exfoliated cancer cells in urine. Cancer 1997; 79: 362.

38. Landman J, Chang Y, Kavaler E, Droller MJ, Liu BC. Sensitivity and specificity of NMP-22, telomerase, and BTA in the detection of human bladder cancer. Urology 1998; 52: 398.

39. Ramakumar S, Bhuiyan J, Besse JA, Roberts SC, Wollan PC, Blute ML, OKane DJ. Comparison of screening methods in detection of bladder cancer. J Urol 1999; 161: 388.

40. Ohyashiki K, Yahata N, Ohyashiki JH, Iwama H, Hayashi S, Ando K, et al. A combination of semiquantative telomerase assay and in-cell telomerase activity measurement using exfoliated urothelial cells for the detection of urothelial neoplasia. Cancer 1998; 83: 2554.

41. Muller M, Krause H, Heicappell R, Tischendorf J, Shay JW, Miller K. Comparison of human telomerase RNA and telomerase activity in urine for diagnosis of bladder cancer. Clin Cancer Res 1998; 4: 1949.

42. Esrig, D, Spruck CH 3rd, Nichols PW, Chaiwun B, Steven K, Groshen S, et al. p53 nuclear protein accumulation correlates with mutations in the p53 gene, tumor grade, and stage in bladder cancer. Am J Pathol 1993; 143: 1389.

43. Cordon-Cardo C, Dalbagni G, Saez GT, Oliva MR, Zhang ZF, Rosai J, et al. p53 mutations in human bladder cancer: genotypic versus phenotypic patterns. Int J Cancer 1994; 56: 347.

44. Lipponen PK. Over-expression of p53 nuclear oncoprotein in transitional-cell bladder cancer and its prognostic value. Int J Cancer 1993; 53: 365.

45. Sarkis AS, Dalbagni G, Cordon-Cardo C, Zhang ZF, Sheinfeld J, Fair WR, et al. Nuclear overexpression of p53 protein in transitional cell bladder carcinoma: a marker for disease progression. J Natl Cancer Inst 1993; 85: 53.

46. Sarkis AS, Zhang ZF, Cordon-Cardo C, Melamed J, Dalbagni G, Sheinfeld J, et al. p53 nuclear overexpression and disease progression in Ta bladder carcinoma. Int J Oncol 1993; 3: 355.

47. Sarkis AS, Dalbagni G, Cordon-Cardo C, Melamed J, Zhang ZF, Sheinfeld J, et al. Association of P53 nuclear overexpression and tumor progression in carcinoma in situ of the bladder. J Urol 1994; 152: 388.

48. Esrig D, Elmajian D, Groshen S, Freeman JA, Stein JP, Chen SC, et al. Accumulation of nuclear p53 and tumor progression in bladder cancer. N Engl J Med 1994; 331: 1259.

49. Sarkis AS, Bajorin DF, Reuter VE, Herr HW, Netto G, Zhang ZF, et al. Prognostic value of p53 nuclear overexpression in patients with invasive bladder cancer treated with neoadjuvant MVAC. J Clin Oncol 1995; 13: 1384.

50. Kuczyk MA, Bokemeyer C, Serth J, Hervatin C, Oelke M, Hofner K, et al. p53 overexpression as a prognostic factor for advanced stage bladder cancer. Eur J Cancer 1995; 31A: 2243.

51. Serth J, Kuczyk MA, Bokemeyer C, Hervatin C, Nafe R, Tan HK, Jonas U. p53 immunohistochemistry as an independent prognostic factor for superficial transitional cell carcinoma of the bladder. Br J Cancer 1995; 71: 201.

52. Stein JP, Ginsberg DA, Grossfeld GD, Chatterjee SJ, Esrig D, Dickinson MG, et al. Effect of p21(WAF1/CIP1) expression on tumor progression in bladder cancer. J Natl Cancer Inst 1998; 90: 1072.

53. Logothetis CJ, Xu HJ, Ro JY, Hu SX, Sahin A, Ordonez N, Benedict WF. Altered expression of retinoblastoma protein and known prognostic variables in locally advanced bladder cancer. J Natl Cancer Inst 1992; 84: 1256.

54. Cordon-Cardo C, Wartinger D, Petrylak D, Dalbagni G, Fair WR, Fuks Z, Reuter VE. Altered expression of the retinoblastoma gene product: prognostic indicator in bladder cancer. J Natl Cancer Inst 1992; 84: 1251.

55. Cote RJ, Dunn MD, Chatterjee SJ, Stein JP, Shi SR, Tran QC, et al. Elevated and absent pRb expression is associated with bladder cancer progression and has cooperative effects with p53. Cancer Res 1998; 58: 1090.

56. Grossman HB, Liebert M, Antelo M, Dinney CP, Hu SX, Palmer JL, Benedict WF. p53 and RB expression predict progression in T1 bladder cancer. Clin Cancer Res 1998; 4: 829.

57. Benedict WF, Lerner SP, Zhou J, Shen X, Tokunaga H, Czerniak B. Level of retinoblastoma protein expression correlates with p16 (MTS-1/INK4A/CDKN2) status in bladder cancer. Oncogene 1999; 18: 1197.

58. Cordon-Cardo C, Zhang Z. F, Dalbagni G, Drobnjak M, Charytonowicz E, Hu SX, et al. Cooperative effects of p53 and pRB alterations in primary superficial bladder tumors. Cancer Res 1997; 57: 1217.

59. Gardiner RA, Walsh MD, Allen V, Rahman S, Samaratunga ML, Seymour GJ, Lavin MF. Immunohistological expression of p53 in primary pT1 transitional cell bladder cancer in relation to tumour progression. Br J Urol 1994; 73: 526.

60. Vet JA, Bringuier PP, Poddighe PJ, Karthaus HF, Debruyne FM, Schalken JA. p53 mutations have no additional prognostic value over stage in bladder cancer. Br J Cancer 1994; 70: 496.
61. Jahnson S, Risberg B, Karlsson MG, Westman G, Bergstrom R, Pedersen J. p53 and Rb immunostaining in locally advanced bladder cancer: relation to prognostic variables and predictive value for the local response to radical radiotherapy. Eur Urol 1995; 28: 135.
62. Jahnson S, Karlsson MG. Predictive value of p53 and pRb immunostaining in locally advanced bladder cancer treated with cystectomy. J Urol 1998; 160: 1291.
63. Tetu B, Fradet Y, Allard P, Veilleux C, Roberge N, Bernard P. Prevalence and clinical significance of HER/2neu, p53 and Rb expression in primary superficial bladder cancer. J Urol 1996; 155: 1784.

7

Pathologic Assessment of Bladder Cancer and Pitfalls in Staging

Christer Busch, MD, PHD, Debra Hawes, MD, Sonny L. Johansson, MD, PHD, and Richard J. Cote, MD

CONTENTS

CLASSIFICATION OF BLADDER TUMORS

The classification of tumors of the bladder falls into three basic categories, histology, patterns of growth (e.g., papillary vs nonpapillary, invasive vs noninvasive), and malignancy grade. The histological tumor types primary to the urinary bladder epithelium are urothelial (transitional), squamous, glandular, and small cell. By far the most common histologic type is urothelial (transitional) (approximately 90%). The bulk of this discussion will therefore deal with this tumor type. However, as they comprise approximately 10% of primary bladder tumors a brief overview of some of the other tumor types is also indicated.

Urothelial Carcinoma (Transitional Cell Carcinoma)

Urothelial (transitional cell, TCC) carcinoma is by far the most common primary tumor of the urothelium, comprising approximately 90% of all cases. In contrast to squamous cell carcinoma and adenocarcinoma,

From: *Current Clinical Urology: Bladder Cancer: Current Diagnosis and Treatment*
Edited by: M. J. Droller © Humana Press Inc., Totowa, NJ

urothelial carcinoma presents as non-muscle invasive (pTA+pT1) disease in 70–80% of new cases *(1)*. The macroscopic appearence at cystoscopy varies regarding size, multiplicity and gross structure of the tumor surface. They most commonly present as papillary lesions, but a fraction appear solid (*see* discussion below). Tumors may be present multifocally throughout the bladder mucosa or are localized in one area. It is important to document the number, size and location of lesions.

Papillary lesions encompass all grades. A branched vascular stroma is also frequently seen in solid tumors. Thus, many may appear solid macroscopically, but are in fact compressed papillary, high grade tumors. Low grade papillary lesions, while often obtaining large sizes, rarely metastasize. Despite their indolent behavior, low grade papillary tumors do tend to recur. The most important prognostic features are depth of invasion, angiolymphatic invasion, grade, associated flat carcinoma *in situ*, multifocality, and a history of prior bladder tumors *(2–4)*. Coexisting flat carcinoma *in situ* is associated with higher progression risk than multifocality of papillomatous tumors. Tumor size may be less important, since large tumors may often be rather well differentiated and non-invasive *(5–8)*. It is vital when dealing with biopsy material from the bladder sufficient tissue be obtained to assess invasion (e.g., by fractionated TUR-B for histopathology). Serious attempts to assess the depth of muscle invasion are critical, and CT-guided transmural core biopsy techniques may provide a new tool for such assessment *(9)*. Likewise, grading the tumor correctly is of utmost importance (*see* below). In contrast, metastasis does occur in higher grade papillary tumors and in corresponding solid lesions. Non-papillary carcinoma *in situ* is almost invariably multicentric and therefore is rarely diagnosed as a solitary entity (less than 10% of the cases) *(10–12)*.

Squamous Cell Carcinoma

This group of tumors, while similar to transitional cell carcinoma, is considered a separate form of cancer due to its unusual geographic distribution and etiology. It is a relatively rare tumor in the Western world, accounting for approximately 3–8% of all malignant bladder tumors *(1)*. Squamous cell carcinoma of the bladder is associated with schistosomiasis, chronic irritation, and inflammation. In endemic areas, most notable in the Nile valley, squamous cell carcinoma comprises two-thirds of all bladder cancer and is the most common form of cancer in males. In the West, squamous cell carcinoma is associated with chronic inflammation and also seen in patients with long-term indwelling Foley catheters (i.e., paraplegics).

Squamous cell carcinoma may be virtually impossible to distinguish from high-grade urothelial carcinoma, especially when it is lacking distinct keratinization. According to Murphy et al. (1994) *(13)* the distinction between mixed urothelial and squamous cell carcinoma in any particular case may be arbitrary. Other individuals are more dogmatic in their opinion, stating that the diagnosis of squamous cell carcinoma should be restricted to pure squamous tumors without any urothelial differentiation *(14)*. Such a strict definition may be biologically wrong and it would appear more reasonable to label cases as squamous cell type carcinoma where the majority of the tumor shows squamous differentiation. The different opinions concerning the proper definitions of squamous cell carcinoma may explain why the reported incidence squamous cell carcinoma varies from 3–8% or even higher *(1)*.

Squamous cell carcinoma is thought to arise from squamous metaplasia of the urothelium. In most cases, the tumor presents as a poorly differentiated tumor and muscle invasion is often present *(15,16)*. Grade I tumors are characterized by keratin pearl formation and only slight nuclear abnormalities *(10)*. Grade II lesions are solid lesions with extensive keratinization and keratin pearl formation *(10)*. Grade III tumors are characterized by keratinization that is largely confined to the individual cell with only scattered pearl formation. Tumors that are comprised of large clear cells are also grade III. Grade IV squamous cell carcinoma is a highly anaplastic tumor with occasional squamous pearls, intercellular bridges and individual cell keratinization *(10)*.

Adenocarcinoma

Primary adenocarcinoma of the urinary bladder is quite rare in its pure form, comprising approximately 1% of all bladder tumors *(17)*. As is the case with squamous cell carcinoma, adenocarcinoma is thought to arise from metaplasia of the urothelium. In contrast to urothelial carcinoma, adenocarcinomas tend to present as solitary lesions *(17–19)*. They may present anywhere in the bladder but some authors have reported a higher percentage occurring in the trigone *(20)*. Others have reported half of the tumors occurring in the dome, most of which are urachal *(21)*. In embryonic life, urachus is present in the wall of the bladder extending to the umbilicus. Urachal rests may become the origin of carcinoma later in life.

The microscopic appearance of adenocarcinoma is often glandular, resembling colonic carcinoma. Mucin containing cells are often seen. Other patterns include signet ring carcinoma, colloid (mucinous) carcinoma, papillary adenocarcinoma and clear cell carcinoma. All of these are extremely rare.

Due ot the infrequency with which these tumors arise in the urothelium, care must be taken to assure that a tumor with the history of adenocarcinoma does not represent a metastasis or direct extension from
another site, e.g., large bowel, uterus or ovary. It is generally not possible
to determine the origin of adenocarcinoma by microscopic examination
(17). As is true in squamous cell carcinoma, adenocarcinoma tends to be
diagnosed as late stage disease with infiltration of the muscularis propria
or beyond. Therefore, adenocarcinomas, like squamous cell carcinomas,
are associated with a poor prognosis, despite the fact that stage for stage
they have similar survival rates *(14,15,22)*.

Small Cell Carcinoma

Small cell carcinoma of the urinary bladder is extremely rare and generally develops in older men. We found an incidence of 0.7% in a prospective study of all bladders diagnosed in western Sweden during a
2 yr period *(24)*. The prevailing theory of the histogenesis of this type of
tumor is that it arises from pluripotential stem cells *(14,23–27)*. The fact
that it often accompanies transitional cell carcinoma and adenocarcinoma supports this theory *(14)*. Although histological identical to its pulmonary counterpart, it seems less aggressive and some patients have been
cured by TUR-B or partial or radical cystectomy combined with radiotherapy, and 5 of 18 patients in our series treated with locoregional therapy
survived more than 5 yr *(24)*.

Histologically, it resembles small cell carcinoma elsewhere in the
body. As with squamous cell and adenocarcinoma arising in the bladder,
it most often presents as locally advanced or metastatic disease *(14)*. In
these cases, it is once again most important to rule out a metastasis from
another site as well as to rule out a lymphoma involving the bladder.
Lymphoma can be excluded by immunohistochemical markers specific
for lymphoid cells (i.e., CD45). When primary disease verses a metastatic process cannot be determined on histologic grounds, clinical correlation may be necessary to establish the site of origin.

DIAGNOSIS AND GRADING
OF UROTHELIAL NEOPLASMS

Histopathology

HISTORY OF HISTOLOGIC GRADING OF BLADDER TUMORS

Bladder carcinoma represents one of the best examples of the old observation that tumor agressiveness correlates with a deviation from normal
both at the tissue architectural and cytological (nuclear morphology) level.

In the early years of pathology, a diagnosis merely of cancer was considered sufficient. However, with increasing knowledge and understanding of disease, it was found that cancers varied in their behavior in association with their gross and microscopic appearance. The concept that tumor cells were derived from normal epithelium by a process of dedifferentiation was advanced by Hansemann *(28)*. This observation led to the study of malignant neoplasms on the basis of cell differentiation. Principles for grading malignant neoplasms on this basis were first published by Broders in the early 1920's *(29)*. Broders did not make a sharp distinction between benign and malignant neoplasms. Rather, tumors that were traditionally known to behave in an indolent or benign fashion were designated as grade 1 lesions. The basis of his grading system was as follows: If an epithelioma showed a marked tendency to differentiate, (i.e., about three-fourths of its structure has differentiated epithelium and one-fourth was undifferentiated), it was graded 1; if the differentiated and undifferentiated epithelium were about equal, it was graded 2; if the undifferentiated epithelium formed about three-fourths of the growth it is graded 3; if there was no tendency of the cells to differentiate, it was graded 4. If the number of mitotic figures *and* the number of cells was large, deeply stained nucleoli, played an important part in the grading *(29)*.

As an extension of this work he went on to publish data that were meant to have a practical bearing on prognosis, or to identify features that were predictive of biologic behaviour *(29)*. It was noted at that time that grade 4 tumors of the bladder differed significantly in survival rate (5.71 yr), from grades 1–3, which were indistinguishable from one another, (8.08, 7.29, and 7.78 yr, respectively). He later showed that prognosis was clearly related to the grade *(30)*. Broders was not alone in the quest to identify prognostically significant factors related to bladder cancer. In 1922 Geraghty *(31)* recorded an association between depth of tumor cell invasion in the bladder wall and the prognosis. Many years later Jewett and Strong *(32)* used depth of invasion as a basis for clinical staging *(see* below).

A grading system proposed by Ash *(33)* in 1940 became widely used. It consisted of four grades (I–IV) and was similar to the subsequent Bergkvist classification *(see* below) *(34)*. The main difference between the two was that the grade I tumors of the Ash system were split into grades 0 (papilloma) and I in the Bergqvist system. The rationale used by Ash was that papillomas were prone to local recurrence *(37,38)*.

In 1950, Franksson outlined a grading system of bladder tumors with seven different grades (34). Tumors that had not breached the basement membrane were considered by some to be benign. Thus, Franksson's system required demonstration of invasion for the diagnosis of cancer.

Using this approach, 30–40% of bladder cancers of today's classification were considered benign. In addition, due to the difficulties in evaluating invasiveness in many biopsy specimens, a high percentage of tumors were placed in Franksson group 3, which implying that invasion and malignancy were suspected but could not be proven.

This proved to be a less than satisfactory method and led Bergkvist and associates to develop a new system of tumor classification in 1965 *(35)*. Their system classified tumors into five groups (grade 0–4) according to the severity of the deviation of the cellular pattern from that of the normal bladder mucosa *(35)*. Grade 0 tumors showed individual papillae covered by normal appearing transitional epithelium, while grade 4 showed severe cellular deviation with anaplasia and complete loss of transitional pattern. Grades 1–3 were progressive gradations of epithelial thickening and cellular atypia. Of significance was their discovery that biopsy samples were easily analyzed for cellular morphology and that there was a good correlation between the degree of cellular atypia and survival rates of patients. Thus, they proposed using the cellular pattern for making the diagnosis of cancer on the basis of grading even in the absence of frank invasion *(35)*. Subsequently, Esposti et al. *(41,42)* concluded that the Bergkvist grade 2 tumor was cytologically benign in about 30% of cases. This prompted the subdivision of grade 2 into 2A and 2B based on cytologic features.

The WHO 1973 Classification

Other grading systems based on nuclear features have been used. For example, the histological grading method described by WHO in 1973 *(36)* was based on the degree of nuclear anaplasia, rather than the relative amount of undifferentiated tumor described by Broders. The WHO 1973 classification text stated that grading was one of the methods used by pathologists for evaluating the degree of anaplasia of tumor cells.

The method proposed by WHO was a simple one that employs three grades. Grade 1 was applied to tumors that had the least degree of cellular anaplasia that was compatible with a diagnosis of malignancy; grade 3 was applied to tumors with the most severe degrees of cellular anaplasia; grade 2 applied to those tumors that lay in between. It was agreed that pathological grading was of clinical value because it had been demonstrated to be related to the survival rate of patients *(36)*.

The Malmstrom et al. Modification of the Bergkvist System

In 1987, Malmstrom et al. developed a modification of the Bergkvist grading system *(37)*. The features used were based on architectural as well as cytological rather than individual nuclear features only. This clas-

Table 1
Malignancy Grading of Bladder Carcinoma: Old and New Systems

Modified Bergkvist 1987	WHO 1973	WHO 1999	WHO/ISUP 1998 Consensus
Papilloma grade 0	Papilloma	Papilloma	Papilloma
Papilloma with atypia grade 1	TCC grade 1	Papillary urothelial neoplasm of low malignant potental	
Urothelial carcinoma grade 2A	TCC grade 1	Urothelial carcinoma, grade I	Urothelial carcinoma, low grade
Urothelial carcinoma grade 2B	TCC grade 2	Urothelial carcinoma, grade II	Urothelial carcinoma, high grade
Urothelial carcinoma grade 3	TCC grade 3	Urothelial carcinoma, grade III	Urothelial carcinoma, high grade

sification subdivided the tumors into grades 0,1, 2A, 2B, and 3, where grade 2A represented low grade, 2B moderate and 3 high-grade carcinoma. Grade 0 corresponded to WHO 1973 papilloma (*see* below) and grade 1 was named urothelial papilloma with slight atypia. As seen below, the Scandinavian grading system is directly translatable into the new WHO/ISUP and WHO 1999 systems *(38,39)* (Table 1).

WHO 1999 AND WHO/ISUP 1998 CONSENSUS CLASSIFICATIONS

In the new grading systems developed by the WHO panel and the WHO/ISUP Consensus Group of uropathologists, the principle of the Scandinavian/Malmstrom modifications of the Bergkvist system *(37,51, 52)*, to use a pattern recognition technique to facilitate grading and make it more reproducible, has been largely accepted and incorporated in both descriptions *(38,39)*. The following represents an attempt to describe criteria to discriminate between categories. The reproducibility is probably best for discrimination between low grade lesions and high grade lesions. It is the position of the WHO/ISUP group that further subclassification in the malignant end of the spectrum is not practically useful. However, the Scandinavian system has demonstrated a significant prognostic difference between their grades 2B and 3 *(37,51,52)*, and the WHO 1999 classification includes a corresponding subdivision of high grade carcinomas into grades 2 and 3 *(39)*. The reproducibility of grading should be tested in quality assurance efforts, however. This could possibly be done via Telematics and Internet in the future.

Grading Principles. (Figs. 1A–F). As a general rule, the overall pattern of a tumor should be assessed in areas of the section where papillae are sectioned perpendicular to the surface and basement membrane with inclusion of the stromal stalk. It is important to avoid obliquely, tangentially or longitudinally cut areas.

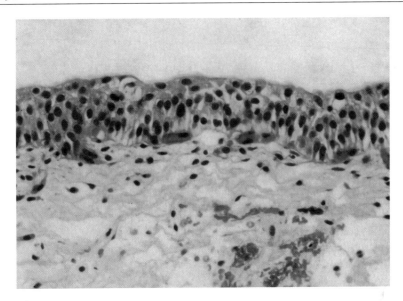

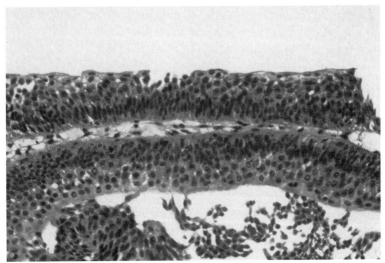

Fig. 1. (A) Normal urothelium; **(B)** urothelial papilloma.

Urothelial Papilloma. *(WHO/ISUP Consensus 1998, WHO 1999).* A urothelial papilloma has urothelium that is of normal thickness, that is, the papillary mucosal lining is indistinguishable from that of normal urothelium. Cellular atypia is not seen and a normal superficial (umbrella) cell layer is present. Mitoses are very rarely seen.

Papillary Urothelial Neoplasm of Low Malignant Potential (PUN-LMP). *(WHO/ISUP 1998, WHO 1999; former Scandinavian grade 1;*

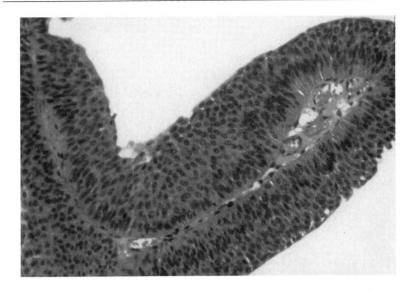

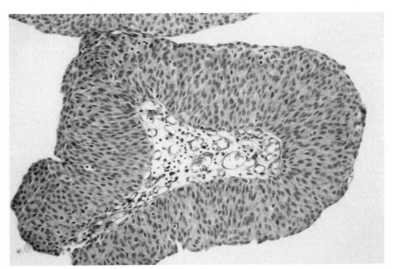

Fig. 1. (C) Papillary urothelial neoplasm of low malignant potential (PUNLMP); **(D)** Papillary urothelial carcinoma, low grade, WHO 1999 grade 1.

best differentiated part of WHO 1973 TCC grade 1). This grade represents a pattern that gives a *predominant impression of order* with *very little variation* of architectural and nuclear features. This pattern evolves from the sum of qualities of individual nuclei, both as individual objects and in their relationships. Thus, there is very slight nuclear atypia some enlargement, but almost no variability in internuclear distances or in the

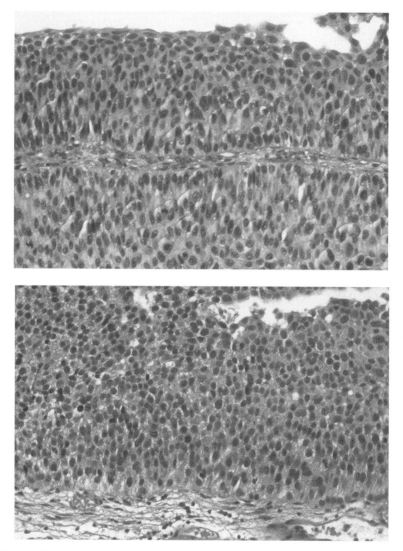

Fig. 1. (E) Papillary urothelial carcinoma, high grade, WHO 1999 grade 2; **(F)** Papillary urothelial carcinoma, high grade, WHO 1999 grade 3. Hematoxylin-eosin, original magnification ↔160.

orientation of nuclear long axes, chromatin texture or form. PUN-LMP is distinguished from papilloma by the fact that there are more cell layers than occur in papilloma. Basal cells frequently show palisading and superficial cell differentiation is evident. Mitoses are rare but are basally orientated when they appear. In such lesions there is generally no progression, no cancer mortality, and a low frequency of recurrence compared with higher grades. In rare cases a patient with this lesion may develop a tumor of higher grade, but this usually occurs only after 10–15 yr *(37,40)*.

Papillary Urothelial Carcinoma, Low Grade. *(WHO/ISUP 1998 urothelial carcinoma,low grade; WHO 1999 grade 1; Scandinavian grade 2A; the more atypical portion of WHO 1973 grade 1 TCC).* As in the PUN-LMP, this pattern yields an *impression of predominant order but in which variation is easily recognized.* The impression of variation emanates from the sum of nuclear features, individually and in neighboring groups (architectural): more evident variation of internuclear distances, long axis orientation, nuclear size, form and chromatin texture. Thus the impression of variability also comes from unevenly spaced nuclei. Basal cell palisading not very pronounced. Superficial cells are distinguishable but are usually more flattened than in normal urothelium. Mitoses are more frequent and closer to the surface. The risk of progression and cancer death rate are low *(37,40)*.

Papillary Urothelial Carcinoma, High Grades.

a. *WHO 1999 grade II; WHO/ISUP 1999 urothelial carcinoma,high grade; WHO 1973 TCC grade 2; Scandinavian grade 2B.* The overall pattern here gives an impression of predominant disorder, but areas of orderly patterns can be distinguished. The pattern emanates from nuclear features and interrelationships as described above, but the variation of each nuclear and architectural quality are more pronounced. Nuclei are larger with more irregular forms and show almost complete loss of polarity. Superficial cell differentiation is rare. Chromatin texture is coarser but also more variable. Mitoses are numerous and irregularly distributed. The progression risk to approximately 20%, and cancer death around 35% in the study by Malmstrom et al. *(37)*.

b. *WHO 1999 grade III; WHO/ISUP 1998 urothelial carcinoma, high grade; WHO 1973 TCC grade 3; Scandinavian grade 3.* The pattern gives *an impression of total structural disorder.* Thus, an orderly pattern is not seen and there is pronounced variation of all nuclear features described above. Mitoses are even more abundant, and irregularly distributed, occur frequently occur in clusters. The progression risk is 40%, and cancer deaths 55% in our material *(37)*.

Comments on Principles of Grading and Prognostic Relevance

As described below *(51,52)* computer assisted analysis studies of bladder cancer have shown that measures of variation are the most important factors for grading. The beauty of the eye-brain connection, i.e.,visual perception or pattern recognition, is that we seem to be well equipped by evolution in our capacity to recognize variation and hence disharmony in patterns and textures. Thus, we can recognize predominant order or

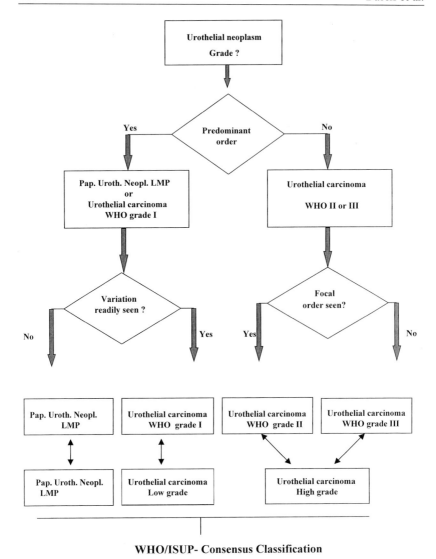

WHO/ISUP- Consensus Classification

Fig. 2. Flow scheme for the decision of histopatholocical malignancy grade in urothelial carcinoma.

disorder in a pattern at a very quick glance. It is possible that both capacities represent survival values and stem from physiological mechanisms evolved to keep us upright and balanced. It is our experience that following the flow chart in Fig. 2 makes grading easier and more reproducible.

Regarding the prognostic relevance of grading, especially of the categories now recognized by the WHO panel and the WHO/ISUP Consensus group, it may be of value to refer to our data from the past *(37)* and to a recent study of PUN-LMP and low grade carcinoma in a population based material from Gothenborg , Sweden *(40)*. Out of 680 patients who were followed for at least 5 yr, 255 had WHO 1973 grade I tumors, stage Ta. These were further subclassified according to WHO and WHO/ISUP Consensus principles into PUN-LMP, (95 patients) and WHO/ISUP 1998 papillary urothelial carcinoma, low grade (=WHO 1999 grade I), (160 patients). The risk of recurrence was significantly lower in patients with PUN-LMP than in those with low grade cancer (35 vs 71%, $p <$ 0.001). Progression to higher stage was seen in 6 patients (2.4%), all with low grade papillary carcinoma (WHO1999 grade I) *(40)*. Thus more than 90% of the WHO 1973 grade 1 tumors had a benign course. This underlines the value of the new classification principles.

Exfoliative Urinary Cytology

Cytology is of little practical value in the initial assessment of primary low grade urothelial tumors of the bladder. Several studies have shown that it is virtually impossible to distinguish histologic grades 0 and 1 from normal transtitional epithelium *(41–44)*. In the early 1960s Johnson and associates stated that highly differentiated papillary tumors of benign histological appearance, which are usually associated with few cellular abnormalities and scanty exfoliation, cannot ordinarily be reliably diagnosed by cytology *(41)*. Similarly Melamed et al. concluded that benign papillomas could not be diagnosed without actual fragments of the tumor being present in the smears *(42)*. These findings were later confirmed in at least two studies by Esposti and associates *(43,44)*. In their study that evaluated 170 primary tumors of the urinary bladder, none of the tumors with histologic grades of 0 or 1 were cytologically reported as carcinoma *(43)*. They also reported in a later study that correlations between histologic and cytologic diagnosis were much stronger in invasive (or suspected invasive) grade 2 carcinoma than in non-invasive grade 2 carcinoma *(44)*. In addition to the drawback of cytology lacking the sensitivity to diagnose low grade lesions, cytologic evaluation has the further disadvantage of not allowing the pathologist to determine the depth of tumor invasion.

It is the consensus of most experts that urine cytology is most effective as a screening tool for recurrent disease in patients with previously diagnosed and treated intermediate and high grade urothelial carcinoma. The cytologic features of urothelial carcinoma include increased nuclear size and irregularity in shape and chromatin texture as well as an increase of the nuclear/cytoplasmic ratio. With increasing malignancy grade these features become more pronounced (Figs. 3A–D).

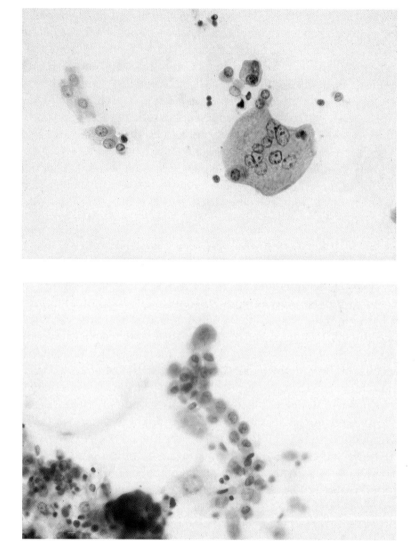

Fig. 3. (A) Normal urothelial cells, superficial and intermediate; **(B)** urothelial cells from a low grade lesion, not diagnostic for malignancy but atypical.

Image Analysis Based Grading

Morphometry

While histopathologic grading of primary bladder cancer has been proved to be of considerable value in predicting clinical outcome, its subjective nature and the rather poor descriptions of the grades in earlier classifications precluded a good reproducibility. As low-grade tumors

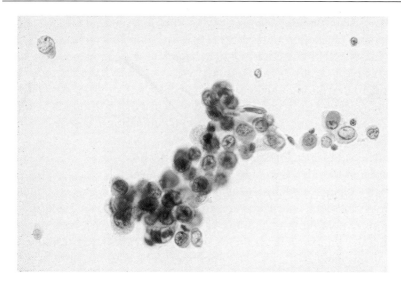

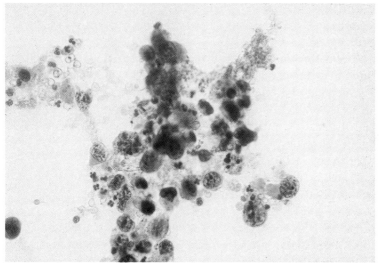

Fig. 3. (C) malignant urothelial cells from a high grade urothelial carcinoma (WHO 1999 grade 2); **(D)** malignant urothelial cells from a high grade urothelial carcinoma (WHO 1999 grade 3).

are generally treated conservatively with either transurethral resection or intravesical chemotherapy, and conversely, high-grade tumors are treated more aggressively, consistent and reproducible methods of grading bladder tumors are needed. Identification of extreme examples of low and high-grade tumors is generally not problematic. However, there are clear difficulties in tumors diagnosed as intermediate grade regardless of the system used. It appears that some behave in a fairly indolent fashion while others are much more aggressive. Therefore, objective methods of grading tumor cells are required. One such method that has been widely studied is morphometry *(45–49)*. It involves, e.g., analysis of the mean and standard deviation of nuclear size in histologic sections *(46,47)*. Early work by Herder and associates *(45)* showed that the WHO grade 2 tumors could be divided into two apparently nonoverlapping groups using cytophotometric measurements. While the number of cases studied *(45)* was insufficient to correlate these findings with clinical outcome, the study supported the idea that objective measurement of nuclear atypia was possible. Similarly, Ooms and associates *(48)* assessed 27 cases of bladder tumors and found the nuclear area to be increased in higher grade tumors, the exception being carcinoma *in situ*. Conversely, Nielsen's groups found that an increased mean nuclear volume indicated recurrence and invasion potential in primary noninvasive bladder tumors (Ta) *(47)*. Recently, a much larger study by Schapers and associates *(50)* involving 294 patients with primary bladder cancer showed that morphometric grade as a single factor was correlated with tumor progression and a poorer overall survival.

The Scandinavian grading system was tested using image analysis in an attempt to develop more objective results by both object and texture based methods. Various levels of structural organization are analysed by this system: individual objects, e.g., nuclei, features relating to individual objects, as well as the entire image contexture. Further work using image texture analysis has shown that it is possible to select a set of morphometric factors based on their combined correlation to subjective grading and to surrogate end points for prognosis, using multivariate statistical methods and so called neural network analysis *(51,52)*.

Flow Cytometry

In addition to morphometry, flow cytometry has been found to be a valuable objective tool in the assessment of human tumors *(53–60)*. Flow cytometric measurements of nuclear DNA content has been widely employed, and there have been several studies that have reported aneuploidy in bladder cancers to be a poor prognostic indicator *(54–58)*. In 1988 Kirkhus et al. *(55)* studied 63 primary transitional carcinoma of the bladder cases using multi-parameter flow cytometry. They showed that WHO 1973 grade II tumors could be divided into two subgroups. One group consisted of diploid tumors that had flow cytometric characteristics similar to grade I lesions. The second group consisted of diploid and aneuploid tumors that were similar to grade WHO 1973 III tumors. They determined that the frequency of infiltration was greater in the latter group, suggesting that these findings could prove to be prognostically significant.

Fluorescence *in situ* hybridization (FISH) studies of chromosomal markers for malignancy. In recent years the availablity of centromere probes as well as probes recognizing specific portions of chromosomes have provoked numerous studies on the usefulness of FISH in diagnosis and monitoring of bladder cancer *(61–64)*. Most commonly, chromosomes X, Y, 1, 7, 8, 9, 11, and 17 have been analysed.

Polysomies of chromosomes 1 and 17 have been indicated to be more frequent in pT1 tumors than in pTa ones, and loss of Y seems to be an early event in the development of bladder tumors *(61)*. Junker et al. using centromere probes for chromosomes 7, 8, 9, and 12, found that the sensitivity of FISH for detecting tumor cells in bladder washings and urine was around 65% compared to 77% and 50% for cytology *(62)*. Thus FISH seemed to enhance the detection possibilities in voided urine but not in bladder washings. Sauter et al. *(63)* using probes for chromosomes X, Y, 1, 7, 9, and 17 similarly found very marked differences between pTa and pT1 tumors.

Validation of the usefulness of FISH analysis in a prospective study has not yet been published. Zhang et al. *(64)* have performed a pilot study designed to determine its clinical potential, define testing limitations, and optimize a panel of probes specific for bladder cancer detection. Correlations with standard cytogenctics and clinicopathological features of bladder cancer were investigated using bladder washings. Their data suggested that FISH and cytology were complementary testing procedures. However, the FISH data provided valuable ploidy and specific genotypic information for recurrent tumors. In addition, chromosomal abberrations defined by FISH were associated with tumor grade and stage (i.e., simple numerical aberrations were associated with low grade tumors, and high grade and invasive tumors exhibited multiple, nonrandom chromosomal aberrations and vast intratumor heterogeneity). Moreover, somatic pairing or homologous centromeric association could give a false-positive result and appeared to be linked to prior therapy. Dual hybridization with reference to gene-specific probes had to be used to control for somatic pairing. Finally, focal deep muscle invasive lesions, with no surface exposure, could yield false negative results. The authors concluded that FISH analysis, with the use of cells from bladder washings may be a powerful technique holding promise for early cancer detection, monitoring treatment outcome, and predicting recurrence of disease *(64)*.

Table 2
Marker Profiles and Prognosis Related
to the WHO/ISUP and WHO 1999 Grading of Bladder Carcinoma[a]

Grade	Stage pTa	Stage pT1	Stage >pT2	Cytology pos	Mitotic frequ.	Tetra- ploidy	Aneu- ploidy	p53-IHC positive
Pap. neop. LMP	100%	0%	0%	0%	14%	0%	0%	0%
WHO 1 (Low gr)	91%	6%	3%	31%	3%	13%	0%	22%
WHO 2 (High gr)	46%	37%	17%	69%	57%	55%	18%	34%
WHO 3	17%	31%	52%	88%	89%	36%	56%	62%

[a] Busch C, Wester K, Malmström P-U, unpublished observations.

Molecular and Immunohistochemical Markers as Prognostic Indicators of Disease

Table 2 demonstrates the correlates between the new WHO/ISUP Consensus and WHO 1999 grades and a range of malignancy markers. It confirms the rationale to subdivide bladder tumors into two broad categories: low and high grade. Thus more than 90% of low grade tumors including the PUN-LMP are stage pTa, i.e., not invasive. There is also a marked difference in proliferation rate between low and high grade as well as in the proportion of tetraploid or aneuploid DNA-patterns. The relative numbers of cytology positive cases are low in low-grade and *in fait* zero in PUN-LMPs. Recently, Helpap and Kellermann have emphasizes the relevance of the new classifications by describing the expression of cytokeratins 34B12, and 20 as well as that of the proliferation marker MIB1 labelling index: PUN-LMPs and low grade carcinomas have a basal cell palisading and show a superficial expression of cytokeratin 20 and basal expression of MIB1 with low labeling index *(65)*.

PROLIFERATION

As in many other tumors, proliferation rate in bladder cancer has been extensively studied and promoted as one of the more important and frequently independent prognostic markers. Flow cytometry S-phase determination, by Ki67 (MIB1) immunohistochemistry, are most commonly used *(60,65)*. A highly standardized method was developed for assessment of mitosis frequency using a computer assisted image analysis algorithm *(66)*. As seen in Table 2 there is a marked difference in mitosis frequency between low and high grade tumors. Regarding Ki67 or MIB1 labeling index assessment, we have to await better standardization of immunohistochemical techniques (by the introduction of external standards accompanying the specimens during histoprocessing, including sectioning and immunostaining).

Such a technique has been developed *(67)*. This system is based on cultured human fibroblasts suspended in an agarose gel hose. The fibroblasts were well characterized as to their cell cycle status and pieces of the hose accompanies the specimen during the histoprocessing and are sectioned with the actual specimen *(67)*.

PROGRESSION

With the advancement of our understanding of biological systems, new and better ways of predicting disease outcome have been developed. Among these have been molecular and immunohistochemical methods of assessing biological markers of disease progression. A number of studies have been undertaken to determine which biological markers have a predictive value for clinical outcome in patients with primary bladder cancer. These have included p53, retinoblastoma (Rb), p21, MDM2, microvessel density (MVD) and epidermal growth factor (EGF) *(68–93)*.

P53 GENE

It has been shown that patients with urothelial (transitional cell) carcinoma of the bladder who demonstrate *p53* gene alterations to have a significantly increased risk of developing tumor metastases and dying of the disease, compared with patients with bladder tumors who lack *p53* alterations*(73,75)*. *p53* nuclear immunoreactivity is strongly associated with mutations in the *p53* gene and with tumor progression *(73)*. Several authors have reported that genetic alteration of *p53* is found to be common in high-grade urothelial (transitional) carcinoma but rarely present in low-grade tumors *(68–71)*. From these data, alterations of the gene have been correlated with tumor grade.

Esrig and associates *(73)* found that in patients with transitional cell carcinoma confined to the bladder, an accumulation of *p53* detected by immunohistochemical methods predicted a significantly increased risk of recurrence and death, independent of tumor grade, stage, and lymphnode status. More recently, Tsutsumi and associates *(68)* tested their theory that *p53* gene alterations might play an active role in malignant progression of superficial bladder cancer. They demonstrated that 3 of 5 cases with malignant progression exhibited allelic loss of the *p53* gene in the initial tumor, and the other two cases did so in recurrent tumors *(68)*. These data suggest the possibility that alteration of the *p53* gene could be a useful marker for the prediction of outcome of superficial bladder cancers. Using immunohistochemistry to identify p53 protein accumulation in the nuclei of tumor cells, and assessing its relationship with lamina propria invasion, Hermann et al. studied 143 patients with T1 bladder cancer and found that *p53* overexpression and the level of lamina propria invasion were significantly associated with survival for patients up to age 75 ($p < 0.05$) *(70)*.

MDM2 GENE

Lianes et al. *(71)*, found that MDM2, a gene that is known to be amplified and over-expressed in sarcomas, was over-expressed in low-stage and low-grade bladder cancers ($p = 0.00050$). They also found a strong statistical association between MDM2 and p53 overexpression, and postulated that aberrant MDM2 along with aberrant p53 phenotypes may be important diagnostic and prognostic markers in bladder cancer *(71)*.

p21 GENE

A primary function of p53 is to be a cell cycle regulatory protein that mediates its effects on the cell cycle through the regulation of p21 WAF1/ CIP1 expression *(80)*. However, it has recently been demonstrated that *p21* expression may also be mediated through p53 independent pathways *(79–88)*. We evaluated *p21* expression using immunohistochemical techniques in bladder tumors from 101 patients who underwent radical cystectomy for invasive bladder cancer *(85)*. All patients had p53 altered tumors *(85)*. Immunohistochemical detection of p21 protein in the nuclei of bladder cancers that showed that altered p53 expression provided important additional prognostic information. The patients with p53 altered and p21 negative urothelial carcinomas of the bladder that were demonstrated a significantly decreased probability of overall survival compared to those with tumors that maintained expression of p21 *(85)*.

RETINOBLASTOMA (*RB*) GENE

The retinoblastoma (*Rb*) gene is considered to be the prototype tumor suppressor gene. The Rb protein interacts with multiple cell cycle regulatory proteins that are involved in the control of cell growth. Rb alterations have been shown to be associated with patient outcome, in that patients with loss of Rb expression have a poorer recurrence-free survival rate than patients with normal Rb expression *(83–85)*.

However, a proportion of tumors showing no alteration in *Rb* also progress; this is true also for *p53 (84)*. Thus, alterations in both *Rb* and *p53* may act in a cooperative or synergistic way to promote bladder tumor progression in humans. Thus, it has been demonstrated that patients with tumors altered in both *p53* and *Rb* had significantly increased rates of recurrence and decreased rates of survival compared with patients with alterations in only one of these proteins. The latter had intermediate rates of recurrence and survival *(85)*. Thus, alterations neither in the *p53* gene, nor in the *Rb* gene alone are mandatory in bladder cancer progression.

A study performed by Cordon-Cardo and associates *(83)* suggested that alterations of *p53* and pRb had a cooperative negative effect on both progression and survival in primary bladder cancer. They postulated that aberrant p53 and pRb expression deregulated cell cycle control by reducing the affected cells' response to programmed cell death. The imbalance produced by an enhanced proliferative activity and a lower rate of apoptosis might determine an aggressive clinical course of tumors with both p53 and pRb alterations *(83)*.

MICROVESSEL DENSITY (MVD)

A majority of studies assessing the prognostic value of assessing tumor angiogenesis through measurement of tumor microvessel density) have found a positive association between increasing microvessel densities and worsening prognosis. The relationship between established prognostic indicators and the extent of tumor-associated angiogenesis was explored in patients with invasive urothelial carcinoma of the bladder *(89)*. The extent of tumor-associated angiogenesis in tumor tissue from 164 patients with urothelial carcinoma was evaluated by immunohistochemical methods using monoclonal antibodies against CD34. We found that microvessel density was significantly and negatively associated with disease-free ($p < 0.0001$) and overall ($p = 0.0007$) survival. Tumor angiogenesis was found to be an independent prognostic indicator when evaluated in association with histologic grade, pathologic stage, and regional lymph node status *(89)*.

EPIDERMAL GROWTH FACTOR (EGF)

Epidermal growth factor (EGF) is normally present in urine. Expression of its receptor (EGFR) on tumor cells has been shown to correlate with grade, and stage and prognosis. In low stage bladder cancer, it correlates with recurrence and progression, while in high stage disease it is correlated to outcome *(90–93)*. In a multivariate analyses, however, it was found not to be independent of stage *(92)*.

STAGING OF BLADDER CANCER

Jewett and Strong were the first to show the importance of staging of bladder cancer *(32)*. They found that the potential curability in patients with bladder cancer was different in patients who demonstrated either no invasion, muscularis propria (detrusor muscle) invasion or perivesical

Table 3
1997 AJCC/TNM Staging of Bladder Cancer

Primary Tumor (T)

TX		Primary tumor cannot be assessed
T0		No evidence of primary tumor
Ta		Noninvasive papillary carcinoma
T1		Tumor invades into lamina propria
T2		Tumor invades the muscularis propria (detrusor muscle)
	T2a	Tumor invades inner half (superficial muscle)
	T2b	Tumor invades outer half (deep muscle)
T3		Tumor invades perivesical tissue
	T3a	Microscopically
	T3b	Macroscopically (extravesical mass)
T4		Tumor invades any of following: prostate, uterus, vagina, pelvic wall, abdominal wall
	T4a	Tumor invades prostate, uterus, vagina
	T4b	Tumor invades pelvic wall, abdominal wall

extension. This 1946 staging system was modified by Marshall in 1952 *(94)* to address superficial invasion and was used extensively until UICC *(95)* and AJCC *(96)* published similar staging systems based on TNM, the latest version of which was published in 1997 (Table 3).

The differences between the 1992 AJCC/UICC staging and the latest version was that in the 1992 system T2 tumors invaded the superficial part of the detrusor muscle and T3 tumors involved the deep muscle or perivesical fat. Support for this new redefinition came from studies by Pearse et al. *(97)*, and Blandy et al. *(98)* They found no significant difference in survival of patients with superficial (1992, T2) or deeply muscle invasive tumors (1992, T3a). It seems more important to determine whether the tumor is organ confined (T2b or less) or not *(98)* (T3a or worse). Furthermore, clinical staging of muscle invasive bladder cancer is even in the confined best of hand only approximately 50%. In addition, pathologists cannot reliably determine whether there is deep or superficial muscle invasion in bladder biopsies or transurethral resection specimens. Therefore, the very presence of muscle invasion rather than its depth determines the mode of treatment in most centers.

Anderström et al. *(3)* studied 177 patients with either noninvasive (stage Ta) (78 patients) or lamina propria invasive (stage T1) (99 patients) bladder cancer who were followed-up for at least 6 yr. Only 1/77 patients without lamina propria invasion died from bladder cancer within five years, regardless of treatment (98% 5 yr survival) while 24/99 of the patients with lamina propria invasion died from their disease (76% 5 yr survival). When these patients were followed for up to 20 yr 9 Ta patients

(11%) and 30 T1 patients (30%) respectively, died of bladder cancer *(100)*. In the initial study *(3)*, there were 22 WHO 1973 grade I tumors, 46 grade II tumors (one of whom died) and 9 grade 3 tumors, all stage Ta. Forty-one of the 99 patients with lamina propria invasion had grade 2 tumors, 48 grade 3 and 10 grade 4. If only grade 2 tumors were evaluated, the five and ten year survival for patients with lamina propria invasion was 83%, compared to 98% and 94% in patients without lamina propria invasion. All 9 patients with noninvasive grade 3 tumors survived five years, while the 5 year survival in grade 3 tumors with lamina propria invasion was only 63%. Similar results were found in a study of 249 patients by the National Bladder Cancer Collaborate Group. Thus, only 30% of the patients with T1 tumors remained tumor free at three years, as compared to about 50% of the patients with Ta tumors. Less than 10% of the Ta tumors progressed, while more than 1/3 of the T1 tumors progressed to deeply invasive tumors *(101)*. These result support that the collective term "superficial cancer" for stage Ta, T1 tumor should be abandoned *(3)*. Staging is a very important predictor for prognosis and is critical in stratifying patients for therapy. Tumor grade cannot be ignored since the progression rate for grade 1–2 tumors is less than 10%, while it is over 50% in grade 3 tumors *(101)*.

The pathological pitfalls in staging include misinterpretation of benign proliferative urothelial lesions such as von Brunns nests, inverted papilloma and nephrogenic metaplasia as invasive lesions. In these lesions and urothelial tumors the problem is made worse by the difficulty to properly orient the specimen. In non-invasive papillary urothelial tumors the stroma epithelial interface is usually smooth and regular. In contrast, in cases of true invasion, there is variable size and shape of the invasive nests. Furthermore, the basement membrane is normally regular in benign or noninvasive tumors and the outline is irregular and is frequently absent in cases of invasion. Invasive tumors usually show a fibroblastic stromal reaction often associated with myxoid stromal change. The invasive tumor cells may present with paradoxical differentiation, which make them appear more differentiated than the overlying noninvasive disease. Major problems in interpreting invasiveness may be associated with a variable degree of squeeze or cautery artifacts. Overinterpretation of muscle invasive disease may be related to unawareness of the presence of muscularis mucosa, thus reading any muscle involvement as detrusor muscle invasion. Generally, it is not difficult to differentiate muscularis mucosa from detrusor muscle because of the larger and more coarse muscle fibers in the latter as compared to the thin wisps of smooth muscle fibers representing the muscularis mucosa. Furthermore, as it was mentioned previously, biopsies and transurethral resection specimens do not allow identification of whether there is superficial or deep muscle invasion. Neither can perivesical invasion be identified with certainty in transurethral resection specimens and biopsies since it is not unusual to see fat both in the lamina propria and interspersed between the detrusor muscle bundles.

Prostatic Involvement

Prostatic involvement by urothelial cancer was first described by Melicow and Hollowell in 1952 (102). The exact incidence of urothelial carcinoma involvement of the prostate remains somewhat uncertain, but numbers varying from 1.5–43% of all prostatic tumors have been reported (103,104). There are some controversies with regard to substaging prostatic involvement. Schellhammer et al. (103), studied 350 cases of patients who underwent radical cystectomy. A subgroup of 38 male patients with involvement of the prostate by transitional cell carcinoma were reported. They described three different patterns of involvement; ductal involvement, with or without stromal invasion, ductal and acinar involvement with or without stromal invasion, and stromal invasion only. Although the numbers of patients were small, patients without stromal invasion seemed to do significantly better than patients with stromal invasion and only two of 11 patients (18%) with ductal and acinar involvement and stromal invasion survived five years. Likewise, only 22% (2/9) patients with stromal invasion only survived five years. The UICC and Marshall staging system in which prostatic involvement is demonstrated as stage IV or D, regardless of involvement makes no provision for differentiating the degree of involvement by urothelial carcinoma in relation to coexisting urothelial carcinoma of the bladder.

Ten years ago, Hardeman and Soloway (105) suggested that prostatic involvement be divided into three groups: 1) tumor (in situ) confined to the prostatic urothelium; 2) tumor involving prostatic ducts or acini without invasion; and 3) tumor invading the prostatic stroma. However, they did not include patients whose tumors extended through the full thickness of the bladder to invade the prostate (pT4a). In a study of 489 cases of bladder cancer treated with radical cystoprostatectomy, 143 had concomitant involvement of the prostate (29.2%) (106). Prostatic involvement of the urothelial epithelium, acini, or ducts did not alter survival, rather survival was determined by primary bladder cancer stage alone. The study clearly demonstrated that P1 bladder tumors with prostatic stromal invasion arising intraurethrally had a higher survival rate than P4a tumors (prostate stromal invasion through the bladder wall) and that a separate designation was required. The majority of P1 tumors had only focal stromal invasion versus the more extensive stromal involvement of P4a tumors, which suggested that they are different biologically, as reflected in their different prognosis. In contrast, P3b primary bladder transitional cell carcinoma with prostate stromal invasion arising intra-urethrally had the same poor prognosis as P4a tumors *(106)*. Similar results were obtained in a study by Pagano et al. *(107)*. Thus, it seems important to determine contiguous versus noncontiguous growth.

In 1983, Dixon and Gosling *(108)* reported on the presence of thin wisps of generally discontinuous muscle fibers in the lamina propria. The called this the muscularis mucosa (MM). These results were confirmed by Ro et al. *(109)*, and Keep et al. *(110)*. In 1990, the first paper describing the substaging of tumors using the MM or large arteries at the level of the MM as the landmark for their substaging, was published by Younes et al. *(111)*. They found that invasion restricted to the area above the MM was associated with a significantly better prognosis than when invasion beyond the layer of the lamina propria was found. Thus, the 5 yr survival for 17 patients with invasion above the MM or to the level of muscularis mucosa was 75% as compared to invasion beyond the MM but not into the muscularis propria, which was associated with a 5 yr survival or 11%. Hasui et al. *(112)*, studies 60 patients and found that their pT1a group, which included 60 patients with invasion above MM had a progression rate of 16.7% as compared to their 28 patients with invasion to or near the MM who had a progression rate of 53.5% ($p = <$ 0.01). Similarly, Angulo, et al. *(113)* studied 99 patients with bladder cancer and found a strong relationship between the depth of lamina propria invasion and prognosis, and this factor was an independent predictor of prognosis ($p < 0.0353$). A study by Holmäng et al. of 113 patients revealed significantly higher progression rate in patients with grade 3 tumors and deep lamina propria invasion. Furthermore, patients with pT1b tumors had twice the risk of dying from bladder cancer as did patients with pT1a tumors *(114)*. Similarly, Hermann et al. *(70)* found that the level of lamina propria invasion was an independent predictor of prognosis in a study of 143 patients with bladder cancer. Five year survival was 70% for patients with superficial lamina propria invasion and 57% for deep lamina propria invasion ($p < 0.005$). Finally Smits et al. *(115)*, in a study of 24 patients with pT1 tumors found a progression rate of 6% in pT1a tumors 33% in pT1b tumors and 55% in pT1c tumors. In the multivariate analysis, only the depth of invasion and the presence of carcinoma *in situ* at or near the tumor was associated with progression. Thus, several studies have supported the value of T1 substaging.

However, the study by Platz et al. *(116)*, found that the microstaging for T1 cancer was technically difficult with poor intraobserver agreement for the level of invasion and that it did not yield separate prognostic separation in the 77 cases studied. One explanation put forward by the authors was that the cases were derived from many different urologists and laboratories. Angelo et al. *(113)* were able to substage 58% of the cases and Holmäng et al. *(114)* over 90% of the cases. The results by Holmäng et al. *(114)*, may have been as good as they were because all of the cases were untreated tumors without previous transurethral dissections and the patients were treated with a TUR-B aimed at removing all the cancer with a minimal of cautery artifact. Thus, substaging of T1 tumors, although difficult, can be done in many cases, and seems to suggest that there are two groups of T1 tumors with different biological potential. However, additional studies are probably needed before it can be recommended that this information be incorporated in the official staging system.

LYMPHOVASCULAR SPACE INVASION

The invasion of lymphovascular spaces in the lamina propria by tumor cells is a further area of controversy in the staging of bladder cancer. We have determined that lymphatic invasion in tumors that were superficially invasive had a significantly worse prognosis than those without such invasion ($p < 0.01$) *(3)*. An even earlier study examining prognosis of patients with blood vessel invasion showed that the five year survival rates were 29% for patients with blood vessel invasion and 51% for patients without *(2)*.

However, identification of vascular invasion can be difficult since artifactual clefting around nests of invasive tumors may mimic invasion. This problem was identified by Larsen and associates *(117)* who used *Ulex europaeus* agglutinin-immunoperoxidase staining as a marker for vascular invasion. They found that only 5/36 patients (14%) had true vascular invasion although on routine H and E histopathologic evaluation, all 36 had been considered positive. A similar study by Ramani et al. *(118)*, diagnosed 5 cases with lymphovascular space involvement by H and E examination, whereas only two were confirmed using Factor VIII immunohistochemical markers. They concluded that lymphovascular space involvement in transitional cell carcinomas may be a rare event and one unlikely to be of value in defining prognostic groups for treatment.

SUMMARY

The nominal diagnosis of bladder tumors normally does not present a significant problem. Consultation in cases with morphological characteristics which are rarely seen can be rapidly made using modern telematics i.e., Internet or telephone line based Telepathology. These techniques make it possible to consult specialists globally in minutes or hours. Also, harmonization of grading systems can be augmented by the use of Tele-pathology in the future.

The areas carrying the highest risk for **subjectivity, leading to inter-pathologist variation** in the assessment of bladder cancer are grading and staging. It is important that care is taken to provide optimal material from the lesions. Small lesions should be resected cold to preserve morphol-ogy. Urologists should be encouraged to provide fractionated resection material to increase the possibility for pathologic staging and transmural biopsies could be encouraged in selected cases.

The new grading systems worked out by WHO/ISUP and the WHO panel provide a new language which we believe will prove simpler to use and more reproducible than previous systems. The only difference between the systems is that WHO 1999 allows subdividing of high grade tumors. Otherwise they are essentially identical.

With regard to staging, the correct assessment of invasion in a pap-illary tumor is notoriously difficult. Pathologists should be encouraged to cut deeper sections in equivocal cases and to be very careful in looking for small foci of invasion in the frequently very complex tissue pattern. Several studies have confirmed that recognition of invasion beneath lamina muscularis mucosae is of prognostic importance. The reproduc-ibility of its assessment has been questioned and is a part of the problem with inadequate biopsy practise. Also, false interpretation of muscularsis mucosae as muscularis propria should be avoided.

The future diagnosis of bladder cancer will undoubtedly incorporate selected molecular markers for malignancy and/or therapeutic sensi-tivity. It is important therefore, that controlled, prospective multicenter studies are performed to assess the relative weight of the various compo-nents of the pathologic assessment of bladder cancer, including molecu-lar markers.

The pathologic assessment of bladder cancer in modern practise is the result of a communicative process between clinicians and the pathologist/cytologist, including a molecular pathologist. It is of utmost importance that each cancer diagnosis is discussed at weekly clinico-pathological conferences ideally with the participation of urologists, uro-oncologists, uroradiologists and uropathologists.

Subspecialisation in uropathology is becoming common and interna-tional groups are being formed and meetings are being held that include representatives of the above mentioned specialties. This enhancement of intensity and quality of interdisciplinary communication will **be criti-cal in providing the best information for the optimal management of the patient**.

REFERENCES

1. Johansson SL, Cohen SM. The pathology of bladder cancer. In: *Bladder Cancer; Biology, Diagnosis and Management* (Syrigos KN, Skinner DG, eds.). Oxford University Press, 1999, pp. 97–123.
2. Bell JT, Burney SW, Friedell GH. Blood vessel invasions in human bladder cancer. J Urol 1971; 105: 675–678.
3. Anderstrom C, Johansson S, Nilsson S. The significance of lamina propria invasion on the prognosis of patients with bladder tumors. J Urol 1980; 124: 23–26.
4. Lopez JI, Angulo JC. The prognostic significance of vascular invasion in stage T1 bladder cancer. Histopathology 1995; 27: 27–33.
5. Loening S, Narayana A, Yoder L, Slymen D, Weinstein S, Penick G, Culp D. Factors influencing the recurrence rate of bladder cancer. J Urol 1980; 123: 29–31.
6. Heney NM, Prppe K Prout GR, Griffin PP, Shipley WU. Invasive bladder cancer: tumor configuration, lymphatic invasion and survival. J Urol 1983; 130: 895–897.
7. Kern WH. The grade and pathologic stage of bladder cancer. Cancer 1984; 53: 1185–1189.
8. Fossa SD, Reitan JB, Ous S, Odegaard A, Loeb M. Prediction of tumor progression in superficial bladder carcinoma. Eur Urol 1985; 11: 1–5.
9. Malmström P-U, Lönnemark M, Busch C, Magnusson A. Staging of bladder carcinoma by computer tomography-guided transmural biopsy. Scand J Urol Nephrol 1993; 27: 193–198.
10. Koss LG. Tumors of the urinary bladder. In: *Atlas of Tumor Pathology Fascicle 11*, AFIP. Bethesda, MD, 1975.
11. Murphy WM. Current topics in the pathology of bladder cancer. In: *Pathology Annual*, vol. 18 (Sommers SC, Rosen PP, eds.). Appleton-Century-Crofts, Norwalk, CT, 1983, pp. 1–25.
12. Nagy GK, Frable WJ, Murphy WM. The classification of premalignant urothelial abnormalities: a Delphi study of the National Bladder Cancer Clinical Collaborative Group A. In: *Pathology Annual,* vol. 17 (Sommers SC, Rosen PP, eds.). Appleton-Century-Crofts, Norwalk, CT, 1982, pp. 219–233.
13. Murphy WM, Beckwith JB, Farrow GM. Tumors of the kidney, bladder and related structures. Third series Fascicle Armed Forces Institute of Pathology. Washington, DC, 1994.
14. Grignon D. Neoplasms of the urinary bladder. In: *Urologic Surgical Pathology* (Bostwick DC, Eble JN, eds.). Mosby, New York, NY, 1997, pp. 184–302.
15. Newman DM, Brown JR, Jay AC, Pontius EE. Squamous cell carcinoma of the bladder. J Urol 1968; 100: 470–473.
16. Rundle JSH, Hart AJL, McGeorge A, Smith JS, Malcolm AJ, Smith PM. Squamous cell carcinoma of the bladder. A review of 114 patients. Br J Urol 1982; 39: 522–526.
17. Johansson SL, Anderstrom CR. Primary adenocarcinoma of the urinary bladder and urachus. In: *Textbook of Uncommon Cancer*, 2nd ed (Raghaven D, Brecher ML, Johnson DH, Meropol NJ, Moots PL, Thigpen JT, eds.). Wiley, 1999, pp. 29–43.
18. Mostofi FK, Thompson RU, Dean AL Jr. Mucinous adenocarcinoma of the urinary bladder. Cancer 1955; 8: 741–758.
19. Nocks BN, Heney NM, Daly JJ. Primary adenocarcinoma of urinary bladder. Urology 1983; 21(1), 26–29.
20. Mostofi FK. Pathological aspects and spread of carcinoma of the bladder. JAMA 1968; 206: 1764–1769.

21. Anderstrom CR, Johansson SL, von Schultz L. Primary adenocarcinoma of the urinary bladder, a clinical pathological prognostic study. Cancer 1983; 52: 1273–1279.

22. Grignon DJ, Ro JY, Ayala AG, Johnson DE, Ordonez NG. Primary adenocarcinoma of the urinary bladder: a clinicopathologic analysis of 72 cases. Cancer 1991; 67: 2165–2172.

23. Davis BH, Ludwig ME, Cole SR, Pastuszak WT. Small cell neuroendocrine carcinoma of the urinary bladder: report of three cases with ultrstructural analaysis. Ultrastruct Pathol 1983; 4: 197–204.

24. Holmang S, Borghede G, Johansson SL. Primary small cell carcinoma of the urinary bladder: a report of 25 cases. J Urol 1995; 153: 1820–1822

25. Kim CK, Lin JI, Tseng CH. Small cell carcinoma of urinary bladder: ultrastructural study. Urology 1984; 24: 384–386.

26. Podesta AH, True LC. Small cell carcinoma of the bladder: report of five cases with immunohistochemistry and review of the literature with evaluation of prognosis according to stage. Cancer 1989; 64: 710–714.

27. Blomjous CE,Vos W, De Voogt HJ, Van der Valk P, Meijer CJ. Small cell carcinoma of the urinary bladder: a clinicopathologic, morphometric, immunohistochemical, and ultrastructural study of 18 cases Cancer 1989; 64: 1347–1357.

28. Hansemann D. Ueber asymmetrische Zelltheilung in Epithelkrebsen und deren biologische Bedeutung. Arch f Path Anat 1890; CXIX: 299–326.

29. Broders AC. Epithelioma of the genitourinary organs. Ann Surg 1922; 75: 574–604.

30. Broders AC. Grading of cancer: its relationship to metastasis and prognosis. Texas State J Med 1933; 29: 520–525.

31. Geraghty JT. Treatment of malignant disease of the prostate and bladder. J Urol 1922; 7: 33–65.

32. Jewett HJ, Strong GH. Infiltrating carcinoma of the bladder. Relation of depth penetration of the bladder wall to incidence wall to incidence of local extension and metastases. J Urol 1946; 55: 366–372.

33. Ash JE. Epithelial tumors of the bladder. J Urol 1940; 44: 135–145.

34. Bergkvist A, Ljungquist A, Moberger G. Classification of bladder tumours based on the cellular pattern. Acta Chir Scand 1965; 130: 371–378.

35. Franksson C. Tumors of the urinary bladder. Acta Chir Scand 1950; 151(Suppl): 1–203.

36. World Health Organization. Histological typing of urinary bladder tumours. International Histological Classification of Tumours. No 10. Geneva, 1973.

37. Malmström P-U, Busch C, Norlen BJ. Recurrence, progression and survival in bladder cancer. Scand J Urol Nephrol 1987; 21: 185–195.

38. Epstein JI, Amin MB, Reuter VR, Mostofi FK, the Bladder Consensus Conference Committee. The World Health Organization/International Society of Urological Pathology Consensus Classification of Urothelial (Transistional Cell) Neoplasms of the Urinary Bladder. Am J Surg Path 1998; 22(12): 1435–1448.

39. World Health Organization. Histological typing of urinary bladder tumours. International Classification of Tumours. No 10. Second Edition. Geneva, 1999.

40. Holmang S, Hedelin H, Anderstrom C, Holmberg E, Busch C, Johansson S. Recurrence and progression in low grade papillary urothelial tumors. J Urol 1999; 162: 702–707.

41. Johnson WD. Cytopathological correlations in tumors of the urinary bladder. Cancer 1964; 17: 867–880.

42. Melamed MR, Koss LG, Ricci A, Whitmore WF. Cytohistological observations on developing carcinoma of the urinary bladder in man. Cancer 1960; 13: 67–74.

43. Esposti PL, Moberger G, Zajicek J. The cytologic diagnosis of transitional cell tumors of the urinary bladder and its histologic basis. A study of 567 cases of urinary-tract disorder including 170 untreated and 182 irradiated bladder tumors. ACTA Cytol 1970; 14: 145–155.

44. Esposti PL, Zajicek J. Grading of transitional cell neoplasms of the urinary bladder from smears of bladder washings. ACTA Cytol 1972; 16(6): 529–537.

45. Herder A, Bjelkenkrantz K, Grontoft O. Histopathological subgrouping of WHO II urothelial neoplasms by cytophotometric measurements of nuclear atypia. Acta Path Microbiol Scand 1982; 90: 405–408.

46. Lipponen, PK, Eskelinen MJ, Kiviranta J, Nordling S. Classic prognostic factors, flow cytometric data, nuclear morphometric and mitotic indexes as predictors in transitional cell bladder cancer. Anticancer Res 1991; 11: 911–916.

47. Nielson K, Petersen SE, Orntoft. A comparison between stereological estimates of mean nuclear volume and DNA flow cytometry in bladder tumours. APMIS 1989; 97: 949–956.

48. Ooms ECM, Kurver PHJ, Veldhuizen RW, Alons CL, Boon ME. Morphometric grading of bladder tumours in comparison with histologic grading by pathologists. Human Pathol 1982; 14(2): 144–150.

49. Sowter C, Sowter G, Slavin G, Rosen D. Morphometry of bladder carcinoma: definition of a new variable. Anal Cell Pathol 1990; 2: 205–213.

50. Schapers FM, Pauwels RPE, Wijnen JTM, Smeets WGB, Bosman FT. Morphometric grading of transitional cell carcinoma of the urinary bladder. J Urol Pathol 1995; 3: 107–118.

51. Choi HK, Vasko J, Bengtsson E, Jarkrans T, Malmstrom P-U, Wester K, Busch C. Grading of transtitional cell bladder carcinoma by texture analysis of histological sections. Anal Cell Pathol 1994; 6: 327–343.

52. Choi HK, Jarkrans T, Bengtsson E, Vasko J, Wester K, Malmstrom P-U, Busch C. Image analysis based grading of bladder carcinoma. Comparison of object, textures and graph based methods and their reproducibility. Anal Cell Pathol 1997; 15: 1–18.

53. Barlogie B, Raber MN, Schumann J, Johnson TS, Drewinko B, Swartzendruber DE, et al. Flow cytometry in clinical cancer research. Cancer Res 1983; 43: 3982–3997.

54. Friedlander ML, Hedley D, Taylor I. Clinical and biological significance of aneuploidy in human tumours. J Clin Pathol 1984; 37: 961–974.

55. Loerum OD, Farsund T. Clinical application of flowcytometry; a review. Cytometry 1981; 2: 1–13.

56. Kirkhus B, Clausen OPF, Fjordvang H, Helander K, Iverson O, Reitan JB, Vaage S. Characterization of bladder tumours by multiparameter flow cytometry with special reference to grade II tumours. APMIS 1988; 96: 783–792.

57. Farsund T, Hoestmark JG, Loerum OD. Relation between flow cytometric DNA distribution and pathology in human bladder cancer: a report on 69 cases. Cancer 1984; 54: 1771–1777.

58. Fossa SD, Kaalhus O, Scott-Knudsen O. The clinical and histopathological significance of Feulgen DNA values in transitional cell carcinoma of the human urinary bladder. Eur J Cancer 1977; 13: 1155–1162.

59. Hemstreet GP 3rd, West SS, Weems WL, Echols CK, McFarland S, Lewin J, Lindseth G. Quantitative fluorescence measurements of OA-stained normal and malignant bladder cells. Int J Cancer 1983; 31: 577–585.

60. Tribukait BT, Gustafson H, Esposti P. Ploidy and proliferation in human bladder tumours as measured by flow cytometric DNA analysis and its relations to histopathology and cytology. Cancer 1979; 43: 1742–1751.

61. Neuhaus M, Schmid U, Ackermann D, Zellweger T, Maurer R, Alund G, et al. Polysomies but not Y chromosome losses have prognostic significance in pTa/pT1 urinary bladder cancer. Hum Path 1999; 30(1): 81–86.

62. Junker K, Werner W, Mueller C, Ebert W, Schubert J, Claussen U. Interphase cytogenetic diagnosis of bladder cancer on cells from urine and bladder washing. Int J Oncol 1999; 14(2): 309–313.

63. Sauter G, Gasser TC, Moch H, Richter J, Jiang F, Albrecht R, et al. DNA aberrations in urinary bladder cancer detected by flow cytometry and FISH. Urol Res 1997; 1(Suppl): S37–S43.

64. Zhang FF, Arber DA, Wilson TG, Kawachi MH, Slovak ML. Toward the validation of aneusomy detection by fluorescence in situ hybridization in bladder cancer:comparative analysis with cytology, cytogenetics , and clinical features predicts recurrence and defines clinical testing limitations. Clin Cancer Res 1997; 3: 2317–2328.

65. Helpap B, Köllermann J. Proliferative patterns of normal and dysplastic urothelium and papillary carcinoma. A contribution to the consensus classification of urothelial tumours of the urinary bladder. Hum Pathol (in press).

66. Vasko J, Malmström P-U, Taube A, Wester K, Busch C. Toward an objective method of mitotic figure counting and its prognostic significance in bladder cancer. J Urol Pathol 1995; 3: 315–326.

67. Wester K, Andersson A-C, Ranefall P, Bengtsson E, Malmstrom P-U, Busch C. Cultured human fibroblasts in agarose gel as a multifunctional control for immunohistochemistry. Standardization of Ki67 (MIB1) assessment in routinely processed tissues. J Pathol (in press).

68. Tsutsumi M, Sugano K, Yamaguchi K, Kakizoe T, Akaza H. Correlation of allelic loss of the p53 gene and tumor grade, stage, and malignant progression in bladder cancer. Int J Urol 1997; 4: 74–78.

69. Cordon-Cardo C, Zhang Z-F, Dalbagni G, Drobnjak M, Charytonowicz E, Hu S-X, et al. Cooperative effects of p53 and pRb alterations in primary superficial bladder tumors. Cancer Res 1997; 57: 1217–1221.

70. Hermann G, Horn T, Steven K. The influence on the level of lamina propria invasion and the prevalence of p53 nuclear accumulation on survival in Stage I bladder cancer. J Urol 1998; 159: 91–94.

71. Lianes P, Orlow I, Zhang Z-F, Oliva MR, Reuter VE, Cordon-Cardo C. Altered patterns of MDM2 and TP53 expression in human bladder cancer. J Natl Cancer Inst 1994; 86(17): 1325–1330.

72. King ED, Matteson J, Jacobs SC, Kyprianou N. Incidence of apoptosis, cell proliferation and bcl-2 expression in transitional cell carcinoma of the bladder: association with tumor progression. J Urol 1996; 155: 316–320.

73. Esrig D, Elmajian D, Freeman JA, Stein JP, Chen S-C, Nichols PW, et al. Accumulation of nuclear p53 and tumor progression in bladder cancer. N Engl J Med 1994; 331: 1259.

74. Malmström P-U, Wester K, Vasko J, Busch C. Expression of proliferative cell nuclear antigen (PCNA) in urinary bladder carcinoma. Evaluation of antigen retrieval methods. APMIS 1992; 100: 988–992.

75. Cote RJ, Esrig D, Groshen S, Jones PA, Skinner DG. p53 and treatment of bladder cancer. Nature 1997; 385: 123–124.

76. Fujimoto K, Yamada Y, Okajima E, Kakizoe T, Sasaki H, Sugimura T, Terada M. Frequent association of p53 gene mutation in invasive bladder cancer. Cancer Res 1992; 52: 1393–1398.

77. Uchida T, Wada C, Ishida H, Wang C, Egawa S,Yokoyama E, et al. p53 mutations and prognosis in bladder tumors. J Urol 1995; 153: 1097–1104.

78. Spruck CH, Ohneseit PF, Gonzalez-Zulueta M, Esrig D, Miyao N, Tsai YC, et al. Two molecular pathways to transitional cell carcinoma of the bladder. Cancer Res 1994; 54: 784–788.

79. Michieli P, Chedid M, Lin D, Pierce JH, Mercer WE, Givol D. Induction of WAF1/CIP1 by a p53-independent pathway. Cancer Res 1994; 54: 3391.

80. Bond JA, Blaydes JP, Rowson J, Haughton MF, Smith JR, Wynford-Thomas D, Wyllie FS. Mutant p53 rescues human diploid cells from senescence without inhibiting the induction of SDI1/WAF1. Cancer Res 1995; 55: 2404.

81. Parker SB, Eichele G, Zhang P, Rawls A, Sands AT, Bradley A, et al. p53-independent expression of p21 Cip1 in muscle and other terminally differentiating cells. Science 1995; 267: 1024.

82. Stein JP, Ginsberg DA, Grossfeld GD, Esrig D, Freeman JA, Dickenson MG, et al. The effect of p21 expression on tumor progression in p53 altered bladder cancer. J Urol 1996; 155(Part 2): 628A, abstract 1270.

83. Cordon-Cardo C, Wartinger D, Petrylak D, Dalbagni G, Fair WR, Fuks Z, Reuter VE. Altered expression of the retinoblastoma gene product: prognostic indicator in bladder cancer. J Natl Cancer Inst 1992; 84: 1251–1256.

84. Logothetis CJ, Xu HJ, Ro JY, Hu SX, Sahin A, Ordonez N, Benedict WF. Altered expression of retinoblastoma protein and known prognostic variables in locally advanced bladder cancer. J Natl Cancer Inst 1992; 84: 1256–1261.

85. Cote RJ, Dunn MD, Chatterjee SJ, Stein S-R, et al. Elevated and absent pRb expression is associated with bladder cancer progression and has cooperative effects with p53. Cancer Res 1998; 58: 1090–1094.

86. Cote RJ, Chatterjee J. Molecular determinants of outcome in bladder cancer. Cancer J 1999; 5(1): 2–15.

87. Cordon-Cardo C. Mutation of cell cycle regulators. Biological and clinical implications of human neoplasia. Am J Pathol 1995; 147: 545.

88. Stein JP, Grossfeld GD, Ginsberg DA, Esrig D, Freeman JA, Figueroa AJ, et al. Prognostic markers in bladder cancer: a contemporary review of the literature. J Urol 1998; 160: 645–659.

89. Bochner BH, Cote RJ, Weidner N, Groshen S, Chen S-C, Skinner DG, Nichols PW. Angiogenesis in bladder cancer: relationship between microvessel density and tumor prognosis. J Natl Cancer Inst 1995; 87(21): 1603–1612.

90. Neal DE, Sharples L, Smith K, Fennel J, Reg R, Hall MS, Harris AL. The epidermal growth factor receptor in the prognosis of bladder cancer. Cancer 1990; 65: 1619–1625.

91. Messing EM. Clinical implications and the expression of the epidermal growth factor receptors in human transitional cell carcinoma. Cancer Res 1990; 50: 2530–2534.

92. Wood DP, Fair WR, Chatanti RSK. Evaluation of epidermal growth factor receptor DNA amplification and mRNA expression in bladder cancer. J Urol 1992; 147: 274–277.

93. Nguyen PL, Swanson PE, Jaszcz W, Aeppli DM, Zhang G, Singleton TP, et al. Expression of epidermal growth factor receptor in invasive transitional cell carcinoma of the urinary bladder. A multivariate survival analysis. Am J Clin Pathol 1994; 101: 166–176.

94. Marshall VF. The relation of the preoperative estimate to the pathologic demonstration of the extent of vesical neoplasm. J Urol 1952; 68: 714–723.

95. UICC International Union Against Cancer. In: *TNM Classification of Malignant Tumours* 4th ed. (Hermanek P, Sobin LH, eds.). Springer-Verlag, Berlin, 1998, pp. 135–137.

96. AJCC. Cancer Staging Manual, Fifth Ed. Lippincott-Raven, Philadelphia, New York, 1997.

97. Pearse HD, Reed RR, Hodges CV. Radical cystectomy for bladder cancer. J Urol 1978; 119: 216–218.

98. Blandy JP, England HR, Evans JW, Hope-Stone HF, Mair GMN, Mantell Beth Shearon, MD, et al. T3 bladder cancer—the case for salvage cystectomy. Br J Urol 1980; 52: 506–510.

99. Hall RR, Prout GR. Staging of bladder cancer. Is tumor, node, metastases system adequate? Semin Oncol 1990; 17: 517–23.

100. Holmäng S, Hedelin H, Anderström C, Johansson SL. The relationship among multiple recurrences, progression and prognosis of patients with stages TA and T1 transitional cell cancer of the bladder followed for at least 20 years. J Urol 1995; 153: 1823–1827.

101. Heney NM, Ahmed S, Flanagan MJ, Frable W, Corder MP, Hafermann MD, Hawkins IR, for National Bladder Cancer Collaborative Group A. Superficial bladder cancer: progression and recurrence. J Urol 1983; 130: 1083–1086.

102. Melicow MM, Hollowell, Wisecarver J. Intra-urothelial cancer: carcinoma in situ, Bowen's disease of the urinary system: discussion of thirty cases. J Urol 1952; 68: 763–772.

103. Schellhammer PF, Bean MA, Whitmore Jr WF. Prostatic involvement by transitional cell carcinoma: pathogenesis, patterns and prognosis. J Urol 1977; 118: 399–403.

104. Wood DP Jr, Montie JE, Pontes JE, Vanderbrug Medendorp S, Levin HS. Transitional cell carcinoma of the prostate in cystoprostatectomy specimens removed fro bladder cancer. J Urol 1989; 141: 346–349.

105. Hardeman SW, Soloway MS. Transitional cell carcinoma of the prostate: diagnosis, stageing and management. World J Urol 1988; 6: 170–174.

106. Esrig D, Freeman JA, Elmajian DA, Stein JP, Chen S-C, Groshen S, et al. Transitional cell carcinoma involving the prostate with a proposed staging classification for stromal invasion. J Urol 1996; 156: 1071–1076.

107. Pagano F, Bassi P, Ferrante GLD, Piazza N, Abatangelo G, Pappagallo GL, Garbeglio A. Is stage pT4a (D1) reliable in assessing transitional cell carcinoma involvement of the prostate in patients with concurrent bladder cancer? A necessary distinction for contiguous or noncontiguous involvement. J Urol 1996; 155: 244–247.

108. Dixon JS, Gosling JA. Histology and fine structure of the muscularis mucosae of the human urinary bladder. J Anat 1983; 136: 265–271.

109. Ro JY, Ayala AG, El-Naggar A. Muscularis mucosa of urinary bladder-importance for staging and treatment. Am J Surg Pathol 1987; 11(9): 668–673.

110. Keep TC, Piehl M, Miller A, Oyasu R. Invasive carcinomas of the urinary bladder-evaluation of tunica muscularis mucosae involvement. AJCP 1988; 9: 575–579.

111. Younes M, Sussman J, True LD. The usefulness of the level of the muscularis mucosae in the staging of invasive transitional cell carcinoma of the urinary bladder. Cancer 1990; 66: 543–548.

112. Hasui Y, Osada Y, Kitada S, Nishi S. Significance of invasion to the muscularis mucosae on the progression of superficial bladder cancer. Urology 1994; 43: 782–786.

113. Angulo JC, Lopez JI, Grignon DJ, Sanchez-Chapado M. Muscularis mucosa differentiates two populations with different prognosis in stage T1 bladder cancer. Urology 1995; 45: 47–53.

114. Holmang S, Hedelin H, Anderstrom C, Holmberg E, Johansson SL. The importance of the depth of invasion in stage T1 bladder carcinoma: a prospective cohort study. J Urol 1997; 157: 800–804.

115. Smits G, Schaafma E, Kiemeney L, Christen C, Debruyne F, Witjes JA. Microstaging of pT1 transitional cell carcinoma of the bladder. Identification of subgroups with distinct risks of progression. Urology 1998; 52: 1009–1015.

116. Platz CE, Cohen MB, Jones MP, Olson DB, Lynch CF. Is microstaging of early invasive cancer of the urinary bladder possible or useful? Mod Pathol 1996; 9: 1035–1039.

117. Larsen MP, Steinberg GD, Brendler CB, Epstein JI. Use of Ulex europaeus agglutinin I (UEAI) to distinguish vascular and pseudovascular invasion in transitional cell carcinoma. Mod Pathol 1990; 3: 83–88.

118. Ramani P, Birch BRP, Harland SJ, Parkinson MC. Evaluation of endothelial markers in detecting blood and lymphatic channel invasion in pT1 transitional carcinoma of the bladder. Histopathology 1991; 19: 551–554.

8

Intravesical Chemotherapy in the Treatment of Superficial Bladder Cancer

Vincent G. Bird, MD, Mark S. Soloway, MD, and Per-Uno Malmström, MD, PHD

CONTENTS

INTRODUCTION
ROLE OF TRANSURETHRAL RESECTION AND INTRAVESICAL
    CHEMOTHERAPY IN THE TREATMENT OF SUPERFICIAL
    BLADDER CANCER
INTRAVESICAL CHEMOTHERAPEUTIC AGENTS
EFFICACY OF INTRAVESICAL CHEMOTHERAPEUTIC AGENTS
THE FUTURE OF INTRAVESICAL CHEMOTHERAPY
SUMMARY
REFERENCES

INTRODUCTION

Bladder cancer has proved to be a great challenge to urologists. This is so in that bladder cancer is a paradigm of malignancy. Some tumors are relatively benign, while others are highly aggressive, making early diagnosis and appropriate treatment critical. Transurethral resection is usually the primary mode of therapy for both diagnosis and treatment. Persistent high grade tumor confined to the urothelium may require further treatment to prevent recurrence or possible progression. Further treatment is usually in the form of intravesical chemotherapy or immunotherapy. This chapter concentrates on the role of intravesical chemotherapy. Its relation to transurethral resection will be discussed. Its use in relation to immunotherapy will also be discussed, but the various

From: *Current Clinical Urology: Bladder Cancer: Current Diagnosis and Treatment*
Edited by: M. J. Droller © Humana Press Inc., Totowa, NJ

forms of immunotherapy will be the subject of another chapter. After review of their characteristics, mechanisms of action, toxicities, and indications for use, the intravesical chemotherapeutic agents will be reviewed in their relation to one another and to immunotherapy. Finally the future directions of intravesical chemotherapy will be discussed.

THE ROLE OF TRANSURETHRAL RESECTION AND INTRAVESICAL CHEMOTHERAPY IN THE TREATMENT OF SUPERFICIAL BLADDER CANCER

Characteristics of Bladder Cancer

Approximately 90% of bladder tumors are of the transitional cell type. Bladder cancer tends to arise at different times and sites in the urothelium. This phenomenon is known as polychronotopicity. Because of this observation bladder cancer has been referred to as a "field change disease," and as such, the entire urothelium is at risk for malignant transformation. Following an initial tumor resection subsequent neoplasms are common. This may be due to neoplastic cells that remained after previous treatment (true recurrence), or to new areas of dysplastic urothelium undergoing malignant transformation (new occurrence). Many molecular studies have been performed, and to date examples of uniclonal and multiclonal origins have been reported (1,2). In summary, it is difficult to know whether a recurrence is due to a uniclonal etiology (true recurrence), polyclonal etiology (field change), or from inadequate resection (3–5).

Transitional cell bladder tumors can generally be divided into two groups; superficial tumors (Tis, Ta and T1), and muscle invasive tumors (T2+). Approximately 60% of all newly diagnosed bladder tumors are well or moderately differentiated superficial papillary transitional cell carcinomas (confined to the mucosa or invading the lamina propria) (6). The majority of these patients will develop a subsequent tumor following initial endoscopic resection (3,7–10). Most "recurrences" appear to be of a well or moderately differentiated type, but as many as 16–25% of such recurrences are high grade (3,8). These new tumors arise from new areas of dysplastic urothelium, from inadequate resection (11), or from implanted tumor cells (12,13). The other 40–45% of bladder tumors are high grade upon presentation, with more than half of these invading the muscularis propria (6). It is important to emphasize that many high grade tumors have a high chance of recurring and progressing to invasive disease (6,14–16). Carcinoma in situ (Tis) is a flat high grade neoplasm confined to the epithelium. This lesion is quite significant in that approximately one half of patients with untreated carcinoma *in situ* develop invasive bladder cancer within 5 yr *(17)*. Indeed these findings illustrate the heterogenous and persistent nature of transitional cell carcinoma. The concept of field change, and the possibility that tumor cells may be left behind, whether it be from implantation or incomplete resection, have lead many urologists to believe that transurethral resection, though effective, will not alone be sufficient treatment for all cases of superficial transitional cell carcinoma. It is in this way that intravesical chemotherapy becomes useful treatment for superficial transitional cell carcinoma. Intravesical chemotherapy is used after transurethral resection to destroy viable tumor cells that may have been left in the bladder, and to possibly destroy nonvisible foci of neoplasia *(18)*. Thus, surgical resection and medical therapy together allow for more intensive treatment.

The Role of Transurethral Resection

Simply stated, transurethral resection is the removal of all obvious tumors. Transurethral resection actually serves a dual purpose; it is both diagnostic and therapeutic.

Transurethral resection is usually adequate therapy for most localized superficial tumors. The incidence of a persistent or inadequately treated localized tumor is low *(19)*. Ablation of bladder tumor may range from simple fulguration of very small low grade appearing tumors to deep resection of an invasive bladder tumor, so that proper histologic evaluation may be performed.

Transurethral resection begins with panendoscopy, which includes visualization of the entire urethra, the prostate, and the entire bladder mucosa *(19)*. A wide-angle lens usually ensures that the survey of the bladder is complete, and that any tumors proximal to the bladder neck are not missed. The number, size, and position relative to bladder landmarks of all bladder tumors should be carefully noted. The papillary or sessile nature of the tumor should be noted and preferably documented. Flat erythematous velvety areas or thickened white areas should be carefully noted as they may represent carcinoma *in situ* or squamous metaplasia. After the bladder, prostate, and urethra have been completely assessed, a logical plan of resection should be formulated, and transurethral resection performed.

Many different types of resectoscopes, sheaths, and accessory equipment are available for transurethral resection of bladder tumors. What is most important is that the resectionist is comfortable and familiar with the equipment. However, a few recommendations can be made. The use of a continuous flow resectoscope sheath may prove useful in that it can maintain constant bladder volume, which allows for safe resection of tumors that are associated with mobile portions of the bladder wall. It is essential that the resectionist is in complete control and has an appreciation of the thickness of the bladder. It is preferable to resect a tumor in a piecemeal fashion so that there will not be difficulty in removing the tumor, as can sometimes happen when a large tumor is resected at its base. It is also necessary to include muscle in the resection of any tumor that appears high grade and possibly invades the lamina propria. After the deep cut has been made muscle fibers should be seen. The appearance of necrotic tissue at this level suggests an invasive bladder tumor *(19)*. If carcinoma *in situ* or high grade bladder tumor is suspected, a biopsy of the prostatic urethra should be considered, as one study demonstrated that 31% of cystectomy specimens with invasive bladder tumor had transitional cell carcinoma of the prostatic urethra *(20)*. This may also be important if cystectomy is planned with the possibility of an orthotopic neobladder as a form of urinary tract reconstruction *(19)*. Biopsy of the prostatic urethra is best accomplished by performing superficial resection at the five or seven o'clock position near the verumontanum *(21)*.

Obese patients may at times be very challenging in terms of resection. In such cases use of long instruments, perineal urethrostomy, or the application of suprapubic pressure by an assistant may be helpful *(19)*.

The **laser** has also been used to ablate bladder tumors. The neodymium:YAG laser has been most commonly used *(22)*. However, the depth of penetration has been shown to be variable *(23)*. One advantage of the laser is that it allows for transmural coagulation without perforation and extravasation. There are also reports of use of the argon laser, mostly with very small tumors *(24)*. The KTP laser *(25)*, and the holmium:YAG laser *(26)* have also been used. Carbon dioxide lasers are not considered suitable for bladder tumor resection, due to the lack of flexible fibers and the need for an air environment to prevent the rapid absorption of energy by water *(19)*. Flexible fibers can usually be inserted through standard cystoscopes, or through cystoscopic equipment appropriately modified for use with laser fibers *(19,27)*. Tumors larger than 2–2.5 cm are difficult to treat with laser energy alone. Lasers are usually reserved for patients with recurrent low grade tumors, as tissue needed for histological evaluation is not usually available *(19)*. It is believed that the lack of biopsy tissue in such circumstances does not compromise patient care, as these lesions are usually low grade Ta lesions *(19)*. A prospective randomized study revealed no difference in recurrence rate between patients treated with either laser energy or electrocautery *(28)*. Other studies suggest a lower rate of local recurrence for laser treated tumors when compared to tumors treated with electrocautery *(23)*. Excellent hemostasis and decreased postoperative voiding symptoms have also been associated with laser treatment. However, bowel perforation remains a serious potential complication in patients treated with a laser *(19,29)*.

A complete evaluation of a patient with bladder cancer includes a bimanual exam in an attempt to assess whether the tumor is palpable and whether there is possible fixation to adjacent structures *(19)*. This exam includes palpation of the prostate for other pathology, e.g., adenocarcinoma.

Role of Intravesical Chemotherapy

As previously stated, a complete preoperative assessment, resection of gross bladder tumor, and staging are the beginning of this process. Analysis of this data will determine if further treatment is needed, possibly in the form of intravesical chemotherapy. When considering the use of intravesical chemotherapy, an understanding of the natural history of the disease, the pharmacology of the chemotherapeutic agents to be used, and the efficacy of the agent are important. This information must be further integrated with an understanding of the patients' age, medical status, and ability to comply with the intended regimen *(30)*.

The fundamental purpose of treatment of superficial bladder cancer with intravesical therapy is threefold: 1) eradicate existing disease; 2) prevention of recurrence; and 3) prevention of tumor progression *(30)*. Prevention of recurrence is an important goal. Prevention of progression may reduce the need for radical cystectomy, thus maintaining and prolonging the patient's quality of life *(31)*. Surgical resection alone is adequate therapy for many patients with superficial bladder cancer. In data compiled from twenty-one prospective randomized trials, Lamm noted that 49% of patients treated with transurethral resection alone remained free of recurrence *(32)*. Thus, it is for those patients who remain at high risk of recurrence, for whom some type of intravesical therapy is reserved, whether it be in the form of intravesical chemotherapy or immunotherapy.

PHARMACOLOGY OF INTRAVESICAL CHEMOTHERAPY

The development of the treatment with intravesical chemotherapeutic agents has been empirical. Simply stated, the dose of an agent was increased if it was found to be effective and tolerable. Dosage has also been guided by the daily parenteral dose that is usually given. Many studies involving these agents do not have standardized regimens, making comparison difficult. However, in recent years, some basic studies have shed light on the nature of these agents *(30,33–39)*.

Penetration of an agent through bladder tissue involves passage through the urothelium and the underlying tissue *(30)*. The urothelium (0–200 μ and 5–10 cell layers thick) does not have capillaries, and rests on the basement membrane *(30,37)*. The cells of the urothelium are bound by

Urothelium: (0–200 μ) **Cdepth = Cu- (Cu-C200/200)(depth)**

Deep tissues: (200–4000+ μ) **Cdepth = (C200- Cb)** e$^{(-0.693/w-\frac{1}{2})(depth-200)}$ **+ Cb**

Fig. 1. Equations describing drug concentration-depth profiles in the bladder wall. Cu is the concentration of drug in the bladder cavity, C200 is the concentration at the interface between the urothelium and the deep tisues, Cb is the concentration in the blood, and w-½ is the half width-the thickness of tissue over which the drug concentration declines by 50% (Dedrick et al., 1982; Flessner et al., 1985; Badalament et al., 1997).

tight junctions, and are covered by a mucopolysaccharide layer. The calculation of diffusion across the urothelium involves the use of Fick's first law. In this calculation the urothelium is considered to be a single homogeneous diffusion barrier, and the decline in concentration of a drug across the urothelium correlates in a linear fashion with depth. The drop off in concentration of the different intravesical chemotherapeutic agents can be calculated using the equation shown here (Fig. 1). It has also been speculated that neoplastic cells, being in a dedifferentiated state and probably having impaired production of membrane plaques, tight junctions, and surface mucopolysaccharide, are likely to be more permeable to intravesical chemotherapeutic agents than normal urothelium. It is likely that bladder inflammation and transurethral resection further augment this process. In vivo studies have shown a higher serum concentration of instilled drugs when introduced into the inflamed bladder compared to intact bladder epithelium *(40)*. In one study the highest plasma concentration of Mitomycin C occurred when the agent was administered during the first three days following transurethral resection (50 ng/mL, compared to less than 1ng/mL during later treatments) *(37)*. The lamina propria is approximately 200–1000 μ thick. The underlying muscularis propria ranges from 1000–10,000 μ in thickness. These two layers are well vascularized, which allow for rapid penetration of an agent into the blood. The decline of an agent across these layers has been demonstrated by Dedrick et al. *(41)* and Flessner et al. *(42)* to occur more in a semilogarithmic fashion. In summation, this means that as the capillary circulation increases with depth, the tissue concentration of the agent levels off until it is equal to the serum concentration *(30)*. A basic understanding of these pharmacokinetic principles explains why an intravesical agent will work best for noninvasive tumors (Ta and Tis). In a similar fashion systemic chemotherapy may be successful in treating invasive disease, but not affect superficial tumors, as the low systemic concentration further decreases as it passes through the lamina propria and urothelium where it eventually comes in contact with urine, where it is significantly diluted again *(30)*.

CHEMICAL PROPERTIES OF INTRAVESICAL CHEMOTHERAPEUTIC AGENTS

Diffusion of an intravesical chemotherapeutic agent will also depend on the agent's molecular weight and lipid solubility. For example, thiotepa has a low molecular weight and is lipophilic, therefore absorption is rapid and extensive. The tissue concentration of thiotepa, however, is offset by its high capillary permeability, thus aiding its removal from the surrounding tissue. On the other hand, mitomycin C and doxorubicin have a higher molecular weight and are relatively hydrophobic, resulting in slower diffusion and less absorption. Their lower capillary permeability, however, will allow for a lower decline of tissue concentration in bladder tissue. In order to compare these agents, they have been assigned a half width (w-1/2), the tissue depth over which the drug concentration declines by 50%. The half width for thiotepa is estimated at 30 µ *(30)*. The half width for mitomycin C and doxorubicin is approximately 500 µ *(39, 43)*. As such, mitomycin C and doxorubicin are better agents for deeper tumors than thiotepa, and, in addition, have less systemic absorption.

Studies on the relationship between osmolality and cytotoxicity suggest that intravesical agents be dissolved in sterile water, rather than saline. In a study performed by Groos *(44)*, urine from patients with bladder cancer before treatment had osmolalities in the range of 187–852 mOsm/kg, and these had decreased by an average of 135 mOsm/kg at the completion of intravesical chemotherapy. Clinical preparations of drugs used for intravesical chemotherapy had osmotic strengths ranging from 65–1038 mOsm/kg. The antitumor activities of the most commonly used drugs (doxorubicin, mitomycin C, thiotepa, epodyl, cis-platin, and epirubicin) were measured with a human bladder cancer cell line by inhibition of colony forming ability. Reducing osmotic strength from 590–125 mOsm/kg significantly increased the in vitro cytotoxicities of thiotepa, mitomycin C, cis-platin, and epirubicin, but not doxorubicin and epodyl. Thus the use of an instillate at the lowest achievable osmotic strength appears to be optimal for the intravesical administration of many chemotherapeutic drugs.

URINE FACTORS

The urine and its composition and characteristics, along with the concentration of the chemotherapeutic agent, are also factors that must be considered. Dalton et al. *(37)* performed many pharmacokinetic studies to explore these issues. The equation describing urine pharmacokinetics, (Fig. 2) demonstrates which factors are important.

Other studies involving computer simulations have demonstrated that the order of importance of different factors is (from most to least): dose, residual urine volume, urine production, urine pH, volume of instillate,

$$C_u = (Dose)(e^{-(ka+kd)t})/V_u$$

Fig. 2. Equation describing urine pharmacokinetics. C_u is the urine concentration, Dose is the dose of the intravesical agent, $V_u = V_0 + (k_0)(t) + V_{res}$, V_u is urine volume at time t, V_0 is the initial volume of instillate, k_0 is the urine production rate constant, V_{res} is the volume of the residual urine in the bladder at the time of instillation, k_a is the apparent absorption rate constant from the bladder (across the bladder epithelium and muscular layers into the capillaries), and k_d is the apparent rate constant of degradation, metabolism, and/or binding to macromolecules (Dalton et al., 1991; Badalament et al, 1997).

Table 1
Pharmacokinetic Variables of Intravesical Mitomycin C[a]

Variable	Estimated improvement factor
Standard regimen	1.0
(Dose = 20 mg, dose vol = 20 mL	
Urine production = 1.5 mL/min	
PH = 5, dwell time = 2 h)	
Drug dose (20–40 mg/20 mL)	2.36
Residual urine volume (32-0 mL/min)	1.93
Urine production (1.5–0.6 mL/min)	1.39
Urine pH (5–7)	1.62
Dosing volume (20–40 mL)	0.77
Dwell time (2–4 h)	1.02

[a]Badalament et al., 1997 *(30)*.

and dwell time *(38)*. Wientjes and Badalament hypothesized that under optimal conditions the efficacy of mitomycin C could be improved by 20%, and that the average recurrence free rate might be increased from 56–76% (Table 1) *(30,38)*.

Analysis of the equation for urine pharmacokinetics and the table showing changes in the pharmacologic variables for intravesical mitomycin C will lead to basic conclusions and recommendations for the use of intravesical chemotherapeutic agents. Dose is of course a major factor. Decreasing the volume of the instillate increases the concentration of the chemotherapeutic agent in the bladder. The relative importance of two variables, drug concentration and period of exposure, in relation to the therapeutic potential of intravesical chemotherapy was examined in an experimental system by Walker *(45)*. A human bladder cancer cell line was exposed to a range of concentrations of four drugs commonly used to treat superficial bladder cancer (doxorubicin, ethoglucid, mitomycin C, and thiotepa) for periods of 30, 60, and 120 min. Cytotoxicity was

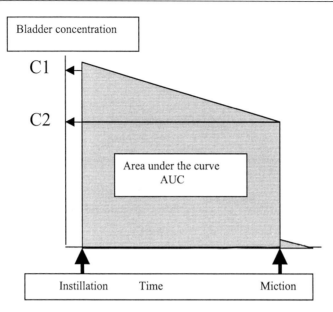

Fig. 3. Variation of bladder concentration during intravesical instillation of anti-cancer drugs. C1 = initial concentration; C2 = final concentration.

proportional to concentration times the period of exposure. These two variables were of equal importance in relation to tumor cell kill, indicating that maximum therapeutic benefit may be obtained by using the highest concentration achievable for as long as the patient can retain the instillate.

Eksborg and coworkers proposed to use the area under a bladder concentration curve (*see* Fig. 3) rather than the amount of instilled drug when optimizing a treatment *(46)*. This is based on the assumption that optimal contact of the drug with the bladder wall is essential. For this reason the drug should be dissolved in the highest possible volume. In this study, clinical tests indicated that diuresis was approximately 50 mL/h if patients restricted fluids 12 h before treatment, and it was then possible to use an instillation volume equal to the bladder capacity minus 50 mL. For a given AUC the amount of drug to be instilled (dose) could be calculated as follows: Dose = AUC (BC−50)/(BC−25). BC is the bladder capacity in mL. The instillation time is one hour. In practical use with adriamycin, this standardized treatment proved to counteract the drastic increase of AUC with decreasing bladder capacity and fixed dosage. A study performed by another group involved the influence of the dose of thiotepa using the AUC concept *(47)*. Each patient received four doses of thiotepa consisting of 30 mg of drug in 30 mL of distilled water, 30 mg/

60 mL, 60 mg/30 mL, and 60 mg/60 mL. Blood and urine were obtained for eight hours following instillation, and thiotepa levels were measured. The AUC (infinity) values (areas under the concentration-time curve, extrapolated to infinity) in plasma were approximately two factors higher at the 60 mg doses. However, the AUC value in the bladder was nearly 70% higher when 60 mg of drug was instilled in 30 mL of distilled water compared with 60 mg in 60 mL. Thus, by decreasing the volume of instillate it was possible to increase the dose rate to the tumor without increasing systemic toxicity. Controversy remains concerning the volume and ultimate concentration of the instillate. A drawback of high volume is poor compliance regarding retention of the drug in the bladder.

Urine pH can have variable effects depending on the agent. Studies have been performed concerning the influence of pH on the sensitivity of a TCC cell line to intravesical chemotherapeutic agents. The colony forming ability of the cell line was lowest at a pH of 5.5 for thiotepa and at a pH of 7.0 for both doxorubicin and mitomycin (48). Jauhainen et al. (49) also investigated the effect of pH on cytostatic activity in vitro and found no change within the limits of physiologic variations for doxorubicin. In this same study the antitumor effect of mitomycin C was impeded at pH less than 6.0 for incubation times over two h. Mitomycin C has also been found to be more rapidly degraded in an acidic environment (50). These findings have lead some urologists to recommend the use of buffer solutions or urinary alkalization when using this drug.

The dwell time of intravesical chemotherapeutic agents has received little attention. In a randomized study (51), bladder cancer patients were treated with intravesical mitomycin C using either a 30 or 60 min dwell time. Recurrence was significantly lower in the 60 min treatment group. In vitro studies done with human tissue show that longer exposure time of an agent increases its efficacy, but its clinical significance is not known (30). As time passes degradation of the agent and ongoing urine production mitigate the advantage of a longer dwell time. Badalament et al. have given some basic recommendations for optimizing the efficacy of intravesical chemotherapeutic agents. These suggestions are listed in Table 2.

Study of the pharmacologic properties and different modes of administration continues, in efforts to find further means of enhancing the efficacy of these agents. There are ongoing trials involving pharmacologically optimized regimens of mitomycin C (38). The interaction of mitomycin C with tumor cells is also being examined, in order to ascertain the status of intracellular reductive enzymes that metabolize mitomycin C to its active form. Special attention is being paid in particular to the enzymes DT diaphorase and NADPH cytochrome P-45 reductase,

Table 2
Recommendations for Optimizing
Efficacy of Intravesical Chemotherapeutic Agents[a]

1. Reserve thiotepa for tumors that are confined to the mucosa of the bladder. It has a small molecular weight, is lipophilic, and has high capillary permeability. Based on pharmacological principles, T1 tumors are best treated with mitomycin C or doxorubicin. From a pharmacological standpoint, there appears to be little difference between mitomycin C and doxorubicin *(43)*.
2. Avoid thiotepa immediately after transurethral resection. Absorption may be increased due to disrupted urothelium and the risk of myelosuppression may be increased.
3. Use the highest dose of intravesical agent with the least amount of diluent. This will facilitate diffusion across the urothelium.
4. Dehydrate patients prior to intravesical therapy; instruct them to take any diuretics later in the day.
5. After catheteterizing a patient for intravesical chemotherapy, but prior to administration of the agent, either have him/her walk around with the catheter in or use a bladder ultrasound machine to document complete drainage of the bladder.
6. Have the patient hold the intravesical therapy in his bladder as long as possible. If the patient is well dehydrated this may be more feasible. Consider anticholinergic administration if the patient is experiencing irritative symptoms in the absence of infection.
7. When using mitomycin C, urinary alkalization will decrease degradation of the drug. Administration of 1300 mg of sodium bicarbonate the evening before and the morning of treatment might be useful. After the patient is catheterized, if the urine pH is still acidic by dipstick testing, administer another 1300 mg of sodium bicarbonate and wait 30–60 min.

[a]Badalament et al., 1997 *(30)*.

cellular enzymes that may be lost due to tumor dedifferentiation *(30)*. Schmittgen et al. noted an interpatient variability of 60 times and 30 times in mitomycin C concentrations needed for 50% and 90% inhibition of tumor cells *(35)*, lending evidence that there may be unknown tumor factors at least partially accounting for such variability. Clinical studies have also corroborated Schmittgen's observations that mitomycin C activity is lower against higher grade and stage tumor cells, as well as rapidly growing tumors *(35,52)*. The use of additional agents and modalities to enhance intravesical chemotherapy will be discussed later in this chapter.

OTHER CONSIDERATIONS

There are also important considerations for the administration of intravesical chemotherapy regarding catheterization. When the bladder

Table 3
Intravesical Agents Used to Treat Bladder Cancer [a]

Compound	Year
Silver nitrate	1903
Trichloroacetic acid	1919
Podophyllin	1948
Thiotepa	1961
Actinomycin C	1965
5-Flourouracil	1965
Mannitol myleran	1966
Methotrexate	1966
Mitomycin C	1967
Etoglucid (Epodyl)	1973
Adriamycin	1977
Bleomycin	1977
Epipodophyllotoxin (VM-26)	1978

[a]Connolly, 1981 (55).

has been emptied with a catheter, the chemotherapeutic agent is instilled with the same catheter. It is imperative to avoid traumatic catheterization, evidenced by hematuria. Systemic absorption may result if the urothelium is damaged in this manner, just as systemic absorption may occur in the presence of cystitis or when intravesical chemotherapy is given immediately after transurethral resection. Anatomic abnormalities, such as a urethral stricture, must be handled with care so that traumatic catheterization does not result. It is recommended that instillation be postponed for one week in cases of trauma or infection (53).

INTRAVESICAL CHEMOTHERAPEUTIC AGENTS

History

The use of intravesical chemotherapy began in the early 1900s (54). Some agents were relatively ineffective, and others were too toxic. Many compounds have been used as intravesical therapy for superficial bladder cancer. As stated by Connolly, "almost any promising chemotherapeutic or antitumor agent, providing it is not too toxic, will be used to treat superficial bladder cancer" (55). Table 3 chronologically lists those agents that have or had been commonly used.

Epirubicin, and more recently AD 32, an anthracycline antibiotic similar to doxorubicin, have been introduced recently. The search for new agents continues, as does study on the determination of the best treatment schedule. The major agents still being used today are discussed here. The following section pertains to the properties, mechanisms of action, specifics of delivery of each agent, and their incidence of side effects, both general and specific. It has been reported that there is a low incidence of developing a secondary hematologic malignancy after intravesical chemotherapy with thiotepa or mitomycin *(56)*. The efficacy of these agents individually, and in relation to one another, is discussed afterward.

Indications for Use
of Intravesical Chemotherapeutic Agents

Obviously, not all patients with superficial bladder cancer require intravesical therapy. Patients who have solitary tumors which pathological examination reveals to be low grade and limited to the mucosa are at low risk for recurrence and progression. In such cases the morbidity and expense of intravesical therapy is not justified *(31)*. When a complete resection has been performed in such patients, and there is no suspicion of residual tumor, these patients can be followed with standard surveillance cystoscopy protocols.

Intravesical therapy is indicated for patients who are at high risk for a new occurrence or recurrence. The risk factors for recurrence of newly diagnosed superficial bladder cancer were analyzed in two large randomized British studies *(57)*. In a multivariate analysis the most important factors were tumor multiplicity and the result of cystoscopy performed three months after the initial transurethral resection. Stage did not independently predict recurrence. New tumor markers are being investigated but have not yet been firmly established. Common indications for intravesical therapy include multiple primary tumors, frequent tumor "recurrence", high grade, stage T1, post resection positive urine cytology, and carcinoma *in situ (31,58)*.

Specific Intravesical Chemotherapeutic Agents

TRIETHYLENETHIOPHOSPHORAMIDE (THIOTEPA)

Thiotepa was first used to treat bladder cancer by J.C. Bateman in 1955 *(59)*. Jones and Swinney were among the first to report the use thiotepa as an intravesical agent to treat superficial bladder cancer *(60)*.

Thiotepa is the oldest of the intravesical chemotherapeutic agents still being actively used today. It is usually inexpensive. Thiotepa is classified as an alkylating agent. Its mechanism of action involves the formation of covalent bonds between DNA, RNA, nucleic acids, and protein *(53)*. The end result is the inhibition of nucleic acid synthesis. It is not a cell cycle specific agent. Weaver et al. *(61)* postulated that thiotepa reduces cell adherence with a direct cytotoxic effect.

Thiotepa is usually given in a dose of 30–60 mg. Studies indicate that 30 mg in 30 mL distilled water is as effective as 60 mg in 60 mL distilled water *(53,55,62)*. Typically six weekly instillations are given. Treatment can be continued thereafter for one year with monthly instillations *(53)*.

Determination of the hematological status of the patient is important prior to each instillation of thiotepa. It is considered best not to begin installation of thiotepa until a week after transurethral resection of bladder tumor, although after resection of small tumors this is not as critical. Treatment should be withheld in the presence of evidence of acute cystitis *(55)*.

Thiotepa has a molecular weight of only 189 Daltons, and as such absorption and systemic toxicity can occur. Early reports indicated that about one third of the instilled dose was absorbed after an instillation period of three hours *(60)*, and that 25% of the patients had leukopenia or thrombocytopenia *(63)*. Other studies on larger numbers of patients suggest that myelosuppression is rare, usually mild, and of short duration *(64)*. Martinez-Pineiro et al. *(65)* noted leukopenia and thrombocytopenia in only 3 and 1 of 56 patients, respectively. The authors noted that 8 of 56 patients had drug induced cystitis.

Mitomycin C

Mitomycin C is an antitumor antibiotic and has demonstrated activity against many human neoplasms. Mitomycin antibiotics were first isolated in 1956 from *Streptomyces caespitosus*, as blue violet crystals *(55, 66)*. It has a molecular weight of 329 Daltons, and it is soluble in water and organic solvents *(53,66)*. Mitomycin C has three potentially active functional groups. After its carbamate group is reduced and its methoxy group lost, it functions as a bifunctional or trifunctional alkylating agent *(67,68)*. Mitomycin C can induce interstrand and intrastrand cross links in many types of DNA, dependent on the base composition of the DNA *(69–71)*. It has also been shown to degrade DNA *(71)* and inhibit DNA synthesis, thus making it effective during the late G1 and S phases of the cell cycle *(68)*.

Due to its molecular weight, Mitomycin C is usually minimally absorbed when given intravesically. There is no standard dose, and it may vary from 20–60 mg per instillation *(53)*.

When Mitomycin C is given as an intravesical agent, the most frequent side effects are chemical cystitis and allergic reactions *(53)*. The usual symptoms of chemical cystitis include dysuria, frequency, and pain. The incidence of chemical cystitis in a number of series ranges between 6% and 41% (mean of 15.8%) *(72)*. Thrasher and Crawford summarized the side effects from 11 series, and noted only a 0.7% incidence of leukopenia and thrombocytopenia *(72)*. There is a report of a patient death due to myelosuppression when 80 mg of Mitomycin C had been given intravesically immediately after transurethral resection *(73)*. Allergic reactions have mainly been noted as skin symptoms, namely a rash *(53)*. One study indicates that up to 9% of patients receiving intravesical mitomycin C experience cutaneous side effects *(74)*. Thrasher and Crawford corroborated these results, finding an incidence of 9.8% (60 of 613) *(72)*. Skin reactions consisted of vesicular dermatitis of the hands and feet, genital dermatitis, and more widespread eruptions. This skin reaction is considered to be a delayed type hypersensitivity reaction *(74,75)*. A few cases involving skin reaction and mitomycin C probably involve contact dermatitis, but most reactions occur after the second instillation of mitomycin C, more consistent with delayed type hypersensitivity *(53)*. Nonetheless patients are instructed to wash thoroughly after treatment. Most of the common side effects of chemical cystitis disappear after cessation of therapy. Some patients may require topical therapy for these lesions.

One large study noted a 0.5% incidence (3 of 538) of contracted bladder *(72)*. Another study with a smaller patient number and a longer period of instillation noted an incidence of 23% (17 of 75) *(76)*. Asymptomatic bladder calcifications have also been reported *(53,77)*.

DOXORUBICIN (ADRIAMYCIN)

Doxorubicin is classified as an anthracycline antibiotic. It acts as an intercalating agent by binding DNA base pairs, and thereby inhibiting the activity of topoisomerase II *(30,53)*. In one experiment *(78)*, in which murine cancer cell line samples were exposed to free doxorubicin, doxorubicin bound to polymeric beads (preventing doxorubicin from entering the cells), and polymeric beads alone, no difference in the dose dependent kill ratios was seen between the bound and unbound doxorubicin. The beads alone had no cytotoxic effect. From this information the authors postulated that a cytotoxic mechanism of action of doxorubicin, not completely understood, might take place at the cell surface. Even though it is classified as a cell cycle phase nonspecific agent, it is most toxic in the S phase *(30,53)*. Doxorubicin is administered in doses ranging from 30–100 mg. It is normally diluted with normal saline to a concentration within the range of 0.5–2 mg/mL. Administration schedules vary from weekly to every three weeks. Dwell time is usually 1–2 h *(30)*.

Systemic reactions, consisting mainly of mild nausea and vomiting, diarrhea, fever, and rarely hypersensitivity, are uncommon after intravesical doxorubicin instillation *(30,53)*. The molecular weight of doxorubicin, 580 Daltons, makes systemic absorption unlikely and correlates well with this finding. Indeed, in two large series totaling more than 600 patients, the Japanese Urological Research Group reported no systemic side effects *(79)*. Local side effects are more common. The most common is chemical cystitis, occurring in approximately 25% of patients *(80)*. In their review of 399 patients Thrasher and Crawford found a mean incidence of 28.8% *(72)*. Other rare side effects consist of allergic reactions (0.3%), gastrointestinal side effects (1.7%), and fever (0.8%) *(53)*. In one study, in which the highest dose of intravesical doxorubicin had been given, (8 × 100 mg) a 16% (7 of 44) incidence of reduced bladder capacity was reported *(81)*. The Japanese Urological Cancer Research Group reported one patient who had a contracted bladder *(82)*. The side effects of doxorubicin and BCG were compared in one large United States study. Irritative bladder symptoms were seen in 49% and 62% of patients receiving doxorubicin and BCG, respectively *(83)*. In a multi center study conducted by Khanna et al. *(84)*, over 80% of patients receiving either agent had side effects, with approximately 25% of side effects in each group considered severe. The most common side effects were urgency, frequency, dysuria, hematuria, nocturia, and passed debris. A significant percentage of patients receiving BCG also experienced fever and chills.

Epirubicin

Like doxorubicin, epirubicin is an anthracycline antibiotic. It is a derivative of doxorubicin, and its mechanism of action involving its anti-tumor effect is believed to be similar to that of doxorubicin *(30,53,77)*.

Epirubicin is usually administered in a dose of 30–80 mg diluted in saline, to make a concentration of 0.6–1.6 mg/mL. One suggested schedule is daily for 3 d, followed by 4 d rest, and then daily for 3 d. Others have used the more conventional schedule of weekly instillations. The dwell time is 1–2 h *(30)*.

Burk et al. *(85)* reviewed the toxicity of epirubicin in 911 patients. The majority of these patients received 8 weekly instillations of 50 mg. There was no systemic toxicity. Chemical cystitis occurred in 14% of patients. This local toxicity appears to be dose related. Many investigators report a reduced incidence of side effects with a lower dose of the drug *(86)*. In a European Organization for Research and Treatment of Cancer (EORTC) *(87)* study, in which a single instillation of 80 mg of epirubicin was given, chemical cystitis was reported in 6.8% of patients. Whelan et al. *(86)* reported minimal complications in high risk group of patients (multiple recurrent superficial tumors) who had been treated with intravesical epirubicin (8 × 30 mg). Melekos et al. *(88)* reported on 43 patients who were treated with six weekly instillations of 50 mg of epirubicin followed by a 2 yr maintenance schedule. There was a 21% incidence of drug induced cystitis. No hematologic toxicity was reported.

The only significant side effect of epirubicin appears to drug induced cystitis, and it may indeed have a lower incidence when compared to other intravesical agents. A recent randomized study indicated that epirubicin had both higher efficacy and lower toxicity than doxorubicin *(89)*. However, data on this agent is still only now being made available, and due to lack of standardization and properly designed studies it is difficult to conclude whether one intravesical chemotherapeutic agent has less side effects.

ETHOGLUCID (EPODYL)

Ethoglucid is a podophyllin derivative. Its mechanism of action is not well understood, though is believed to act on cellular division in a manner similar to that of alkylating agents *(30)*.

When administered, 100 mL of 1% solution is instilled weekly, usually for 4–12 wk. This can be followed with monthly maintenance therapy *(30)*.

Ethoglucid has a molecular weight of 262 Daltons, and as such systemic toxicity is rare. In fact, during its early use no significant side effects were reported *(90)*. However, in later studies local and systemic side effects were reported. Robinson et al. *(91)* reported bone marrow depression in two patients. Local toxicity usually manifests itself as chemical cystitis. In their review Badalament and Farah report a frequency of cystitis ranging from 3–56%. Robinson et al. *(91)* reported drug induced cystitis in 59% of patients. These authors also reported a small capacity bladder in 10 patients (two of whom required cystectomy). There appears to be conflicting data regarding the toxicity of ethoglucid, with reports of low incidence of both local and systemic toxicity, to higher incidence of such effects at times necessitating discontinuation of treatment *(92,93)*.

OTHER AGENTS

There are other intravesical chemotherapeutic agents that have been used, though less routinely. **Intravesical cis-platin** was tested in an EORTC randomized trial *(94)*. It was compared to thiotepa and doxorubicin. Seven of the sixty eight patients receiving cis-platin experienced an anaphylactic reaction with hypotension, resulting in termination of this treatment arm. Another study *(95)* involved the use of 50–150 mg of intravesical cis-platin in high risk superficial bladder cancer patients. Only 3 of 24 patients (13%) achieved complete remission. One patient experienced an anaphylactic reaction.

Mitoxantrone is effective against human cancer cells. It was used in 22 patients with recurrent tumors who had failed previous intravesical chemotherapy *(96)*. 5–10.5 mg were given in 6 weekly instillations. The most common side effect was chemical cystitis, which appeared to be more common when a higher dosage was used. A contracted bladder was reported in one patient. A 50% CR rate have been found in a ablative study but in another controlled study the recurrence rate was similar to an untreated controlgroup *(97,98)*.

Cytosine arabinoside, an agent that functions as an antimetabolite, has been used in combination with both mitomycin and doxorubicin *(99,100)*. The agent appeared to have a beneficial effect. The limited use of this agent and other recently tested agents limit what is known concerning side effects caused by them.

EFFICACY OF INTRAVESICAL CHEMOTHERAPEUTIC AGENTS

Therapeutic Efficacy

Chemotherapy has mostly been used for prophylaxis, however the assessment of efficacy is better defined and clarified when used for treatment of residual cancer. The EORTC Genito-Urinary Group has documented the feasibility and safety of the marker lesion model *(101)*. A well-defined tumor (marker lesion) is left in the bladder after transurethral resection (TUR) in patients with multiple primary or recurrent Ta-T1 bladder cancer for the objective evaluation of the antitumor activity of intravesically administered drugs.

The next issue to consider when evaluating the efficacy of a drug is the dose. In general dose-response studies are a basis for establishing an optimal dose after considering toxicity. Unfortunately there are few randomized dose-response studies with a sufficient number of patients. In a randomized trial thiotepa was administered at two dose levels (30 and 60 mg). No difference in efficacy was observed *(62)*. Epirubicin has been tested at various dose levels (30–80 mg). No differences in recurrence rate was observed between the two treatment groups in one study *(89)*. Another study *(100)* involving a small patient population with carcinoma *in situ* showed more promising results with an 80 mg dose.

In marker lesion studies a complete response (CR) was observed in half the cases treated with mitomycin C and in one third of cases treated with doxorubicin *(101)*. Epirubicin appears to have an efficacy similar to doxorubicin. In a recent marker lesion study comparing different doses of interferon to mitomycin C the CR rate for mitomycin C was 72% (40 mg/60 mL water/2 h × 8) (Malmström personal communication).

Adjuvant Efficacy

Twenty-three placebo controlled trials (Table 4), enrolling more than 4500 patients, comparing resection with and without intravesical chemo-

Table 4
Recurrence Rate in Controlled Adjuvant Intravesical Chemotherapy Trials[a]

Drugs	No. Pts	Recurrence rate (%) Control	Chemo.	P value	Reference
Ethoglucid	209	59	28	0.0004	Kurth, 1985
Mitomycin C	58	50	7	0.01	Huland, 1983
Mitomycin C	278	62	57	NS	Niijima, 1983
Mitomycin C	298	33	24	NS	Akaza, 1987
Mitomycin C	397	65	51	0.001	Tolley, 1988
Mitomycin C	43	82	81	NS	Kim, 1989
Mitomycin C	83	42	35	NS	Rubben, 1990
Mitomycin C	261	45	29	<0.05	Minervini, 1996
Thiotepa	51	97	58	0.001	Burnand, 1976
Thiotepa	86	60	47	0.016	Byar, 1977
Thiotepa	42	64	65	NS	Nocks, 1979
Thiotepa	134	41	40	NS	Ashai, 1980
Thiotepa	93	66	39	0.02	Koontz, 1982
Thiotepa	209	69	59	NS	Schulman, 1982
Thiotepa	58	71	30	0.002	Zinke, 1983
Thiotepa	90	76	64	0.05	Prout, 1983
Thiotepa	367	37	40	NS	MRC, 1985
Doxorubicin	436	62	45	0.05	Niijima, 1983
Doxorubicin	59	71	32	0.01	Zinke, 1983
Doxorubicin	217	59	35	0.006	Kurth, 1985
Doxorubicin	220	61	56	NS	Rubben, 1988
Doxorubicin	457	33	25	NS	Akaza, 1992
Epirubucin	399	41	29	0.0152	Oosterlink, 1993

[a]Adapted with permission from Sten Nilsson. Chemotherapy for Cancer, 2001.

therapy, have so far been reported in the English literature *(102–124)*. The studies vary considerably with respect to parameters such as inclusion criteria, treatment regimens, followup, and data analysis methods. The cumulative result from the above studies shows a short term 15% decrease in tumor recurrence rate when adjuvant chemotherapy is given following transurethral resection. Eleven of these trials included progression data; none found a statistically significant difference.

A combined analysis on 2244 patients has been performed by the EORTC and the Medical Research Council (MRC) *(125)*. It was found that for prophylaxis the short term (2–3 yr) recurrence rate is 14% lower with chemotherapy than in controls. The long term protection from tumor recurrence was more difficult to evaluate but was calculated to be 7%. No effect on progression was proven.

In most comparative studies with chemotherapy, no agent has proved more effective than the other *(94,126–128)*. An exception is a recent randomized study that demonstrated that epirubicin had better efficacy and lower toxicity than doxorubicin *(100)*. This was in contrast to an earlier study, comparing the drugs at lower doses, that reported no difference in efficacy *(129)*.

The timing and duration of therapy has been extensively studied. For a long time urologists have used single dose chemotherapy as an adjuvant after transurethral resection, but the experience was largely anecdotal. The rational for this is the risk of implantation of tumor cells in scar tissue in the bladder. Five randomized controlled studies adressing this issue have been reported in the literature. The first two were quite small but clearly indicated the value of this approach *(130,131)*. More recently three large studies have verified these earlier studies. The MRC performed a multicenter randomized clinical trial involving 502 patients with newly diagnosed superficial bladder cancer *(132)*. After complete resection patients were randomized into 1 of 3 treatment arms: no further treatment; 1 instillation of mitomycin C at resection; and 1 instillation at resection and at 3-mo intervals for 1 yr (total 5 instillations). The dose of mitomycin C used was 40 mg/40 mL water. After median followup of 7 yr, 1 and 5 instillations of mitomycin C resulted in decreased recurrence rates and increased recurrence-free interval. The benefit of mitomycin C was observed in patients at low, medium, and high risk for subsequent recurrence. It was suggestive but not conclusive evidence that 5 instillations of mitomycin C offered a slight advantage over 1 instillation.

The EORTC group randomized a total of 431 eligible patients with solitary, primary or recurrent stages Ta and T1 transitional cell carcinoma of the bladder to compare a single intravesical instillation of 80 mg epirubicin with water given immediately after resection *(13)*. The interval to initial recurrence was significantly better in favor of the epirubicin group. After a mean followup of 2 yr it became evident that the recurrence rate after a single epirubicin instillation was decreased by nearly half with the same trend being found in all subgroups examined. Toxicity was mainly restricted to bladder irritation in approximately 10% of the cases. An Egyptian study *(133)* included 168 evaluable patients that were assigned to three groups after transurethral resection of bladder tumour (TURBT) and histological confirmation of its superficial nature (pTa and pT1). In group 1, patients received a single dose of 50 mg epirubicin in 50 mL normal saline immediately after TURBT; group 2 received 50 mg epirubicin in 50 mL normal saline 1–2 wk after TURBT, instillations were repeated for 8 wk and thereafter monthly to complete

1 yr of treatment: group 3 (control group) received no adjuvant therapy after TURBT. The recurrence rate was significantly lower in the patients treated with epirubicin than in the control group (24, 25 and 52%, respectively; $p = 0.001$). In those receiving epirubicin, the rates of recurrence were statistically comparable ($p = 0.9$). In all these studies all risk groups seemed to benefit from the single, early instillation of the cytotoxic agent.

The role of maintenance therapy has been controversial. Prospective studies have not shown any difference in the recurrence-free interval and long term recurrence rate compared to no maintenance (134–136). Two parallel prospective randomized studies by the EORTC indicate an advantage for early instillations (for 6 or 12 mo) or those having prolonged treatment (either immediate or delayed) (127).

Chemotherapy and BCG

Marker studies with BCG have usually reported a complete response in two thirds of the patients (137), indicating that BCG may provide an initially higher response rate than cytostatics. Different strains of BCG have been tested and there seems to be no major difference in their antitumor activity.

Direct randomized comparisons have been performed comparing BCG with thiotepa, doxorubicin, or mitomycin C. Studies with thiotepa or doxorubicin have shown that BCG is superior (137). Seven randomized studies compared mitomycin C with BCG. The results have not been as conclusive as the studies with other chemotherapy agents (138–144). Six of these studies are shown in Table 5. Some trials included all risk categories, but others only high-risk patients. Most studies included patients with Tis but the numbers were usually small. The difference in BCG strain, mitomycin C dose and concentration, and instillation schedule make comparisons difficult. For example, the concentration of mitomycin C varied more than twofold between studies (Table 6). Three of the trials found BCG to be more effective in lowering the number of recurrences, two reported no difference, while one trial with two different BCG strains found mitomycin C superior to one of the strains but equal to the other strain. The progression rate was generally quite low due to few high-risk patients and short followup. An exception is the study by Malmström et al. (141) that was designed to include high risk patients. There was a 19% progression rate at 5 yr despite long term treatment. Another study with long followup reported less progressions in the mitomycin C arm among patients without carcinoma in situ (142). A longer followup than 5 yr is however necessary to fully evaluate progression and survival in those with this disease entity.

Table 5
Results of Treatment in Randomized Prospective Studies
Comparing Intravesical Instillations of Mitomycin-C and BCG

BCG strain/ dosage	MMC dosage	Treatment duration	Conclusion	Reference
Pasteur F 6×10^8	20–40 mg	Both 24 mo	BCG superior	Rintala, 1991 (140)
Tice and RIVM 5×10^8	30 mg	MMC 6 mo BCG: 1–2 × 6 weekly	RIVM and MMC superior to Tice	Vegt, 1995 (139)
RIVM 5×10^8	30 mg	MMC 6 mo BCG: 1–2 × 6 weekly	No difference MMC superior reg. progression in Tis negative	Witjes, 1998 (142)
Tice 5×10^8	20mg	Both 12 mo	BCG superior	Lamm, 1995 (137)
Connaught 1×10^9	20mg	MMC 24 mo BCG: 6 weekly + 4 mo	No difference	Krege, 1996 (138)
Pasteur D 1×10^9	40 mg	Both 24 mo	BCG superior	Malmström, 1999 (141)

Combination Treatment

Combination chemotherapy combines agents that differ in both the way they act and in their side effects. Combining drugs may effectively eliminate cancer cell resistance. Promising results have been reported after intravesical mitomycin C and doxorubicin sequential therapy for carcinoma *in situ (145)*, and also with mitomycin C followed by BCG in a marker lesion study *(146)*. A later controlled study did not find any major difference in toxicity or treatment efficacy with intravesical mitomycin C and the sequential use of BCG or mitomycin C for intermediate and high risk superficial papillary bladder cancer *(147)*.

In a study from Finland the combination of epirubicin and interferon-α gave promising results *(148)*. A Japanese randomized study evaluated the combination of doxorubicin and oral 5-fluorouracil (5-FU) in a trial *(149)*. There was no indication of a synergistic effect between these drugs.

Second-Line Retreatment with the Same Chemotherapeutic Agent, Another Chemotherapeutic Agent, and Intravesical Chemotherapy After BCG

Retreatment with the same drug may be worthwhile in patients with low risk for progression *(150)*. In the literature 42–60% respond to

Table 6
Results of Treatment in Randomized Prospective Studies
Comparing Intravesical Instillations of Mitomycin-C and BCG[a]

MMC dos	Vol/sol/dur	Concentration mg/mL	Reference
20–40 mg	AUC/ph.buf./NA	variable	Rintala, 1991 (140)
30 mg	50 mL/NaCl/NA	0.6	Vegt, 1995 (139)
30 mg	50 mL/NaCl/NA	0.6	Witjes 1998 (142)
20 mg	20 mL/H2O/2 h	1.0	Lamm, 1991 (137)
20 mg	50 mL/NaCl/2 h	0.4	Krege, 1996 (138)
40 mg	50 mL/ph.buf./2 h	0.8	Malmström, 1999 (141)

[a]Dosing of mitomycin-C in randomized prospective studies.

second line chemotherapy after failure to previous chemotherapy (128, 151–153).

Chemotherapy may also be helpful in BCG failures. In one of the above randomized trials (141) the protocol recommended cross-over treatment for non responders. This was administered in 60 patients, 39 patients received BCG after failure with mitomycin C, and 21 patients received mitomycin C after failure with BCG. 19 of the 60 patients (32%) remained free of recurrences; 15/39 (39%) with second line BCG and 4/21 (19%) with second line mitomycin C (Fig. 4).

THE FUTURE OF INTRAVESICAL CHEMOTHERAPY

Tumor Markers

Tumor markers able to better predict recurrence and progression in patients with newly diagnosed tumors and thus select cases for early and aggressive instillation therapy are needed, especially in cases with T1 disease. Also, markers that can predict which patients may respond to intravesical chemotherapy would be useful. DNA ploidy assessments have been discussed for more than a decade as a possible prognostic and predictive factor. In a recent report, the predictive value of ploidy was assessed in the context of a large clinical trial comparing mitomycin C and BCG (154). The predictive information of DNA ploidy was not additive to treatment arm and grade for recurrence or progression. P53 protein overexpression has been evaluated by several groups, but the data is contradictory (155–157). Results from the Swedish-Norwegian BCG/mitomycin C study (141) indicate a predictive role for p53 status for risk of progression but not for recurrence (see Fig. 5). Recently several urinary tests have been introduced for screening and monitoring of disease. If these tests are able to detect preclinical disease, therapy can be instituted at the time of minimal tumor burden and hopefully be more effective.

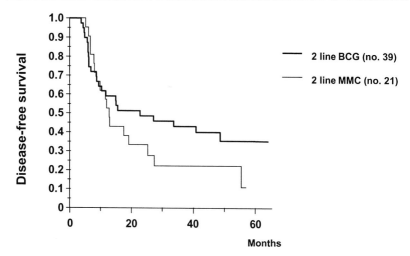

Fig. 4. Disease-free survival after cross-over treatment. MMC, mitomycin-C.

New Chemotherapeutic Drugs

Manipulation of the basic pharmacological and chemical parameters of intravesical chemotherapeutic agents has usually not resulted in any remarkable differences in the action of these agents. More recent efforts have focused on the addition of other agents or supplemental treatments in an attempt to increase efficacy.

Recently several new chemotherapeutic drugs have been shown to produce good results in pilot studies.

Suramin is a polysulfonated naphthylurea which has a broad range of antitumor activity. The mechanism of action of suramin is not completely understood, although it is known to inhibit enzymes in all cellular compartments, inhibit steroidogenesis, and interfere with ligand-receptor binding. Suramin's large molecular size and negative charge make it poorly absorbed through the bladder mucosa, a desired characteristic for an intravesical chemotherapeutic agent. In vitro studies have demonstrated suramin's significant efficacy against transitional cell carcinoma cell lines at relatively low doses (156). Humans treated with similar doses delivered in a systemic fashion have experienced no bladder toxicity. Suramin has been shown to block the binding of epidermal growth factor (EGF) to its receptors, which are found in large amounts in bladder cancers. Because a significant association has been found between the number of EGF receptors on a bladder cancer cell and its sensitivity to suramin, transitional-cell carcinoma could potentially be very responsive to such therapy. On the basis of these findings, a phase I escalating-suramin-dose study is currently being conducted.

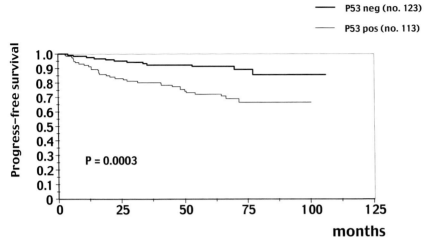

Fig. 5. Progress-free survival by initial p53 status.

Paclitaxel (taxol), an antimicrotubular drug, has been investigated in vitro *(157)*. Histocultures of surgical specimens from patients were used and the effect of paclitaxel on partial inhibition of DNA precursor incorporation and apoptosis was studied. The results indicated that a 2-h paclitaxel treatment was sufficient to produce antiproliferation and apoptosis in 70–90% of human bladder tumors. The apoptotic effect appeared to be linked to proliferation and occurred after DNA synthesis. The effects of intravesical administration of paclitaxel in vivo have also been studied *(158)*. Two cell lines, derived from MBT-2 cells, were employed in these experiments. The T50 line (obtained by many passages in mice) was much more aggressive in vivo than the T5 line. In vivo paclitaxel treatment for 3 d after T5 implantation resulted in a considerable retardation of tumor growth, whereas under the same conditions the T50 line was less affected. When treatment was started one day after tumor implantation, both tumor cell lines were affected by paclitaxel to the same extent.

Paclitaxel is absorbed across the urothelium better than mitomycin C and doxorubicin *(159)*. However, the systemic concentration resulting from intravesical treatment was insignificant. Intravesical paclitaxel appears to be a reasonable candidate drug for intravesical therapy.

Tamoxifen, a hormonal agent, has also been evaluated in vitro *(160)*. It significantly enhanced the cytotoxicity of three chemotherapeutic agents to two cell lines, however; tamoxifen alone caused significant toxic effects. Although cytotoxic levels of tamoxifen ($>50 \mu M$) can be achieved easily in the intravesical model, further study is necessary before tamoxifen can be used clinically as intravesical chemotherapy.

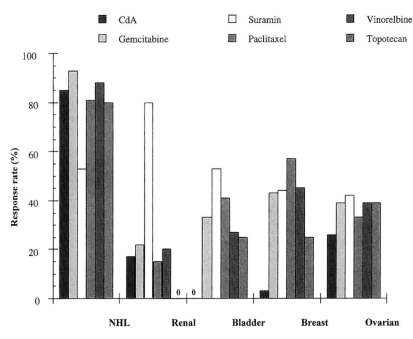

Fig. 6. Response rates, i.e., the fraction of samples with a survival index below the median for all samples investigated, for the indicated investigational drugs at the in vitro concentrations indicated in materials and methods. 0; no responder.

Cytotoxic Resistance

In vitro tumor models analyzing cytotoxic resistance could be supportive in the process of development of new cytotoxic drugs and in selection of suitable drugs for the individual patient.

The clonogenic survival of MGH-U1 human bladder carcinoma cells treated with melphalan, cisplatin, mitomycin-C, adriamycin, vincristine and 5- fluorouracil was measured to assess the relative cytotoxic effects of these agents *(161)*. Mitomycin C, adriamycin and melphalan were found to be the agents with the greatest efficacy.

Testing of tumor cells from patients with urinary bladder carcinoma in a fluorometric microculture cytotoxicity assay (FMCA) as a means of providing clinically relevant data for these tumor types has been investigated *(162)*. Bladder carcinomas were essentially as sensitive as carcinomas of the breast and ovary but had a steeper dose-response relationship. Among the investigational drugs, paclitaxel, gemcitabine and suramin showed promising activity *(see* Fig. 6).

Another study examined in vitro proliferation and mitomycin C sensitivity of patient bladder tumors as a function of the tumor pathobiology

(163). The data indicated that the proliferation of tumor histocultures paralleled the tumor aggressiveness in vivo. Also the data indicated a large difference in sensitivity of human bladder tumors to mitomycin C, with greater sensitivity for well differentiated superficial tumors and lesser sensitivity for undifferentiated, invasive tumors.

Multidrug Resistance

Unfortunately, the efficacy of chemotherapy is often hampered by multi-drug resistance. Multidrug resistance can be either intrinsic or acquired, and can be caused by several mechanisms. The so-called classical multi-drug resistance mediated by the MDR1 gene product P-glycoprotein has been held mainly responsible for inferring the multidrug resistance phenotype. The resistance is mediated through the expression of the P-glycoprotein, which acts as an energy dependent drug efflux pump. However, several other multidrug resistance pathways have been identified. Multi-drug resistance can be caused by a membrane-bound multidrug resistance associated protein, a detoxifying glutathione metabolism, the antiapoptotic protein BCL2, and changes in levels or activity of topo-isomerase enzymes. Strategies to overcome multidrug resistance have arisen with the better understanding of the biologic and molecular mecha-nisms of multidrug resistance, and have been studied in experimental and clinical settings.

The clinical significance of immunohistochemically detected multi-drug resistance associated proteins has been investigated. Nakagawa et al. *(164)* found that the multidrug resistance associated protein, as well as P-glycoprotein mediated multidrug resistance, may be induced after chemotherapy for bladder tumors. However, the presence of P-glyco-protein before chemotherapy did not predict clinical outcome in patients with bladder cancer. Nargrund et al. *(165)* studied the effect of intravesi-cal chemotherapy on P-glycoprotein status in chemoresistant and recur-rent superficial tumors which progressed to metastasis or needed further treatment. The P-glycoprotein expression was not related to histological grading or clinical progression of bladder tumors. Thus, attempts to use analysis of multidrug resistance in clinical setting has not been rewarding.

Nevertheless, applications of novel therapies to reverse multidrug resis-tance and to increase efficacy of chemotherapy have been pursued. Verap-amil, a calcium channel blocker which has been shown to reverse multi-drug resistance in vitro in other neoplasms, was tested in a multidrug resistant human bladder transitional cell carcinoma cell line *(166)*. Ver-apamil reversed resistance to doxorubicin in vitro. This mechanism was further characterized by Duffy et al. *(167)*. They used confocal micro-scopy in the study of resistance to epirubicin to determine the effect of temperature, viability, and a resistance-reversing agent on the intracellular distribution of this drug in sensitive and resistant derivatives of a superficial bladder cancer cell line. Viable and nonviable adherent cells were incubated in epirubicin solutions under various conditions. After incubation, the distribution of intracellular epirubicin fluorescence was visualized using confocal microscopy and a 50× magnification water-immersion lens. There was a striking and consistent difference between resistant and sensitive cells in the intracellular distribution of the drug. In addition to having greater overall levels of epirubicin fluorescence, sensitive cells accumulated epirubicin predominantly in the nucleus. Epirubicin fluorescence in resistant cells was cytoplasmic and granular in appearance. The resistance-reversing agent verapamil appeared to cause reversion of the resistant to the sensitive phenotype. Thus, confocal microscopy allowed epirubicin-sensitive and resistant cultured tumor cells to be differentiated reliably. It also provided information about the mechanism of action of epirubicin, and the development of resistance. Applying this technique to clinical specimens should enable patients who have the resistant phenotype to be detected. Experiments in vivo were performed to investigate the systemic and local absorption after intravesical verapamil administration *(166)*. Verapamil was found in high concentrations in the mucosa, less in the adventitia, and was absent in venous blood. The intravesical use of verapamil thus appeared to be safe, and could prove to be a useful adjunct in the intravesical therapy of some bladder tumors.

This was tested in a study reported by Naito et al. *(168)*. Patients were randomized after transurethral resection (TUR) of superficial bladder cancer into two groups: one group received an intravesical instillation of doxorubicin (30 mg) plus verapamil (15 mg) after TUR of superficial bladder cancer, and the other group received doxorubicin alone on the same treatment schedule. The doxorubicin plus verapamil instillation group showed a significantly higher nonrecurrence rate than the doxorubicin-only instillation group. The incidence and severity of bladder irritative symptoms was not significantly different between the two groups.

Immunochemotherapy

Antibodies or peptides linked to cytotoxic agents have been proposed. Doxorubicin has been conjugated via a dextran bridge method to a murine IgG3 monoclonal antibody, 1G3.10, directed against human bladder cancer. The drug-antibody conjugate retained essentially the original immunological activity. The in vitro and in vivo results suggested that the conjugate could be useful as a potentially cytotoxic agent in immunochemotherapy of human bladder cancer *(169)*. A conjugate of mitomycin C and a monoclonal antibody for specific chemotherapy have also been developed and tested in other tumor types *(170)*.

Drugs to Affect Absorption

Several drugs have been proposed to enhance the permeability of the bladder wall in order to increase the local drug concentration. These include dimethyl sulfoxide, Tween 80 and hyaluronidase.

Dimethyl sulfoxide (DMSO) is a dipolar solvent that is instilled into the bladder for interstitial cystitis. An in vivo study indicated that pretreatment with DMSO increased the absorption of chemotherapy instilled afterwards *(171)*. There is also evidence that DMSO can increase the anti-cancer activity of chemotherapeutic drugs. This was studied using a human bladder cancer cell line *(172)*. However, the addition of 4% DMSO to four drugs frequently used for intravesical chemotherapy (adriamycin, epodyl, mitomycin C, and thiotepa) did not increase tumor cell kill in vitro. Concern about the risk of initiating carcinogenesis with this drug has been raised after in vivo studies *(173)*.

Tween 80, a surface active detergent, has been shown to enhance the cytotoxic activities of chemotherapeutic drugs (adriamycin, epodyl, mitomycin C, and thiotepa) frequently administered to treat superficial bladder cancer *(174)*. Pharmacokinetic studies with a combination of thiotepa and Tween 80 showed statistically significant increases in mean peak plasma levels compared to controls *(175)*.

Hyaluronidase, an enzyme that splits mucopolysacharides containing hyaluronic acid, has been tested clinically. The effect of intravesical instillation of 200,000 IU hyaluronidase in addition to mitomycin C as chemoprophylaxis of superficial bladder cancer was evaluated in a randomized trial. Patients in the group receiving hyaluronidase had less recurrences *(176)*. It appears that additive hyaluronidase enhances the local effect in the intravesical chemoprophylaxis of bladder cancer, presumably by improving diffusion into the bladder mucosa and catalyzing the breakdown of a hyaluronic acid contained in a protective halo around malignant urothelial cells.

Other Methods to Affect Absorption

Electromotive drug administration has been recently explored. A comparative study evaluated the efficacy of electromotive administration (EMDA) of intravesical mitomycin C at a current of 15 mA for 20 min once a wk for 8 wk *(177)*. No difference in efficacy was noted compared to a control group.

Hyperthermia has been instituted in combination with intravesical chemotherapy. Early studies demonstrated that it was safe, well tolerated, and that neoplastic tissue was selectively destroyed *(178)*. Later studies then examined its use as adjuvant therapy, given simultaneously with mitomycin C in a controlled marker tumor study *(179)*. The system consisted of a computerized 915 MHz microwave source that directly heats the bladder wall (within a temperature range of 42.5–45.5°C) using a transurethral catheter. In this study patients were randomly assigned to receive combined neoadjuvant intravesical chemotherapy with or without local hyperthermia. A pathological complete response was documented in a higher frequency after microwave induced hyperthermia. The complete response rate, 66% vs 22%, was significantly higher for the mitomycin C-hyperthermia group versus the mitomycin C alone group.

Gene Therapy

Gene therapy is well suited for intravesical administration. Several protocols have been shown to be effective in animal models. Gene correcting and tumor vaccination studies have been performed. In one study the aim was to evaluate the effects of introduction of wild-type p53 or p21WAF1/CIP1 (p21) on chemosensitivity of bladder cancer cells *(180)*. A human bladder cancer cell line, which contained mutant *p53* and *p21* genes, was used in this study. The effects of adenoviral-mediated *p53* or *p21* gene transfer on sensitivity of cells to cis-platin were analyzed both in vitro and in vivo. The introduction of wild-type *p53* gene markedly enhanced the sensitivity to cis-platin in vitro. Direct injection of the *p53*-adenoviral vector into subcutaneous tumors established in nude mice, followed by intraperitoneal administration of cis-platin, induced massive apoptotic destruction of the tumors. In contrast, the sensitivity to cis-platin was not increased by the introduction of the *p21* gene either in vitro or in vivo. These findings suggest that the combined regimen of gene replacement and chemotherapy may become an efficient and powerful tool for treatment of bladder cancer.

SUMMARY

When considering the use of intravesical chemotherapy, an understanding of the natural history of the disease, the pharmacology of the chemotherapeutic agents to be used, and the efficacy of the agent are important.

In most comparative studies with chemotherapy, no agent has proved more effective than the other.

The recurrence rate is lower with chemotherapy than in controls. No effect on progression has been proven.

Single dose chemotherapy as an adjuvant after transurethral resection is effective. The role of maintenance therapy has been controversial.

REFERENCES

1. Jones PA. Molecular basis for disease-transitional cell carcinoma. Presented at Society of Urologic Oncology Annual Meeting, San Francisco, CA, May 14. J Urol 1994; 151: 63A.

2. Messing EM, Catalona W. In: *Urothelial Tumors of the Urinary Tract* (Walsh PC, Retik AB, Vaughan ED, Wein AJ, eds.). WB Saunders Company, Philadelphia, PA, 1998, pp. 2327–2410.

3. Prout GR, Barton BA, Griffin PP, Friedell G. Treated history of noninvasive grade 1 transitional cell carcinoma. J Urol 1992; 148: 1413–1419.

4. Thompson RA, Campbell EW Jr, Kramer HC, et al. Late invasive recurrence despite long term surveillance for superficial bladder cancer. J Urol 1993; 149: 1010–1011.

5. Messing EM, Young TB, Hunt VB, et al. Hematuria home screening: repeat testing results. J Urol 1995b; 154: 57–61.

6. Messing EM, Young TB, Hunt VB, et al. Comparison of bladder cancer outcome in men undergoing hematuria home screening versus those with standard clinical presentations. Urology 1995c; 45: 387–396.

7. Althausen AF, Prout GR Jr, Daly JJ. Noninvasive papillary carcinoma of the bladder associated with carcinoma in situ. J Urol 1976; 116: 575–580.

8. Gilbert HA, Logan JL, Lagan AR, et al. The natural history of papillary transitional cell carcinoma of the bladder and its treatment in an unselected population on the basis of histologic grading. J Urol 1978; 119: 486–492.

9. Fitzpatrick JM, West AB, Butler MR, et al. Superficial bladder tumors (stage pTa, grades 1 and 2): the importance of recurrence pattern following initial resection. J Urol 1986; 135: 920–922.

10. Malmstrom PU, Busch C, Norlen BJ. Recurrence, progression, and survival in bladder cancer: a retrospective analysis of 232 patients with greater than or equal to 5-year follow-up. Scand J Urol Nephrol 1987; 21: 185–195.

11. Klan R, Loy V, Huland H. Residual tumor discovered in routine second transurethral resection in patients with stage T1 transitional cell carcinoma of the bladder. J Urol 1991; 146: 316–318.

12. Page BH, Levison VB, Curwen MP. The site of recurrence of noninfiltrating bladder tumors. Br J Urol 1978; 50: 237–242.

13. Oosterlinck W, Kurth KH, Schroder F, et al. A prospective European Organization for Research and Treatment of Cancer Genitourinary Group randomized trial comparing transurethral resection followed by a single intravesical instillation of epirubicin or water in single Ta, T1 papillary carcinoma of the bladder. J Urol 1993; 149: 749–752.

14. Cookson MS, Sarosdy MF. Management of stage T1 superficial bladder cancer with intravesical bacillus Calmette-Guerin therapy. J Urol 1992; 148: 797–801.

15. Norming U, Tribukait B, Nyman CR, et al. Prognostic significance of mucosal aneuploidy in stage Ta/T1 grade 3 carcinoma of the bladder. J Urol 1992, 148: 1420–1426.

16. Freeman JA, Esrig DE, Stein JP, et al. Radical Cystectomy for high risk patients with superficial bladder cancer in the era of orthotopic urinary reconstruction. Cancer 1995a; 76: 833–839.

17. Wolf H, Melsen F, Pederson SE, Nielson KT. Natural history of carcinoma in situ of the urinary bladder. Scand J Urol Nephrol 1994; 157: 147–151.

18. Soloway MS. Rationale for intensive intravesical chemotherapy for superficial bladder cancer. J Urol 1980; 123: 461–466.

19. Smith JA. Surgical management of superficial bladder cancer. Semin Surg Oncol 1997; 13: 328–334.
20. Matzkin H, Soloway MS, Hardeman S. Transitional cell carcinoma of the prostate. J Urol 1991; 146: 1207–1212.
21. Sakamoto N, Tsuneyoshi M, Naito S, Kumazawa J. An adequate sampling of the prostate to identify prostatic involvement by urothelial carcinoma in bladder cancer patients. J Urol 1993; 149: 318–321.
22. Smith JA Jr. Endoscopic applications of laser energy. Urol Clin North Am 1986; 13: 405–419.
23. Smith JA Jr, Landau S. Neodymium: YAG laser specifications for safe intravesical therapy. J Urol 1989; 141: 1238.
24. Smith JA Jr, Dixon JA. Argon laser phototherapy of superficial transitional cell carcinoma of the bladder. J Urol 1984; 131: 655–666.
25. Benson RC. Laser treatment. In: *High Tech Urology: Technological Innovations and Their Clinical Applications* (Smith JA Jr, ed.). WB Saunders, Philadelphia, PA, 1992, pp. 47–49.
26. Johnson DE. Use of the holmium: YAG (ho: YAG) laser for treatment of superficial bladder carcinoma. Lasers Surg Med 1994; 14: 213–218.
27. Milam DF. Surgical laser fibers and right angle laser techniques. In: *Lasers in Urologic Surgery* (Smith JA Jr, ed.), 3rd ed. Mosby-Year Book, St. Louis, MO, 1994, pp. 26–31.
28. Beisland HO, Seland P. A prospective randomized study on neodymium: YAG laser irradiation versus TUR in treatment of urinary bladder cancer. Scand J Urol Nephrol 1986; 20: 209–212.
29. Sander S, Beisland HO. Superficial bladder cancer. In: *Lasers in Urologic Surgery* (Smith JA Jr, ed.). Mosby Year Book, St. Louis, MO, 1994, pp. 126–134.
30. Badalament RA, Farah RN. Treatment of superficial bladder cancer with intravesical chemotherapy. Semin Surg Oncol 1997; 13: 335–341.
31. Lamm DL, Griffith G, Pettit LL, Nseyo UO. Current perspectives on diagnosis and treatment of superficial bladder cancer. Urology 1992; 39(4): 331–341.
32. Lamm DL. Long term results of intravesical therapy for superficial bladder cancer. (Review). Urol Clin North Am 1992; 19: 573–580.
33. Schmittgen TD, Au JL, Wientjes MG, et al. Cultured human bladder tumors for pharmacodynamic studies. J Urol 1991; 145: 203–207.
34. Wientjes MG, Dalton JT, Badalament RA, et al. A method to study drug concentration-depth profiles in tissues: mitomycin C in dog bladder wall. Pharmaceut Res 1991: 8: 168.
35. Schmittgen TD, Wientjes MG, Badalament RA, Au JL. Pharmacodynamics of mitomycin C in cultured human bladder tumors. Cancer Res 1991; 51: 3849–3856.
36. Wientjes MG, Dalton JT, Badalment RA, et al. Bladder wall penetration of intravesical mitomycin C in dogs. Cancer Res 1991; 51: 4347–4354.
37. Dalton JT, Wientjes MG, Badalament RA, et al. Pharmacokinetics of intravesical mitomycin C in superficial bladder cancer patients. Cancer Res 1991; 51: 5144–5152.
38. Wientjes MG, Badalament RA, Au JL. Use of pharmacologic data and computer simulations to design an efficacy trial of intravesical mitomycin C therapy for superficial bladder cancer. Cancer Chemother Pharmacol 1993: 32: 255–262.
39. Wientjes MG, Badalament RA, Wang RC, et al. Penetration of mitomycin C in human bladder. Cancer Res 1993; 53: 3314–3320.
40. Schmidbauer CP, Porpaczy P, Georgeopoulos A, et al. Absorption of doxorubicin-hydrochloride and mitomycin C after instillation into noninfected and infected bladders of dogs. J Urol 1984; 131(4): 818–821.

41. Dedrick RL, Flessner MF, Collins JM, Schultz JS. Is the peritoneum a membrane? ASAIO J 1982; 5: 1.

42. Flessner MF, Dedrick RL, Schultz JS. A distributive model of peritoneal-plasma transport: Analysis of experimental data in the rat. Am J Physiol 1985: 248: F413–F424.

43. Wientjes MG, Badalament RA, Au JL. Penetration of intravesical doxorubicin in human bladders. Cancer Chemother Pharmacol 1996; 37: 539–546.

44. Groos E, Masters JR. Intravesical chemotherapy: studies on the relationship between osmolality and cytotoxicity. J Urol 1986; 136: 399–402.

45. Walker MC, Masters JR, Parris CN, Hepburn PJ, English PJ. Intravesical chemotherapy: in vitro studies on the relationship between dose and cytotoxicity. Urol Res 1986; 14(3): 137–140.

46. Eksborg S, Nillson S, Edsmyr F. Intravesical instillation of adriamycin; a model for standardization of the chemotherapy. Eur Urol 1980; 6: 218–220.

47. Masters JR, McDermott BJ, Harland S, Bibby MC, Loadman PM. ThioTEPA pharmacokinetics during intravesical chemotherapy: the influence of dose and volume of instillate on systemic uptake and dose rate to the tumour. Cancer Chemother Pharmacol 1996; 38(1): 59–64.

48. Tarkington M, Sommers, CL, Gelmann EP, Tefft MC, Lynch JH. The effect of pH on the in vitro colony-forming ability of transitional cell carcinoma cells treated with various chemotherapeutic agents: implications for in vivo therapy. J Urol 1992; 147: 511–513.

49. Jauhiainen K, Kangas L, Nieminen AL, Kapyla H, Alfthan O. Optimising mitomycin C activity during intravesical instillation. Urol Res 1983; 11(2): 59–62.

50. Yen WC, Schmittgen T, Au JL. Different pH dependency of mitomycin C activity in monolayer and three- dimensional cultures. Pharm Res 1996; 13(12): 1887–1891.

51. De Bruijn EA, Sleeboom HP, van Helsdingen PJ, van Oosterom AT, Tjaden UR, Maes RA. Pharmacodynamics and pharmacokinetics of intravesical mitomycin C upon different dwelling times. Int J Cancer 1992; 513): 359–364.

52. Heney NM, Koontz WW, Barton B, et al. Intravesical thiotepa versus mitomycin C in patients with Ta, T1, and Tis transitional cell carcinoma of the bladder: a phase III prospective randomized study. J Urol 1988; 140: 1390–1393.

53. Witjes JA, Oosterhof GON, Debruyne FMJ. In: *Comprehensive Textbook of Genitourinary Oncology* (Vogelzang NJ, Scardino PT, Shipley WU, Coffey DS, eds.). Williams and Wilkins, Philadelphia, PA, 1996, pp. 416–427.

54. Hamdy FC, Hastic KJ, Kerry R, Williams JL. Mitomycin-C in superficial bladder cancer. Is long-term maintenance therapy worthwhile after initial treatment? Br J Urol 1993; 71: 183–186.

55. Connolly JG. Chemotherapy of superficial bladder cancer. In: *Carcinoma of the Bladder* (Connolly JG, ed.). Raven, New York, NY, 1981, pp. 165–175.

56. Sonneveld P, Kurth KH, Hagenmyer A, et al. Secondary hematologic neoplasm after intravesical chemotherapy for superficial bladder carcinoma. Cancer 1990; 65: 23–25.

57. Parmar MK, Freedman LS, Hargreave TB, Tolly DA. Prognostic factors for recurrence and followup policies in the treatment of superficial bladder cancer: report from the British Medical Research Council Subgroup on Superficial Bladder Cancer (Urological Cancer Working Party). J Urol 1989; 142: 284–288.

58. Rubben H, Lutzeyer W, Fischer N, et al. Natural history and treatment of low and high risk superficial bladder tumors. J Urol 1988; 139: 283–285.

59. Bateman JC. The chemotherapy of solid tumors with triethylene thio phosphoraminde (Thiotepa). N Engl J Med 1955; 252: 879.

60. Jones HC, Swinney J. Thiotepa in the treatment of tumors of the bladder. Lancet 1961; 2: 615.

61. Weaver D, Khare N, Haigh J, et al. The effect of chemotherapeutic agents on the ultrastructure of transitional cell carcinoma in tissue culture. Invest Urol 1980; 17: 288–292.

62. Koontz WW Jr, Prout GR, Smith W, et al. The use of intravesical thiotepa in the management of non-invasive carcinoma of the bladder. J Urol 1981; 125: 307–312.

63. Hollister D, Coleman M. Hematological effects of intravesical thiotepa therapy for bladder carcinoma. JAMA 1980; 244: 2065–2067.

64. Soloway MS, Ford KS. Thiotepa induced myelosupression: a review of 670 bladder instillations. J Urol 1983; 130: 889–891.

65. Martinez-Pineiro JA, Jimenez Leon J, Martinez-Pineiro L Jr, et al. Bacillus Calmette-Guerin versus doxorubicin versus thiotepa: a randomized prospective study in 202 patients with superficial bladder cancer. J Urol 1990; 143: 502–506.

66. Crooke ST. Mitomycin C: an overview. In: *Mitomycin C Current Status and New Developments* (Carter SK, Crooke ST, eds.). Academic, New York, NY, 1979, pp. 1–4.

67. Phillips FS, Schwartz HS, Sternberg SS. Cancer Res 1960; 20: 1354.

68. Schwartz HS, Sternberg SS, Philips FS. Cancer Res 1963; 23: 1125.

69. Iyer VN, Szybalski W. Proc Natl Acad Sci 1963; 50: 355.

70. Iyer VN, Szybalski W. Science 1964; 145: 55.

71. Lown SW, Weir G. Studies related to antitumor antibiotics. Part XIV. Reactions of mitomycin B with DNA. Can J Biochem 1978; 56: 296.

72. Thrasher JB, Crawford ED. Complications of intravesical chemotherapy. Urol Clin North Am 1992; 19: 529–539.

73. Zein TA, Friedberg N, Kim H. Bone marrow suppression after intravesical mitomycin C treatment. J Urol 1986; 136: 459–460.

74. de Groot AC, Meijden APM vd, Conemans JMH, Maibach HI. Frequency and nature of cutaneous reactions to intravesical instillation of mitomycin for superficial bladder cancer. Urology 1992; 40(Suppl): 16.

75. Colver GB, Inglis JA, McVittle E, et al. Dermatitis due to intravesical Mitomycin C: a delayed type hypersensitivity reaction? Br J Dermatol 1990; 122: 217–224.

76. Eijstein A, Knonagel H, Hotz E, et al. Reduced bladder capacity in patients receiving intravesical chemoprophylaxix with mitomycin C. Br J Urol 1990; 66: 386.

77. Drago PC, Badalament RA, Lucas J, Drago JR. Bladder wall calcifications after intravesical Mitomycin-C treatment of superficial bladder cancer. J Urol 1989; 142: 1071–1072.

78. Tritton TR, Yee G, Wingard B Jr. Immobilized adriamycin: a tool for separating cell surface from intracellular mechanisms. Fed Proc 1983; 42: 284–287.

79. Akaza H, Isaka S, Koiso K, et al. Comparative analysis of short-term and long-term prophylactic intravesical chemotherapy of superficial bladder cancer. Cancer Chemother Pharmacol 1987; 20: S91–S96.

80. Crawford ED, Mc Kenzie D, Mansson W, et al. Adverse reactions to the intravesical administration of doxorubicin hydrochloride: a report of six cases. J Urol 1986; 136: 668–669.

81. Lundbeck F, Mogenson P, Jeppeson N. Intravesical therapy of noninvasive bladder tumors (stage Ta) with doxorubicin and urokinase. J Urol 1983; 130: 1087–1089.

82. Matsumura Y, Akaze H, Isaka S, et al. The 4th study of prophylactic intravesical chemotherapy with adriamycin in the treatment of superficial bladder cancer: the experience of the Japanese urological cancer research group for adriamycin. Cancer Chemother Pharmacol 1992; 30: S10.

83. Lamm DL, Blumenstein BA, Crawford ED, et al. A randomized trial of intravesical doxorubicin and immunotherapy with bacillus Calmette-Guerin for transitional cell carcinoma of the bladder. N Engl J Med 1991; 325: 1205–1209.

84. Khanna OP, Son DL, Mazer H, et al. Multicenter study of superficial bladder cancer treated with intravesical bacillus Calmette-Guerin or adriamycin. Urology 1991; 38(3): 271–279.

85. Burk K, Kurth KH, Newling D. Epirubicin in treatment and recurrence prophylaxis of patients with superficial bladder cancer. Prog Clin Biol Res 1989; 303: 423–434.

86. Whelan P, Cumming JA, Garvie WHH, et al. Multicentre phase II study of low dose intravesical epirubicin in the treatment of superficial bladder cancer. Br J Urol 1991; 67: 600–602.

87. Oosterlinck W, Kurth KH, Scroder F, et al. A prospective European Organisation for Research and Treatment of Cancer Genitourinary Group randomized trial comparing transurethral resection followed by a single intravesical instillation of epirubicin or water in single Ta, T1 papillary carcinoma of the bladder. J Urol 1993; 149: 749–752.

88. Melekos MD, Dauaher II, Fokaefs E, et al. Intravesical instillations of 4-epidoxorubicin (epirubicin) in the prophylactic treatment of superficial bladder cancer: results of controlled prospective study. J Urol 1992; 147: 371–375.

89. Ali-el-dein B, el-Baz M, Aly AN, et al. Intravesical epirubicin versus doxorubicin for superficial bladder tumors (stages pTa and pT1): a randomized prospective study. J Urol 1997; 158 (1): 68–74.

90. Riddle PR. The management of superficial bladder tumors with intravesical epodyl. Br J Urol 1973; 45: 84–87.

91. Robinson MRG, Shelty MB, Richards B, et al. Intravesical epodyl in the management of bladder tumors: combined experiences of the Yorkshire Urological Cancer Research Group. J Urol 1977; 118: 972–973.

92. Flamm J, Bucher A. Adjuvant topical chemotherapy versus immunotherapy in primary superficial transitional cell carcinoma of the bladder. Br J Urol 1991; 67: 70–73.

93. Hoetl W, Hasun R, Albrecht W. Prospective randomized trial to evaluate high- versus low-dose interferon-alpha 2b versus conventional chemotherapy in prevention of the recurrence of superficial transitional cell carcinoma of the urinary bladder. Anticancer Drugs 1992; 3(Suppl 1): 29.

94. Bouffioux C, Denis L, Oosterlinck W, et al. Adjuvant chemotherapy of recurrent superficial transitional cell carcinoma: results of an European Organisation for Research on Treatment of Cancer randomized trial comparing intravesical instillations of thiotepa, doxorubicin, and cisplatin. J Urol 1992; 148: 297–301.

95. Blumenreich MS, Needles B, Yagoda A, et al. Intravesical cisplatin for superficial bladder tumors. Cancer 1982; 50: 863–865.

96. Stewart DJ, Green R, Futter N, et al. Phase I and pharmacology study of intravesical mitoxantrone for recurrent superficial bladder tumors. J Urol 1990; 143: 714–716.

97. Ricos Torrent JV, Monros Lliso JL, Iborra Juan I, Casanova Ramon-Borja JA, Dumont Martinez R, Solsona Narbon E. (Mitoxantrone (MTX) versus mitomycin C (MMC) in the ablative treatment of Ta, T1 superficial bladder tumors. Phase III, randomized prospective study). (Article in Spanish) Arch Esp Urol 1992; 45(7): 647–652.

98. Maffezzini M, Simonato A, Zanon M, Raber M, Carmignani G. Up-front intravesical chemotherapy for low stage, low grade recurrent bladder cancer. J Urol 1996; 155(1): 91–93.

99. Omoto T, Masaki Z, Kano M, et al. Postoperative prophylactic intravesical instillation of cytosine arabinoside and mitomycin c in superficial bladder tumor. A follow-up study. Urology 1982; 20: 510–514.

100. Togashi M, Shinihara N, Toyota K, et al. Prophylactic chemotherapy for primary and recurrent superficial bladder cancer: preliminary results. Cancer Chemother Pharmacol 1992; 30: S21–S25.

101. Bono AV, Hall RR, Denis L, Lovisolo JA, Sylvester R. Chemoresection in Ta-T1 bladder cancer. Members of the EORTC Genito-Urinary Group. Eur Urol 1996; 29(4): 385–390.

102. Kurth K, Vijgh WJF, Fibo TK, et al. Phase study of intravesical epirubicin in patients with carcinoma in situ of the bladder. J Urol 1991; 146: 1508–1513.

103. Richie JP. Intravesical chemotherapy. Treatment selection, techniques, and results. Urol Clin North Amer 1992; 19: 521.

104. Kurth KH, Debruyne FJ, Senge T, Carpentier PJ, Riedl H, Sylvester R, et al. Adjuvant chemotherapy of superficial transitional cell carcinoma: an E.O.R.T.C. randomized trail comparing doxorubicin hydrochloride, ethoglucid and TUR-alone. Prog Clin Biol Res 1985:135–142.

105. Huland H, Otto U. Mitomycin instillation to prevent recurrence of superficial bladder carcinoma. Results of a controlled, prospective study in 58 patients. Eur Urol 1983; 9(2): 84–86.

106. Niijima T, Koiso K, Akaza H. Randomized clinical trial on chemoprophylaxis of recurrence in cases of superficial bladder cancer. Cancer Chemother Pharmacol 1983; 11(Suppl): 79–82.

107. Akaza H, Isaka S, Koiso K, Kotake T, Machida T, Maru A, et al. Comparative analysis of short-term and long-term prophylactic intravesical chemotherapy of superficial bladder cancer. Prospective, randomized, controlled studies of the Japanese Urological Cancer Research Group. Cancer Chemother Pharmacol 1987; 20(Suppl): 91–96.

108. Tolley DA, Hargreave TB, Smith PH, Williams JL, Grigor KM, Parmar MK, et al. Effect of intravesical mitomycin C on recurrence of newly diagnosed superficial bladder cancer: interim report from the Medical Research Council Subgroup on Superficial Bladder Cancer (Urological Cancer Working Party). Br Med J (Clin Res Ed) 1988; 296(6639): 1759–1761.

109. Kim HH, Lee C. Intravesical mitomycin C instillation as a prophylactic treatment of superficial bladder tumor. J Urol 1989; 141(6): 1337–9; discussion 1339–1340.

110. Rubben H, Graf-Dobberstein, Ostwald R, et al. Prospective randomized study of adjuvant therapy after complete resection of superficial bladder cancer; mitomycin C vs BCG Connaught vs TUR alone. In: *Immunotherapy of Urological Tumors* (deKernion JB, Mazema E, eds.). Churchill Livingstone, New York, NY, 1990, pp. 27–36.

111. Minervini R, Felipetto R, Viganoa L, Pampaloni S, Fiorentini L. Recurrences and progressions of superficial bladder cancer following longterm intravesical prophylactic therapy with mitomycin C instillation: 48 month follow-up. Urol Int 1996; 56: 234–237.

112. Burnand KG, Boyd PJ, Mayo ME, Shuttleworth KE, Lloyd-Davies RW. Single dose intravesical thiotepa as an adjuvant to cystodiathermy in the treatment of transitional cell bladder carcinoma. Br J Urol 1976; 48(1): 55–59.

113. Byar D, Blackard C. Comparisons of placebo, pyridoxine, and topical thiotepa in preventing recurrence of stage I bladder cancer. Urology 1977; 10(6): 556–618.

114. Nocks BN, Nieh PT, Prout GR Jr. A longitudinal study of patients with superficial bladder carcinoma successfully treated with weekly intravesical thio-tepa. J Urol 1979; 122(1): 27–29.

115. Asahi T, Matsumura Y, Tanahashi T, Yoshimoto J, Kaneshige T, Fujita Y, et al. The effects of intravesical instillation of Thio-Tepa on the recurrence rate of bladder tumors. Acta Med Okayama 1980; 34(1): 43–49.

116. Koontz WW Jr, Prout GR Jr, Smith W, Frable WJ, Minnis JE. The use of intravesical thio-tepa in the management of non-invasive carcinoma of the bladder. J Urol 1981; 125(3): 307–312.

117. Schulman CC, Robinson M, Denis L, Smith P, Viggano G, de Pauw M, et al. Prophylactic chemotherapy of superficial transitional bladder carcinoma. An EORTC randomized trial comparing thiotepa, an epipodophyllotoxin (VM26) and TUR alone. Eur Urol 1982; 8: 207–212.

118. Zincke H, Utz DC, Taylor WF, Myers RP, Leary FJ. Influence of thiotepa and doxorubicin instillation at time of transurethral surgical treatment of bladder cancer on tumor recurrence: a prospective, randomized, double-blind, controlled trial. J Urol 1983; 129(3): 505–509.

119. Prout GR Jr, Koontz WW Jr, Coombs LJ, Hawkins IR, Friedell GH. Long-term fate of 90 patients with superficial bladder cancer randomly assigned to receive or not to receive thiotepa. J Urol 1983; 130(4): 677–680.

120. The effect of intravesical thiotepa on the recurrence rate of newly diagnosed superficial bladder cancer. An MRC Study. MRC Working Party on Urological Cancer. Br J Urol 1985; 57(6): 680–685.

121. Zincke H, Utz DC, Taylor WF, Myers RP, Leary FJ. Influence of thiotepa and doxorubicin instillation at time of transurethral surgical treatment of bladder cancer on tumor recurrence: a prospective, randomized, double-blind, controlled trial. J Urol 1983; 129(3): 505–509.

122. Rubben H, Lutzeyer W, Fischer N, Deutz F, Lagrange W, Giani G. Natural history and treatment of low and high risk superficial bladder tumors. J Urol 1988; 139(2): 283–285.

123. Akaza H, Koiso K, Kotake T, Matsumura Y, Isaka S, Machida T, et al. Long-term results of intravesical chemoprophylaxis of superficial bladder cancer: experience of the Japanese Urological Cancer Research Group for Adriamycin. Cancer Chemother Pharmacol 1992; 30(Suppl): 15–20.

124. Oosterlinck W, Kurth KH, Schroder F, Bultinck J, Hammond B, Sylvester R. A prospective European Organization for Research and Treatment of Cancer Genitourinary Group randomized trial comparing transurethral resection followed by a single intravesical instillation of epirubicin or water in single stage Ta, T1 papillary carcinoma of the bladder. J Urol 1993; 149(4): 749–752.

125. Pawinski A, Sylvester R, Kurth KH, et al. A combined analysis of European Organization for Research and Treatment of Cancer, and Medical Research Council randomized clinical trials for the prophylactic treatment of stage TaT1 bladder cancer. European Organization for Research and Treatment of Cancer Genitourinary Tract Cancer Cooperative Group and the Medical Research Council Working Party on Superficial Bladder Cancer. J Urol 1996; 156: 1934–1940.

126. Huland H, Kloppel G, Feddersen I, Otto U, Brachmann W, Hubmann H, et al. Comparison of different schedules of cytostatic intravesical instillations in patients with superficial bladder carcinoma: final evaluation of a prospective multicenter study with 419 patients. J Urol 1990; 144(1): 68–71; discussion 71–72.

127. Buffioux C, Kurth KH, Bono A, et al. Intravesical adjuvant chemotherapy for superficial transitional cell bladder carcinoma: results of two European Organization for Research and Treatment of Cancer randomized trials with mitomycin C and doxorubicin comparing early versus delayed instillations and short term versus long term treatment. European Organization for Research and Treatment of Cancer Genitourinary Group. J Urol 1995; 153: 934–941.

128. Zinke H, Benson RC Jr, Hilton JF, et al. Intravesical Thiotepa and Mitomycin C treatment immediately after transurethral resection and later for superficial (stages Ta and Tis) bladder cancer: a prospective, randomized, stratified study with crossover design. J Urol 1985; 134: 1110–1114.

129. Bonfante V, Villani F, Bonnadonna G. Toxic and therapeutic activity of 4' epidoxorubicin. Tumori 1982; 68: 105–111.

130. Abrams PH, Choa RG, Gaches CG, et al. A controlled trial of single dose intravesical adriamycin in superficial bladder tumors. Br J Urol 1981; 53(6): 585–587.

131. Burnand KG, Mayo ME, Shuttleworth KE, et al. Single dose intravesical thiotepa as an adjuvant to cystodiathermy in the treatment of transitional cell bladder carcinoma. Br J Urol 1976; 48(1): 55–59.

132. Tolley DA, Parmar MK, Grigor KM, et al. The effect of intravesical mitomycin C on recurrence of newly diagnosed superficial bladder cancer: a further report with 7 years of follow up. J Urol 1996; 155: 1233–1238.

133. Ali-el-Dein B, Nabeeh A, el-Baz M, Shamaa S, Ashamallah A. Single-dose versus multiple instillations of epirubicin as prophylaxis for recurrence after transurethral resection of pTa and pT1 transitional-cell bladder tumours: a prospective, randomized controlled study. Br J Urol 1997; 79(5): 731–735.

134. Flamm J. Long-term versus short-term doxorubicin hydrochloride instillation after transurethral resection of superficial bladder cancer. Eur Urol 1990; 17(2): 119–124.

135. Okamura K, Kinukawa T, Tsumura Y, Otani T, Itoh H, Kobayashi H, et al. A randomized study of short-versus long-term intravesical epirubicin instillation for superficial bladder cancer. Nagoya University Urological Oncology Group. Eur Urol 1998; 33(3): 285–288.

136. Nseyo UO. Immunotherapy of bladder cancer. Semin Surg Oncol 1997; 13(5): 342–349.

137. Lamm DL, Riggs DR Traynelis CL, et al. Apparent failure of current intravesical chemotherapy prophylaxis to influence the long-term course of superficial transitional cell carcinoma of the bladder. J Urol 1995; 153(50): 1444–1450.

138. Krege S, Giani G, Meyer R, et al. A randomized multicenter trial of adjuvant therapy in superficial bladder cancer: transurethral resection only versus transurethral resection plus mitomycin C versus transurethral resection plus bacillus Calmette-Guerin. Participating Clinics [see comments]. J Urol 1996; 156: 962–966.

139. Vegt PD, Witjes JA, Witjes WPJ, et al. A randomized study of intravesical Mitomycin C, Bacille Calmette-Guerin Tice and Bacille Calmette-Guerin RIVM treatment in pTa-pT1 papillary carcinoma and carcinoma in situ of the bladder. J Urol 1995; 153: 929–933.

140. Rintala E, Jauhianien K, Alfthan O, et al. Intravesical chemotherapy (MMC) versus immunotherapy (BCG) in superficial bladder cancer. Eur Urol 1991; 20: 19–25.

141. Malmstrom PU, Wijkstrom H, Lundholm C, Wester K, Busch C, Norlen BJ. 5-year followup of a randomized prospective study comparing mitomycin C and bacillus Calmette-Guerin in patients with superficial bladder carcinoma. Swedish-Norwegian Bladder Cancer Study Group. Br J Urol 1999; 161(4): 1124–1127.

142. Witjes JA, van der Meijden AP, Sylvester LC, Debruyne FM, van Aubel A, Witjes WP. Long-term follow-up of an EORTC randomized prospective trial comparing intravesical bacille Calmette-Guerin-RIVM and mitomycin C in superficial bladder cancer. EORTC GU Group and the Dutch South East Cooperative Urological Group. European Organisation for Research and Treatment of Cancer Genito-Urinary Tract Cancer Collaborative Group. Urology 1998; 52(3): 403–410.

143. Lamm DL. BCG in perspective: advances in the treatment of superficial bladder cancer. Eur Urol 1995; 27(Suppl 1): 2–8.

144. Zhang S, Li H, Cheng H. The preventive recurrent results of postoperative intravesical instillation therapy in bladder cancer. Chung Hua Wai Ko Tsa Chih 1995; 33(5): 304–306.

145. Sekine H, Fukui I, Yamada T, et al. Intravesical mitomycin C and doxorubicin sequential therapy for carcinoma in situ of the bladder : a longer followup result. J Urol 1994; 151(1): 27–30.

146. Witjes JA, Caris CTM, Mungan NA, et al. Results of a randomized phase III trial of sequential intravesical therapy with mitomycin C and bacillus Calmette-Guerin versus mitomycin C alone in patients with superficial bladder cancer. J Urol 1998; 160: 1668–1671.

147. Van der Meijden AP, Hall RR, Macaluso MP, et al. Marker tumour responses to the sequential combination of intravesical therapy with mitomycin-C and BCG-RIVM in multiple superficial bladder tumours. Report from the European Organisation for Research and Treatment on Cancer-Genitourinary Group (EORTC 30897). Eur Urol 1996; 29(2): 199–203.

148. Raitanen MP, Lukkarinen O. A controlled study of intravesical epirubicin with or without alpha 2b-interferon as prophylaxis for recurrent superficial transitional cell carcinoma of the bladder. Finnish multicentre study group. Br J Urol 1995; 76(6): 697–701.

149. Obata K, Ohashi Y, Akaza H, et al. Prophylactic chemotherapy with intravesical instillation of adriamycin and oral administration of 5-flourouracil after surgery for superficial bladder cancer. The Japanese Urological Cancer Research Group for Adriamycin. Cancer Chemother Pharmacol 1994; 35(Suppl): S88.

150. Mukamel E, DeKernion JB. Conservative treatment of diffuse carcinoma in situ of the bladder with repeated courses of intravesical therapy. Br J Urol 1989; 64(2): 143–146.

151. Prout GR Jr, Griffin PP, Nocks BN, et al. Intravesical therapy of low stage bladder carcinoma with mitomycin C: comparison of results in untreated and previously treated patients. J Urol 1982; 127(6): 1096–1098.

152. Issel BF, Prout GR, Soloway MS, et al. Mitomycin C intravesical therapy in non-invasive bladder cancer after failure on thiotepa. Cancer 1984; 53(5): 1025–1028.

153. Milani C, Bassi P, Meneghini A, et al. Mitomycin C in multiple superficial bladder tumors: short term therapy, long term results. Urol Int 1992; 48(2): 154–156.

154. deVere White RW, Ditch A, Tesluk H, et al. Prognostic significance of DNA ploidy in Ta/T1 bladder cancer: a southwest oncology group study. Uro Oncol 1996; 2: 27.

155. Lee E, Park I, Lee C. Prognostic markers of intravesical Bacillus Calmette-Guerin therapy for multiple, high-grade, stage T1 bladder cancers. Int J Urol 1997; 4: 552–556.

156. Lebret T, Becette V, Barbagelatta M, et al. Correlation between p53 overexpression and response to Bacillus Calmette-Guerin therapy in a high risk select population of patients with T1G3 bladder cancer. J Urol 1998; 159: 788–791.

157. Oveson H, Horn T, Steven K. Long term efficacy of intravesical Bacillus Calmette-Guerin for carcinoma in situ: relationship of progression to histological response and p53 nuclear accumulation. J Urol 1997; 157: 1655–1659.

158. Walther MM, Figg WD, Linehan WM. Intravesical Suramin: a novel agent for the treatment of superficial transitional-cell carcinoma of the bladder. World J Urol 1996; 14: 8–11.

159. Au JL, Kalns K, Gan Y, et al. Pharmacologic effects of paclitaxel in human bladder tumors. Cancer Chemother Pharmacol 1997; 41(1): 69–74.

160. Nativ O, Aronson M, Medalia O, et al. Antineoplastic activity of paclitaxel on experimental superficial bladder cancer; in vivo and in vitro studies. Int J Cancer 1997; 70(3): 297–301.
161. Song D, Wientjes MG, Au JL. Bladder tissue pharmacokinetics of intravesical taxol. Cancer Chemother Pharmacol 1997; 40(40): 285–292.
162. Pu YS, Hsieh TS, Cheng AL, et al. Combined cytotoxic effects of tamoxifen and chemotherapeutic agents on bladder cancer cells: a potential use in intravesical chemotherapy. Br J Urol 1996; 77(1): 76–85.
163. Erlichman C, Vidgen D, Wu A. Antineoplastic drug cytotoxicity in a human bladder cancer cell line: implications for intravesical chemotherapy. Urol Res 1987; 15(1): 13–16.
164. Nygren P, Csoka K, Larsson R, Busch C, Wester K, Malmstrom PU. Activity of standard and investigational cytotoxic drugs in primary cultures of tumor cells from patients with kidney and urinary bladder carcinomas. J Urol 1999; 162(6): 2200–2204.
165. Schmittgen TD, Weaver JM, Badalament RA, et al. Correlation of human bladder tumor histoculture proliferation and sensitivity to mitomycin C with tumor pathobiology. J Urol 1994; 152: 1632–1636.
166. Nagawa M, Emoto A, Nasu N, et al. Clinical significance of multi-drug resistance associated protein and P-glycoprotein in patients with bladder cancer (see comments). J Urol 1997; 157(4): 1260.
167. Nargund VH, Lowe J, Flannigan GM, et al. Role of P-glycoprotein in chemoresistant superficial bladder tumors. Eur Urol 1997; 31(2): 160–162.
168. Long JP Jr, Prout GR Jr, Wong YK, et al. The effect of verapamil on a multi-drug resistant bladder carcinoma cell line and its potential as an intravesical chemotherapeutic agent. J Urol 1990; 143(5): 1053–1056.
169. Duffy PM, Hayes MC, Gatrell SK, et al. Determination and reversal of resistance to epirubicin intravesical chemotherapy. Br J Urol 1996; 77(6): 824–829.
170. Naito S, Kotoh S, Omoto T, et al. Prophylactic intravesical instillation chemotherapy against recurrence after a transurethral resection of superficial bladder cancer: a randomized controlled trial of doxorubicin plus verapamil versus doxorubicin alone. The Kyushu University Urological Oncology Group. Cancer Chemother Pharmacol 1998; 42(5): 367–372.
171. Yu DS, Chu TM, Yeh MY, Chang SY, Ma CP, Han SH. Antitumor activity of doxorubicin-monoclonal antibody conjugate on human bladder cancer. J Urol 1988: 140(2): 415–421.
172. Tanaka J, Sato E, Saito Y, et al. Preparation of a conjugate of mitomycin C and anti-neural cell adhesion molecule monoclonal antibody for specific chemotherapy against biliary tract carcinoma. Surg Today 1998; 28(11): 1217–1220.
173. Hashimoto H, Tokunaka S, Sasaki M, et al. Dimethylsulfoxide enhances the absorption of chemotherapeutic drug instilled into the bladder. Urol Res 1992; 20(3): 233–236.
174. Walker L, Walker MC, Parris CN, Masters JR. Intravesical chemotherapy: combination with dimethyl sulfoxide does not enhance cytotoxicity in vitro. Urol Res 1988; 16: 329–331.
175. Ohtani M, Miyanaga N, Naguchi R, et al. Promotive effects of intravesical instillation of dimethylsulfoxide on bladder carcinogenesis in mice. Nippon Hinyokika Gakkai Zasshi 1992: 83(9): 1423.
176. Parris CN, Masters JR, Walker MC, Newman B, Riddle P: Intravesical chemotherapy: combination with Tween 80 increases cytotoxicity in vitro. Urol Res 1987; 15: 17–20.

177. Masters JR, McDermott BJ, Jenkins WE, et al. ThioTEPA pharmacokinetics during intravesical chemotherapy and the influence of Tween 80. Cancer Chemother Pharmacol 1990; 25(4): 267–273.

178. Maier U, Baumgartner G. Metaphylactic effect of mitomycin C with and without hyaluronidase after transurethral resection of bladder cancer: randomized trial. J Urol 1989; 141(3): 529–530.

179. Brausi M, Campo B, Pizzocaro G, et al. Intravesical electromotive administration of drugs for treatment of superficial bladder cancer: a comparative phase II study. Urology 1998; 51(3): 506–509.

180. Rigatti P, Lev A, Colombo R. Combined intravesical chemotherapy with mitomycin-C and local bladder microwave-induced hyperthermia as a preoperative therapy for superficial bladder tumors. A preliminary clinical study. Eur Urol 1991; 20: 204–210.

181. Colombo R, Da Pozzo LF, Lev A, et al. Neoadjuvant combined microwave induced hyperthermia and topical chemotherapy alone for superficial bladder cancer. J Urol 1996; 155(4): 1227–1232.

182. Miyake H, Hara I, Gohji K, et al. Enhancement of chemosensitivity in human bladder cancer cells by adenoviral-mediated p53 gene transfer. Anticancer Res 1998; 18(4C): 3087–3092.

9

Use of Intravesical BCG in Treatment of Superficial Bladder Cancer

Michael A. O'Donnell, MD

CONTENTS

INTRODUCTION

The Idealized Goals of Intravesical Therapy

Ideally, intravesical therapy should safely eradicate residual bladder cancer and prevent tumor recurrence thus ultimately averting the serious consequences of muscle invasion and metastasis. Unfortunately, while a wide array of topical chemo- and immunotherapeutic drugs exist, the perfect agent is not yet available. Although intravesical chemotherapy results in reasonable short-term cancer response rates, the durable net benefit for tumor recurrence is marginal *(1)*. Furthermore, multiple well-designed intravesical chemotherapy studies have not shown a favorable alteration in tumor progression rate or survival *(2)*. The immunotherapeutic agent, BCG comes closest to meeting these ideals with high early and durable complete response rates. However, while several studies

From: *Current Clinical Urology: Bladder Cancer: Current Diagnosis and Treatment*
Edited by: M. J. Droller © Humana Press Inc., Totowa, NJ

Table 1
Effective BCG Substrains for Bladder Cancer Immunotherapy

Strain	Country	Dose	Ref. year
Pasteur	France	150 mg	1961
Armand frappier	Canada	120 mg	1937
Connaught	Canada	81 mg	1948
Tice	USA	50 mg	1934
Evans	UK	75 mg	1961
RIVM	Netherlands	~10^9 CFU	1921
Danish 1331 (WHO reference)	Denmark	120 mg	1931
Moreau	Brazil	100 mg	1924
Tokyo 172	Japan	80 mg	1925

have demonstrated a decrease in disease progression, there are no long-term studies that are sufficiently statistically powered to provide conclusive demonstration of a survival advantage to BCG. Toxicity with BCG can also be significant making appropriate patient selection based on risk/benefit analysis very important. Yet, strict clinical criteria have not been able to reliably identify patients pretreatment that will benefit from this therapy. The purpose of this chapter is to critically examine the accumulated information on the use of BCG in superficial bladder cancer to provide not only a realistic assessment of its clinical utility but also to identify potential areas for future investigation and improvement.

A Brief History of BCG

In response to the successful development and application of bacterial and antiviral vaccines such as vaccinia for smallpox at the turn of the nineteenth century, coworkers Albert Calmette and Camille Guerin in 1921 at the Pasteur Institute in France succeeded in attenuating the cow tuberculosis bacillus, *Mycobacterium bovis (3)*. Despite the loss of much of its virulence, this bacillus of Calmette and Guerin (BCG) retained enough strong antigenicity to become an effective vaccine for the prevention of human tuberculosis *(4)*. Relatively inexpensive to produce and in high demand, seed lots from the Pasteur Institute were sent to and propagated in many parts of the world ultimately forming the basis for most of the clinical substrains of BCG in use today (Table 1). Genetic drift over time plus differences in culture conditions and preparation, (e.g., surface pellicle growth vs deep culture; lyophilized vs frozen preparations), undoubtedly has resulted in subtle differences between substrains, the clinical significance of which is not entirely clear *(5)*. It has been estimated that over 2.5 billion people have now been vaccinated with BCG. Hot spots for widespread immunization include Asia, Europe, and South America while the United States and Canada have consciously opted against a program of mass vaccination.

The idea that BCG might have potential as a therapeutic agent against cancer probably emerged out of the observations and subsequent application by Coley of bacterial products for cancer therapy. By inciting severe inflammation at the site of injection, these "Coley's Toxins" could induce local regression of various cancers *(6)*. Coupled with the autopsy observations of Pearl that patients with tuberculosis had an apparent lower incidence of cancer, Holmgren in 1935 was the first to report the use of BCG inoculations against cancer. Due to concerns of toxicity subsequently linked to virulent Tb contamination of a BCG lot (the so-called "Lubeck Disaster"), it was not until the late 1950s and 1960s that experimental and clinical studies generated more enthusiasm for its use against cancer. In 1969 a significant antitumor effect of BCG was showed by Mathe and Hadsiev in acute leukemia and bronchial carcinoma respectively *(7,8)*. The following year Morton reported good results with direct injection of BCG into melanoma nodules *(9)*. The advent of modern chemotherapy and radiation therapy plus difficulty in replicating earlier clinical results with BCG eventually led to abandonment of its use for all except melanoma.

BCG's potential for use in bladder cancer sprang out of the work of Coe and Feldman demonstrating that the bladder was an immunocompetent organ responsive to topical BCG and out of the observations by Zbar and colleagues that close contact between BCG and a limited tumor volume in immunocompetent animals was required for efficacy *(10, 11)*. In 1976, Morales reported on the first successful treatment of 7 of 9 patients with recurrent superficial stage Ta/T1 transitional cell carcinoma (TCC) using 6 wk of sequential intravesical BCG plus simultaneous intradermal inoculation *(12)*. It is noteworthy to realize, however, that the choice of dose, interval, dwell time, and number of treatments was arbitrary without the benefit of Phase I and Phase 2 optimization studies. Other subsequent techniques of BCG delivery via intradermal administration alone, direct intratumoral injection, or oral administration did not yield reproducibly high efficacy results and/or were associated with greater toxicity *(13,14)*. Neither was BCG shown to provide any clear therapeutic benefit for patients with muscular invasive disease *(15)*. Use of BCG against nontransitional cell carcinomas of the bladder has not been recommended *(16)*. After verification of efficacy of the Morales regimen against TCC by both the South West Oncology Group (SWOG). and Memorial Sloan Kettering in the early 1980s, this treatment scheme became accepted during the ensuing 2 decades of clinical use *(17,18)*. The only unquestioned modification was the elimination of coincident intradermal injection *(19–22)*.

MODERN CLINICAL TRIALS
OF BCG USE FOR SUPERFICIAL BLADDER CANCER

Considerations in Interpreting Intravesical Therapy Trials

BCG may be used in three specific therapeutic modalities: (1) prophylaxis after definitive resection of papillary bladder tumors (Stages Ta and T1); (2) adjuvant therapy to eliminate non-resectable residual papillary transitional cell carcinoma (pTCC); and (3) primary therapy to eradicate carcinoma *in situ* (CIS). Due to its diffuse and macroscopically indistinct appearance, CIS is presumed to be unresectable by surgery alone. While many of the early reports on BCG efficacy grouped these categories together, differences in the state of the disease at study entry makes direct comparisons difficult and potentially erroneous *(23)*. Thus, the term *complete response* is only appropriate when evaluating ablation of extant disease after TUR (residual pTCC and CIS) while *recurrence rate* (percent of patients with any recurrence by a given time), *recurrence index* (number of recurrence episodes per patient month) and *time to first recurrence* are only strictly meaningful in the prophylactic setting or after a complete response has been already achieved. Kaplan-Meier analysis is often used in these different treatment groups to provide estimates of *percent freedom from disease* or *percent disease free survival* over time. However, while this statistical technique does compensate for dropouts (censoring) and differential time of follow-up, caution must be exercised in interpreting projections well beyond the median follow-up where few numerical study subjects may exist. Defining the start and end-points can also be problematic. For prophylactic treatment, the appropriate start time is the time of definitive TUR, while the start time in the adjuvant or primary therapy setting may be assigned to the first evaluatory point or to the midpoint between start of therapy and first evaluation. Endpoints for failure may be similarly ambiguous: does one chose the time of documented failure, the last point of no evidence of disease, or some point in between? *Freedom from disease progression (>= Stage T2)* and *survival* (preferably disease-specific) are clinically meaningful endpoints for each subgroup and may be appropriately compared, however, since these are relatively rare events, only the very long range studies are able to provide this information. Recently, the concept of *worsening free survival* has emerged as a surrogate endpoint to reflect the clinical decision to definitively alter therapy even without clear pathological evidence of disease progression *(24)*. Thus, time to cystectomy, radiation therapy, and systemic chemotherapy might all be counted as appropriate "worsening" events.

Since all of these outcome determinations depend heavily on time, it is vital to know the degree of follow-up. To properly interpret clinical trials of tumor prophylaxis, a randomized prospective control group for reference comparison is needed as well as a breakdown of clinical parameters that define the risks for recurrence and progression. Differences in treatment regimen including use of retreatment, cross-over, and maintenance therapy must likewise be critically considered.

Intravesical BCG for Prophylaxis after TURB

Multiple clinical trials directly comparing TURB alone to BCG plus TURB for tumor prophylaxis (i.e., no CIS) have demonstrated a statistically significant benefit in reduction of bladder cancer recurrence rate ranging between 20–57% at median follow-ups of 2–7 yr (25–32) (Table 2). In aggregate, this amounts to an estimated net benefit of over 30% vs surgery alone, an amount over twice that reported for intravesical chemotherapy by Lamm using a similar comparison technique (2). Interestingly, the greatest clinical benefits appear to be derived by those patients with more recurrent or aggressive disease, including prior chemotherapy failures (22,25,26). Median disease free interval increases may exceed 100% while recurrence index is generally reduced 3–4 fold. However, while several prophylaxis studies have shown a trend in reduction of progression rate, only Pagano could demonstrate a statistically significant reduction albeit with relatively short follow-up (26).

BCG for Residual Disease

One of the most demonstrable examples of intravesical BCG's anticancer activity is its ability to ablate existing bladder tumors either following incomplete TURB (residual tumor) or in place of TURB as primary therapy (33–42) (Table 3). While the ablative effect of one course of BCG on residual papillary tumors varies between 15–70%, a significant and consistent total salvage rate of approximately 60% is found if at least one additional course of therapy is included. By comparison, similar intravesical chemotherapy trials have reported complete response rates for residual disease of between 30–50% (43). Those BCG studies providing 1–3 yr follow-up show only a marginal drop off over time but this is difficult to interpret given the tendency to institute various regimens of maintenance therapy. Results from these trials also suggest it is prudent to: 1) perform debulking TURB whenever possible especially if tumor burden exceeds 3 cms; 2) institute therapy soon after TURB (within 10–21 d); and 3) use caution when treating residual T1 grade 2–

Table 2
Tumor Recurrence After TURB With or Without BCG (Non-CIS)

Author	Year	Number	TURB	BCG	Net Benefit	Followup	Statistics	BCG regimen	Tumor type	Remarks
Lamm	1985	57	52%	20%	32%	30 Mo	$p < 0.008$	qwk ×6; late addition maint BCG q3–6 Mo	Recurrent ×1 pTa, T1; gr 2	Crossover for ~1/3 control; Median relapse 24 vs 48 mo; Musc. progr. 8% vs 3% (NS)
Pagano	1991	133	83%	26%	57%	21 Mo	$p < 0.001$	qwk ×6; repeat if NR; qMo × 1Yr; q4Mo × 1Yr	Recurrent < 2yr ~40% chemo failures	1/2 Dose BCG; Musc. progr. 17% vs 4% BCG ($p < 0.005$)
Melekos	1993	94	59%	32%	27%	32 Mo	$p < 0.05$	qwk ×6 + 4 (high risk); q 3Mo × 2Yr; q6Mo	~2/3 primary, solitary Ta gr 1–2	Musc. progr. 12% vs 3% BCG (NS); Stage progr. 22% vs 7% ($p = 0.07$)
Yang	1994	97	65%	34%	31%	70 Mo	Favor BCG	Not specified	Not specified	
Zhang	1995	160	46%	18%	28%	1–7 Yr	Favor BCG	Not specified	Not specified	
Krege (NS)	1996	224	46%	26%	20%	20 Mo	$p < 0.05$	qwk ×6; qMo ×4	~3/4 Ta gr 1–2	Musc. progr. 6% vs 4.5% BCG
Tkachuk	1996	180	43%	13%	30%	3 Yr	Favor BCG	qwk x8; qMo x1yr	~1/2 primary/solitary	
Iantorno	1999	146	100%	62%	38%	55 Mo	$p < 0.05$	qwk x6; qMo x1Yr	Recurrent pTCC	1/2 Dose BCG; Musc. progr. 10% for both (NS)
TOTAL		1091	61%	29%	32%					

Table 3
BCG for Tumor Ablation

Author	Year	Number	% CR	BCG regimen	Tumor type	Remarks
Douville	1978	6	67%	qwk ×6	Recurrent pTCC	59% by 9 mo's; mean f/u 19 mo's
Morales	1981	17	70%	qwk ×6	Incomplete TURB Ta, T1, gr 2–3	6/6 recurrent gr 3 failed
Brosman	1984	27	15% 6 wks 44% 12 wks 63% 18 wks	qwk ×6 repeat if NR × 2	Recurrent pTCC < 3cm No CIS	No benefit after 18 wks CR's kept on maintenance
DeKernion	1985	22	36%	qwk ×6	Ta gr 1–2; no CIS 86% thiotepa failures	1/1 pt responded to 2nd course (43%) CR evaluated at 13 mo's
Heney	1986	98	41%	qwk ×6	Mixed pTCC & CIS (22%)	~1/3 cases w/ large tumor burden
Schellhammer	1986	22	55% 6 wks 64% add'tl	qwk ×6	Mixed recurrent, multiple ~1/2 failed thiotepa, 1/2 CIS	2/2 pt w/ partial response NED after additional 3–5 q mo treatment
Pansadora	1987	47	53% 6 wks 66% 12 wks	qwk ×6 repeat if NR	pTCC gr 2–3, CIS (20%) 1/3 resid TURB; 2/3 chemorec	Minimal benefit to 3rd course (1/16 CR)
Kavoussi	1988	17	41% 6 wks 65% 12 wks	qwk ×6 repeat if NR × 1–4	Recurrent Ta, T1; gr 1–3	Initial CR 59%; results @ 20 mo's No benefit after 2nd treatment
Khanna	1990	53	70% aggregate	qwk ×6 repeat if NR	No CIS 60% Ta, gr 1–2	
Akaza	1995	125	66%	qwk ×8	Ta, T1 no TURB	~23% relapse at 4 year f/u
TOTAL		434	59% (optimized)			

231

3 disease since these tumors appears to be less responsive to BCG ablation alone.

BCG for Carcinoma In Situ

With its high progression rate and inaccessibility to complete surgical
resection, CIS represents the prototype disease indication for intravesical therapy. Numerous BCG therapy trials for CIS have been reported
previously and essentially demonstrate aggregate complete response rates
between 70–75% if up to 2 induction cycles are used *(44)*. Similar results
have been reported with multiple different BCG strains worldwide and
exceed those reported for chemotherapy trials which range between
38% for thiotepa to 53% for mitomycin C making BCG the initial therapy
of choice for CIS *(45)*. Excellent results have been obtained for primary
CIS, secondary CIS, and concomitant CIS *(46)*. Over half of complete
responders remain disease free over 5 yr out from start of therapy resulting in a substantial reduction in the need for alternative therapy, primarily cystectomy *(47–49)*.

Comparative Clinical Trials of BCG Versus Chemotherapy

Most studies suggest BCG is superior to chemotherapy for tumor
prophylaxis after TURB *(27,29,30,49–58)* (Table 4). However, there
remains controversy regarding Mitomycin C with 3 trials favoring BCG
and 4 trials showing no significant difference. Two independent Dutch
trials *(56,57)*, in particular, suggest equivalence if not superiority for Mitomycin over BCG for recurrent tumors in the absence of CIS. The reason
for this discrepancy is not entirely clear. Treatment schedules for both
BCG and Mitomycin were different and patient selection was more biased
toward lower risk patients in the Dutch studies where the superiority of
BCG may not be so clear. Noncontroversial was the observation that
fewer and less severe side effects were found in Mitomycin treatment
arms. Given the current ambiguity, it would appear that both Mitomycin
and BCG remain appropriate first line therapeutic options in low to intermediate risk patients but that BCG may be preferred for higher risk
groups, especially against stage T1 grade 3 tumors.

Large comparative trials of BCG versus chemotherapy for CIS are
relatively few but strongly support BCG as first line therapy. The South
West Oncology Group (SWOG) study comparing BCG to adriamycin
showed initial complete response rates of 70% vs 34%, respectively that
decreased to 45% and 18% by 5 yr ($p < 0.001$) *(49)*. Similarly, Malmstrom
reported 55% freedom from disease at 5 yr for BCG vs 26% for Mitomycin C ($p = 0.04$) *(58)*.

Table 4
Comparative Clinical Trials of Tumor Recurrence After BCG or Chemotherapy (Non-CIS)

Author	Year	Number	TURB	Thiotepa	Adr/Epi	MMC	BCG	Followup	Statistics	Remarks
Brosman	1982	44		47%			0%	>24 Mo	p < 0.01	Intensive 2 yr regimens
Tachibana	1989	77			73% (A)		27%	3 Yr	p < 0.002	? Randomized trial
Martinez	1990	176		36%	43% (A)		13%	3 Yr	p < 0.004	~3 × decrease recurrence index
Rintala	1991	91				62%	35%	24 Mo	p < 0.01	~3 × decrease recurrence index
Lamm	1991	131			83% (A)		63%	65 Mo	p = 0.015	Median relapse 10 vs 23 mo's
Lamm	1995	377				54%	40%	30 Mo	p < 0.02	Median relapse 18 vs 36 mo's
Zhang	1995	385		31%		30%	18%	1–7 Yrs	Favor BCG	? Randomized trial
Melekos	1993/96	161	46%		46% (E)		35%	33 Mo	NS	BCG greatest benefit for T1 Gr3
Krege	1996	337	59%			27%	25%	20 Mo	NS	2 Year Rx w/ MMC; 6 Mo w/ BCG
Vegt	1995	387	46%			43%	46% RIVM 64% TICE	36 Mo	NS p = 0.01	MMC × 6 Mo w/ 3 Rxs for recurrence BCG qwk × 6; repeat if recur < 6 mos
Witjes	1998	344				47%	54%	7.2 Yrs	NS	Weighted toward lower stage and grade
Malmström	1999	167				66%	57%	64 Mo	NS	Intensive 2 year course for MMC and BCG 67% vs 45% (BCG) recurrence for Gr3

233

Long-Term Results with BCG
on Tumor Recurrence, Progression and Survival

With several independent clinical BCG trials maturing since the early to mid 1980s, it is now possible to provide reliable 5, 10, and even 15 yr data on the fate of patients treated with BCG *(40,47–49,56–63)* (Table 5). It is clear that the greatest number of recurrences occur within the first year, often at the time of the first cystoscopic evaluation even despite various retreatment and maintenance schedules. Among medium to high risk patients with recurrent or aggressive disease, this amounts to a remarkably consistent 30–35% initial failure rate. By 5 yr roughly half of all the originally treated patients have relapsed. Beyond 5 yr there appears to be continued dropouts albeit at a slower rate of under 4% per year. The longest term study to date by Herr and colleagues suggests this levels off between 10–15 yr with roughly 1/3 of patients completely free of disease but 1/2 experiencing disease progression *(63)*. The updated results from the Washington University group show that, in general, the earlier the relapse, the more likely the disease is to be life-threatening *(48)*. This is especially true for relapses within the first 3–6 mo that are accompanied by positive cytology or stage/grade progression *(60)*. Indeed, such features portend an ominous prognosis with unrecognized muscle invasion, metastasis, and reduced survival *(64)*. This increased risk of progressive bladder cancer persists even up to 5 yr out from the onset of successful BCG therapy while recurrences beyond 5 yr tend to be more manageable although occasionally these too can be significant *(48)*. For original tumors with accompanying multifocal CIS, sites outside the bladder vault such as the upper tracts and prostatic ducts may be the source of occurrence in up to 20% of cases *(63)*. These collective observations substantiate the need for close surveillance of both upper and lower tracts during the first 5–10 yr and an aggressive policy for recurrences displaying high grade features.

Whether BCG decreases tumor progression in the long term or merely delays inevitable failure cannot be determined with confidence from the studies to date. Small numbers, low intrinsic progression rates and insufficient follow-up in part may be responsible but it is noteworthy that even in several aforementioned larger comparative BCG/TURP/chemotherapy trials no absolute differences, let alone statistical differences, have been observed in progression to muscle invasive disease. Where apparent improvements in progression have been reported, statistical significance was either not achieved *(25,27,52)*, or follow-up was too short *(26)*. The SWOG study randomizing BCG to adriamycin did not show a difference in progression or survival but 3 times as many patients

Table 5
Long Term Effects of BCG on Recurrence, Progression, and Survival

Author	Year	Med f/u	Tumor type	Freedom from disease	Progression	Dz Sp survival	Crude survival	Remarks
Lamm	1991	65	CIS	74% (1 yr); 45% (5 yr)		72% (5 yr)	59% (5 yr)	7/127 cystectomies for BCG vs 21/135 for ADR
			Ta, T1	62% (1 yr); 37% (5 yr)		79% (5 yr)	70% (5 yr)	Composite analysis 6 trials
DeJager	1991	47	CIS	65% (1 yr); 39% (5 yr)				
Malmstrom	1999	64	CIS	68% (1 yr); 55% (5 yr)	16% (5 yr) composite	88% (5 yr) composite	75% (5 yr) composite	No difference in progression or survival BCG vs MMC
			Ta, T1	68% (1 yr); 46% (5 yr)				
Witjes	1998	86	CIS	56% (1 yr); 45% (5 yr) 45% (10 yr)	10% (5 yr) 17% (10 yr) composite	91% @ med f/u composite	73% @ med f/u composite	pTCC progression favor MMC 11.5% vs 3% (p = 0.006)
			Ta, T1	69% (1 yr); 49% (5 yr) 45% (10 yr)				No survival difference
Vegt	1995	36	Mixed	70% (1 yr); 54% (5 yr)	5% @ med f/u			No difference BCG vs MMC
Kavoussi	1988	20	Ta, T1	69% (20 m); 69% (48 m)	13% (20 m)	94% (20 m)	87% (20 m)	Includes best results
Coplen	1990	48	CIS	72% (20 m); 59% (48 m)	17% (48 m)	85% (74 m)	71% (74 m)	of 1 or 2 treatments
Nadler	1994	74	Residual	65% (20 m); 59% (48 m)	28% (74 m)			
			All	70% (20 m); 59% (48 m) 54% (74 m)	composite			
Herr	1988	72	CIS + Ta, T1	37% (6 yr) vs 0% TUR	28% (6 yr) vs 35% TUR	86% (6 yr) vs 60% TUR		Worsening: cystectomy, prog or mets 28% vs 58% TUR
Herr	1992	12 yr	CIS + Ta, T1	31% (12 yr)	41% (12 yr)	80% (12 yr)	77% (12 yr)	Includes original 43 pt (above) + 18 early crossover controls addt'l BCG courses given in 1/3 progressed after 5 yrs
Herr	1995	10–14 yr	CIS + Ta, T1		38% (10 yr) vs 63% TUR	75% (10 yr) vs 55% TUR		~20% recurrence in prostate and upper tracts each
Cookson	1997	15 yr	CIS + Ta, T1		53% (15 yr) both BCG and TUR	62% combined NS between groups	40% combined NS difference	

underwent cystectomy in the adriamycin group suggesting a practical benefit in reducing "disease worsening" *(49)*. The strongest published evidence has come from the aforementioned study performed by Herr et al. in a randomized series of 86 patients with aggressive superficial bladder cancers, 57% of which had coincident CIS *(61)*. In this very high risk group, BCG therapy delayed tumor progression and prolonged short-term survival. At 6 yr, progression to muscle invasion/metastasis was significantly improved from 58% in TURB controls to 74% in BCG treated patients. Cystectomy was performed in 42% of control patients vs 26% of BCG treated patients at a median of 8 and 24 mo, respectively. Survival was also superior: 64% vs 84%, respectively. Unfortunately, these benefits were ultimately lost due to later recurrence and/or progression occurring over the next 10 yr of follow-up, often outside the bladder vault *(62,63)*. While it can be argued that crossover of TURB controls to BCG treatment, additional unscheduled BCG retreatments, non-optimized BCG regimens, and alternative therapies make definitive conclusions impossible, the fact remains that the burden of proof showing BCG alters ultimate progression and disease specific bladder cancer survival has not yet been met.

The Role of BCG Maintenance Therapy

Many modern BCG treatment programs incorporate some form of time-limited continuous retreatment with BCG for patients for which no demonstrable disease is present with the implicit assumption that this will help maintain a tumor-free status. This practice probably finds its origin from:

1. The historical use of maintenance intravesical chemotherapy (incidentally not proven to be effective);
2. The recognized benefit of additional courses of BCG reinduction therapy *(26,35,39,40,65)*;
3. The steady relapse rate of initial complete responders over time; and
4. The uncertainty in knowing whether all disease is eliminated or simply at a subclinical level of detection.

With many uncontrolled trials showing good overall results with this strategy, there has been little impetus for change. However, until recently there has not been any clear proof that such a policy has any real clinical benefit. Two early randomized controlled studies using either 1 dose of BCG q 3 mo or 1 dose monthly for 2 yr failed to demonstrate a statistical advantage to this approach *(66,67)*. In the former case, 42 evaluable patients split between maintenance and no maintenance had essentially identical Kaplan-Meier disease-free survival curves when followed out over 2 yr. In the latter case 93 randomized patients had the same mean number of tumors per month, equivalent disease free recurrence rates at 2 yr, and equivalent progression rates. Furthermore, in both trials additional local toxicity attributable to BCG was found. Studies from other countries have been similarly disappointing. Tachibana reported on 44 patients randomized to no maintenance, 12 monthly treatment or 18+ monthly treatment and did see more favorable results in the latter but statistical significance was not achieved *(51)*. Interestingly, while Akaza could not demonstrate any advantage to 12 monthly maintenance treatments for patients achieving a complete ablative response to BCG, a statistically significant difference of 37% at 1 yr and 41% at 3 yr was seen for patients having only a partial response requiring completion TURB *(42)*. Palou reported in a large randomized Spanish trial no benefit to routine additional 6 wk courses q 6 mo for 2 yr in patients with no evidence of disease after TUR plus BCG *(68)*.

Recently, the long-awaited results of the SWOG 8507 trial specifically intended to answer the maintenance question have been released indicating an alternative schedule may be useful *(69)*. Using 3 weekly miniseries administered at 3, 6, 12 mo then biannually to 3 yr, statistically significant differences in favor of maintenance therapy have been found over a 10 yr followup. For 233 randomized patients with CIS, 84% ultimately achieved a complete response with maintenance vs 68% without ($p = 0.004$) with durable benefits beyond 5 yr. Patients not free of disease at the first 3 mo evaluation appeared to benefit most, demonstrating this schedule also possesses ablative activity. For 254 patients with original papillary disease NED at the time of randomization, 87% were disease free at 2 yr in the maintenance arm compared to 57% without maintenance. At least a 20% differential persisted up to 5 yr then was gradually lost by 10 yr at which point less than 20% were NED and/or alive in both arms. For combined CIS plus papillary groups median recurrence free survival was roughly doubled from 36 to 77 mo while worsening free survival was reduced by a 6% differential even at the 10 yr mark ($p = 0.04$). An overall 5% survival differential favoring maintenance approached statistical significance ($p = 0.08$). Not surprisingly, maintenance therapy did not come without a price. One quarter of patients on maintenance experienced significant grade 3 toxicity, and less than half completed more than 3 cycles with only 16% completing all 7 planned cycles. On the basis of these results it has been argued that even more extended treatments should be given, perhaps indefinitely, to prevent the inexorable drop-off in response with time. Alternatively, the maintenance group as a whole benefited even without most patients completing a full 3 yr of therapy suggesting maximum benefit may have been achieved earlier. At this time, one can only say that this schedule should be regarded as the new benchmark to which other maintenance schedules should be compared.

Dose Reduction Strategies

Efforts to decrease BCG toxicity while maintaining or enhancing efficacy are currently under study. Several recent clinical trials have shown than decreasing the dose of BCG to one-half or one-third in the induction phase will lower the local toxicity by a 20-30% differential but controversy exists as to whether efficacy is sacrificed especially in the more high risk CIS and stage T1 grade 3 patients (26,70–80) (Table 6). In certain studies, cancer results were worse but in other cases they were actually better. Some of this discrepancy may be due to differences in various patient population sensitivity to BCG either genetically or from prior BCG immunization. US and Canadian populations, for instance, are rarely vaccinated with BCG while this practice had been or still is commonly used throughout much of the world. The routine use of rein-duction courses and extended maintenance regimens may also make up for a weaker induction course. However, until this controversy is resolved, a more sensible approach may be to reduce the dose during the mainte-nance phase to increase treatment tolerability, an option that still awaits formal clinical testing. Finally, there is at least one preliminary report (81) that every other week BCG dosing for low-intermediate risk patients may be as effective as the conventional every week dosing scheme but with reduced side effects.

RECOGNIZING
AND TREATING BCG TOXICITY

The toxic effects of BCG may occur both locally and systemically. The vast majority of patients experience a self-limited cystitis associ-ated with marked frequency, urgency and dysuria that escalates with later treatments (82–85). Symptoms usually begin 2–4 h after instillation, peak between 6-10 h and resolve rapidly over the next 24–48 h. Microscopic hematuria and pyuria are common while occasional gross hematuria and passage of "tissue" (actually white cell clots) occur in up to one-third. Systemic manifestation of the inflammatory response follow a similar timecourse and include fevers, chills, a flu-like malaise and occasional arthralgias. During reinduction or maintenance cycles, all of these symp-toms tend to be more intense, occur sooner after the instillation, and

Table 6
BCG Dose Reduction Trials

Author	Year	Number	BCG strain	Dose-std	Dose-low	Followup	Efficacy @ f/u	Toxicity	BCG schedule	Remarks
Uncontrolled trials										
Rintala	1989	36 Ta/T1 10 CIS	Pasteur	N/A	75 mg (1/2)	26 Mo (mean)	7 fold decr preRx Recr Rate 40% CR for CIS	dropout 19% no BCGitis	qwk ×4; qMo x2Yr	Better than MMC for Ta/T1 Not superior to MMC for CIS
Blumenstein	1990	136 CIS	Connaught	120 mg	N/A	65 Mo (med)	45% NED @ 5 Yrs	not specified	qwk ×6; q3Mo x2; q6Mo × 2Yr	No efficacy difference despite 23 fold variation in lot CFUs
Pagano	1991	70 Ta/T1 pap 12 T1 nodular 44 CIS	Pasteur	N/A	75 mg (1/2)	21 Mo (mean)	74% NED vs 17% TUR 33% NED 64% NED	Severe cystitis 5% Temp >102 17% No BCGitis	qwk ×6; repeat if NR; qMo × 1Yr	2nd course effective in 50–69% of first failures
Rivera	1993	108 T1 Gr2,3	Japanese	N/A	1 mg (1/80th)	37Mo (mean)	81% NED	None severe	qwk ×4; q2wk ×4; q Mo × 1Yr	Very low dose; no CIS
Mack	1995	25 Ta/T1 "high-risk"	Connaught	N/A	27 mg (1/3)	31 Mo (mean)	84% NED	No systemic toxicity Occasional severe local	qwk ×6; qMo × 1Yr	
Hurle	1996	51 T1 Gr3	Pasteur	N/A	75 mg (1/2)	33 Mo (med)	55% NED	Severe cystitis 4% Fever 14%, no BCGitis	qwk ×6; repeat if NR; qMo × 1Yr	2nd course effective in 54% 14% progression
Lebert	1998	35 T1 Gr3	Pasteur	N/A	75 mg (1/2)	45 Mo (mean)	71% NED	Not specified	qwk ×6; repeat if NR	2nd course effective in 4/11 29% disease worsening
Controlled trials										
Morales	1992	97 Ta/T1/CIS	Armand-Frappier	120 mg	60 mg (1/2)	21 Mo (mean)	67% NED std dose 37% NED low dose	Decreased toxicity from 33% to 12% w/ low dose	qwk ×6	Low dose especially worse for CIS with Ta
Takasi	1995	74 Ta/T1	Tokyo 172	80 mg	40 mg (1/2)	NS	Untreated BTs-no difference Pretreated BTs-std better	Lower toxicity w/ lower dose	qwk ×8	Retrospective study
Martinez	1995	381 Ta/T1 33 CIS	Connaught	81 mg	27 mg (1/3)	19 Mo (mean)	Std/Low 82% vs 80% NED CIS: 92% vs 69% NED Prog 2.4% vs 4.8%	Severe local 23% vs 4% Fever 27% vs 13% Pulmonary 2.3% vs 0.4%	qwk ×6; q 2wk ×6	Caution urged for low dose BCG use in CIS & Gr3 disease with ~2 fold increase in progression
Pagano Bassi	1995 1999 (update)	210 Ta/T1/ CIS	Pasteur	150 mg	75 mg (1/2)	59 Mo (med)	Std vs low: NED Ta: 58% vs 56% T1: 44% vs 53% CIS: 30% vs 62% ($p = 0.006$)	Std vs low Cystitis: 57% vs 32% Fever: 33% vs 18% Hematuria: 26% vs 13%	qwk ×6; repeat if NR; qMo × 2Yr	No difference in progression

239

reach the highest level by the 2nd or 3rd treatment. Most symptoms can be controlled with the appropriate use of acetaminophen, nonsteroidal anti-inflammatories (NSAIDs), urinary analgesics and antispasmodics. The practice of routinely administering antibiotics with catheterization is to be discouraged. If clinically indicated for non-BCG infection, penicillins, cephlosporins, trimethoprim/sulfa, and nitrofurantoin are preferred while fluoroquinolones, azithromycin and doxycycline are to be avoided since they are cidal to BCG and could affect efficacy *(86,87)*. Conversely, in a controlled study, short courses of anti-BCG specific antibiotics such as isoniazid (INH) have not been shown to diminish either the associated symptomatology or the incidence of serious BCG infection *(88)*. However, neither did they affect anticancer efficacy. Importantly, despite most patients experiencing some temporary toxicity from BCG therapy, two studies have shown that this does not adversely affect their overall long-term quality of life *(89,90)*.

Clinical signs of a more serious process, such as BCG intravasation into the blood stream (BCGosis), include exaggerated manifestations of the above systemic effects particularly if they occur early during the initial course of induction therapy, within 2 h after BCG instillation, or in the setting of traumatic catheterization. In the extreme case, a picture resembling gram negative sepsis may emerge with the rapid and sequential appearance of chills, rigors, high temperatures (often over 103°F) and hypotension likely as a result of high levels of bioactive inflammatory mediators known as cytokines released directly into the bloodstream. The estimated incidence for this life-threatening event is 0.4% *(91)*. Prompt fluid resuscitation measures should be instituted as well as antipyretics, antituberculosis antibiotics, and systemic steroids which has been shown to be life-saving in such instances *(see below) (92,93)*.

While any fever over 102.5°F associated with chills or rigors is cause for concern, this in itself is not a definite sign of BCGosis, especially if it occurs at the expected peak time and resolves within 24 h. This may represent a leak or spillover of bioactive cytokines from the bladder into the systemic circulation. In fact, higher therapeutic responses in such patients have been reported *(21)*. Such patients may be retreated with NSAID prophylaxis (e.g., ibuprofen 600 mg q 6 h × 3 beginning 2 h prior to therapy) and at a reduced dose of BCG (O'Donnell, unpublished data). Conversely, fevers that begin after 24 h, persist more than 48 h, or relapse in a diurnal pattern (usually in the early evening) are more indicative of an established BCG infection (BCGitis). Organ-specific manifestations may be present suggesting epididymal-orchitis, pneumonitis, and hepatitis that occur with a cumulative incidence of 2–3% *(94)*. CT scans may show a pattern typical of miliary spread in the liver or lung. These patients usually require hospitalization and the administration of double or triple drug therapy such as INH (300 mg/d), rifampin (600 mg/d) +/− ethambutol (1200 mg/d). A second or third generation fluoroquinolone may be added or substituted since it covers most gram negative infections and has moderate activity against BCG. BCG is resistant to both pyrizidimide and cycloserine. It is reasonably sensitive to amikacin but less to gentamicin or tobramycin *(87)*. Failure to improve on such therapy within a week or significant clinical deterioration should prompt institution of systemic steroids (e.g., prednisone 40 mg/d tapered over 2–6 wk) *(95)*. Antituberculosis drugs should be continued for 3, 6 or 12 mo depending on the severity of the presenting illness. Liver enzyme monitoring is required for INH and rifampin.

Prolonged symptomatic BCG cystitis and/or prostatitis (often associated with granulomas) can become a troubling problem during therapy and in the post BCG observation period. This is particularly more likely to occur during retreatment or prolonged maintenance therapy. This situation is best avoided by withholding BCG treatment until all significant symptoms from the prior instillation have subsided. A 1–2 wk delay has not been shown to reduce BCG efficacy in such a setting *(25,50)*. Reinstitution of BCG at a lower dose or premature termination of further treatment for this cycle may also be appropriate. If localized severe cystitis does occur and conservative symptomatic treatment measures fail, this condition can be treated with oral fluoroquinolones (3–12 wk) or oral INH. A short 2–3 wk oral steroid taper sandwiched in between antibiotic coverage has also been shown to be helpful in refractory cases *(96)*. The incidence of permanent bladder contracture after BCG is estimated as under 2% *(82,91)*. Other very rare events include a noninfectious hypersensitivity Reiter's type syndrome (urethritis, arthritis, conjunctivitis) and frank anaphylactic reactions *(97,98)*. Both require immediate and permanent cessation of further therapy.

BCG MECHANISM OF ACTION

BCG Is a Pleiotropic Immune Stimulator Oriented Toward Cellular Immunity

Mycobacteria have long been known to be potent stimulators of the immune response. Mycobacterial cell walls are widely used in complete Freund's adjuvant *(3,6)*. BCG has been shown to activate macrophages, NK cells, B cells, and various T cells (CD4$^+$, CD8$^+$ and γδ-T cells) in vitro and in vivo *(99–108)*. T helper type 1 cells (Th1), which are restrictive for cell-mediated immunity, appear more accessible to BCG than Th2 cells that are restrictive for humoral/allergic immunity *(109,110)*.

This is not surprising because BCG is an obligate intracellular pathogen and can only be effectively cleared by a cell mediated process. Analysis of cytokine production from murine splenocyte cultures, human peripheral blood mononuclear cell (PBMC) cultures and human urine during BCG treatment has demonstrated that BCG can stimulate the expression of interleukins IL-1, 2, 4, 6, 8, 10 and 12, TNF-α, GMCSF, IP-10, and IFN-γ *(111–127)*. Of these, IFN-γ appears to be a critical mediator of anti-mycobacterial immunity as both mice and humans with defective IFN-γ production or IFN-γ receptors are susceptible to overwhelming mycobacterial infection *(128,129)*. Furthermore, Th1/Th2 polarity is directly responsible for effective pathogen elimination that manifests itself in the case of leprosy as either a pathogen-poor tuberculoid form (Th1) or a pathogen-rich lepromatous form (Th2) *(110)*.

BCG Antitumor Therapy Appears to Depend on a Cell-Mediated Th1 Immune Response

Although the exact mechanism of BCG action in bladder cancer remains incompletely understood, it appears to rely on cell-mediated immunity. Within 4–6 h after a late induction cycle BCG instillation there is massive pyuria containing neutrophils and mononuclear cells *(101, 104)*. Parallel with this cellular exudate, Th1 cytokines (IL-2, IFN-γ and TNF-α) appear in patient urine at the time when bladder cancer cytology reverts from malignant to nonmalignant *(130)*. A typical delayed type hypersensitivity response (DTH) in the bladder can be histologically observed after clinical BCG instillation, showing a mononuclear cell infiltration into the superficial layers of the bladder associated with edema, denudation, and granuloma formation *(101,112,131–133)*. Immunohistologically, the major types of infiltration cells can be identified to be CD4[+] (helper) and CD8[+] (cytotoxic) T cells, macrophages, and a minor amount of NK cells *(101,102,133–135)*. A phenomenon of elevated expression of MHC class I and II antigens on urothelium is also apparent that persists for 3–6 mo after BCG treatment *(102,136)*. Augmented peripheral blood lymphocyte responses to BCG persist for a similar period of time before eventually waning *(137)*.

The relationship between measured cytokines and tumor responses in patients receiving BCG remains incompletely defined but suggests a benefit to Th1 vs Th2 orientation. Patients with high urinary IL-2 expression are more likely to have durable bladder cancer responses *(111,120, 138)*. In contrast, bladder cancer patients whose PBMCs during active BCG therapy show a depressed ability to make IL-2 mRNA have much lower clinical cancer responses *(139)*. IL-2 production is strongly linked to IFN-γ production in vitro and in vivo and both tend to rise in parallel in the urine during initial induction therapy *(113,119,120,140)*. The clinical utility of urinary IFN-γ levels has been controversial, possibly due to the inherent instability of this molecule in acidic urine, but generally higher levels have been associated with a better prognosis *(113, 115,127,141)*. On the other hand, patients with elevations in serum antibody to BCG or elevated urinary IL-6, typical of Th2 immune responses, are less likely to be cured of their bladder cancer by BCG *(142,143)*. Moreover, the potent Th1 suppressing cytokine IL-10 is readily assayable in the urine of patients after BCG treatment typically rising after the peak of IFN-γ and IL-2 suggesting it may play a role in shutting down the Th1 response *(144)*.

While multiple cytokines are induced by BCG, direct antitumor effects have been linked primarily to IFN-γ and TNF-α . Both inhibit bladder tumor proliferation as well as upregulate the expression of major histocompatibility complex (MHC) class I and II antigens and adhesion molecules on bladder cancer cells *(102,145–149)*. This change in surface phenotype increases the likelihood that tumor cells will be recognized by CD4+ T cells or CD8+ cytotoxic T lymphocytes (CTLs) *(150–153)*. TNF-α and IFN-γ also induce Fas receptor (a homologue to the TNF receptor) expression on bladder cancer cells providing a mechanism for apoptotic destruction by Fas ligand positive activated T cells that are not MHC restricted but usually associated with a Th1 response *(154–156)*. BCG-activated killer (BAK) cells, an unique subpopulation of IFN-γ dependent killer cells, are also expanded by BCG stimulation and exhibit cytotoxicity against NK-resistant bladder cancer cells *(157, 158)*. It has also been found that BCG induces a hostile environment for endothelial cell proliferation through its induction of IFN-γ, TNF-α, and the anti-angiogenic chemokine IP-10 *(125)*.

Studies on animal bladder tumor models have further reinforced the requirement of Th1 cells for BCG anticancer efficacy. In these models, the ability to either prevent or retard the outgrowth of tumor with BCG has been shown to be T-cell dependent *(159,160)*. Similarly, immunocompetent mice lose the capacity to reject bladder tumors after BCG treatment if they are first depleted in vivo of either CD4+ or CD8+ T cells *(132)*. IFN-γ and IL-2 mRNA are upregulated in the bladder tissue of mice treated with intravesical BCG *(161)* and potentiated in genetically altered IL-10 knockout mice suggesting IL-10 is a functional Th1 inhibitor *(162)*. Taken together, these observations strongly imply that both T cell subsets and a cell-mediated immune response characteristic of Th1 are required for BCG antitumor immunity.

A Model of the BCG Antitumor
Mechanism Based on the Th1 Hypothesis

STEP 1: INVASION

BCG initiates its action by establishing a localized infection in the bladder that involves both attachment and internalization. BCG binds to the urothelium largely via a fibronectin dependent attachment process previously defined by Ratliff and colleagues (163). Antibodies or peptide mimics to a recently cloned BCG fibronectin attachment protein (FAP) specifically reduces BCG attachment and subsequent anti-cancer activity in the intravesical mouse bladder cancer model using the transplantable cell line MB49 (164). Once attached, BCG is internalized into urothelial cells (both malignant and normal) via an energy dependent process involving integrin receptors (154,165). It is not known if cancer cells preferentially ingest BCG more than normal urothelium or if this is important for the anti-cancer mechanism.

STEP 2: DANGER SIGNAL GENERATED

According to a new paradigm largely championed by Polly Matzinger, productive immune responses require an inciting threatening or damaging event that acts as a signal for immune cell recruitment and activation (166). In the case of BCG, there must be some specificity to this signal in order to recruit the characteristic submucosal monocytic and T-cell infiltration seen with BCG treatment. While the complete details are not known, certain chemokines such as IL-8, MCP-1 and RANTES have been found in the urine early after BCG treatment and likely originate in part directly from the urothelium (121,167).

STEP 3: RECRUITMENT OF LEUKOCYTES INTO THE BLADDER

The net effect of chemokine signals is an escalating recruitment of monocytic and granulocytic leukocytes into the bladder with each successive weekly BCG instillation. While neutrophils dominate acutely in the urine, T cells eventually establish residence in the submucosa in scattered forms or as more defined granulomata likely as a result of the later production of active T-cell chemokines such as IP-10 (125). The importance of T cells is further suggested by late tumor elimination found in ~20% of patients an additional 3 mo after cessation of active BCG treatment (64,69). A similar process of neutrophilic replacement with activated T cells has been documented during the successful elimination of the intracellular parasite Listeria, a process that requires Th1 cells. IFN-γ knockout mice succumb to overwhelming Listeria infection in this model without any T cell replacement (168).

STEP 4: ACTIVATION OF RECRUITED LEUKOCYTES

The activation process for recruited leukocytes has partly been eluci-dated through the study of in vitro mononuclear cell subsets. Monocyte-macrophages or the recently identified resident CD1a+ dendritic cells (DC) of the bladder are likely crucial in orchestrating T-cell activation *(169)*. These professional antigen presenting cells (APCs) can display BCG antigens on major histocompatibility complexes (MHC) I and II while providing necessary co-stimulatory signals through B7-1 and B7-2 as well as important cytokine co-activators such as IL-12, IL-15, IL-18, and TNF-α *(170,171)*. While it has been shown that murine tran-sitional cell cancers themselves may present BCG antigen, this is less likely to occur in humans since co-stimulatory B7 molecules have not been found on normal or malignant human urothelium *(150,172)*. IFN-γ can strongly potentiate APC activity and may possibly first be expressed by early infiltration of NK and $\gamma\delta$ T cells whose antigen activation require-ments are much less stringent than $\alpha\beta$ T cells. Once this process is initi-ated, a proliferative and activating Th1 cascade ensues in which repetitive antigen exposure elaborates IL-2 which synergizes with IL-12 and TNF-α to make more IFN-γ which activates APCs to make more IL-12 and so forth. Simultaneously, there is the potential for NK & T-cell activation by IL-2 and IL-12, fas ligand induction on CD4+ and CD8+ cells by repe-titive T-cell receptor engagement with BCG antigens, BCG activated killer (BAK) cell induction (an IL-12 dependent process), and non-spe-cific activation of macrophages and neutrophils by IFN-γ and TNF-α .

STEP 5: ALTERATION OF LOCAL CANCER PHENOTYPE BY CYTOKINE MILIEU TO MAKE BETTER TARGETS FOR IMMUNE ELIMINATION

The elaboration of high levels of bioactive cytokines in the urine that bathes the local tumor is likely responsible for the observed marked long-lasting elevation of MHC Class I and II molecules, ICAMs, and Fas seen on the urothelium of patients after BCG therapy. IFN-γ, TNF-α, and IP-10 also directly inhibit bladder cancer proliferation and/or angio-genesis *(125)*. Theoretically these changes should make the tumor cell a better target for immune recognition and elimination, however, no conclusive proof for this requirement yet exists. Indeed, intravesical clinical use of either recombinant IFN-γ or TNF-α has not demonstrated significant anti tumor activity, suggesting these cytokines by themselves are not sufficient for tumor killing *(173,174)*.

STEP 6: EFFECTOR CELL KILLING OF MALIGNANT CELLS

This is the LEAST understood of all the BCG mechanistic processes. Indeed, the identity of the actual effector cell(s) directly responsible for tumor killing is unknown. While there is strong evidence for a T-cell dependent process as discussed above, there is no direct evidence for classic tumor-specific cytotoxic T cells (CTLs). In murine bladder cancer models, elimination of a local tumor will not prevent outgrowth of a distant tumor. Similarly, in humans tumor persistence in the isolated ureters or prostatic ducts is common despite clearance of all cancer in the bladder. Compatible effector mechanisms thus include:

1. Direct killing of BCG infected bladder cancer cells by BCG-specific CTLs.
2. Direct killing by MHC non-restricted NK cells, γδ T cells or the BAK cell subset.
3. Direct killing by tumoricidal macrophages.
4. Bystander killing of Fas+ bladder cancer by Fas ligand+ BCG-specific T cells.
5. Direct killing of ICAM1+ bladder cancer by activated neutrophils expressing the cognate LFA-1 receptor *(175)*.

Step 7: Restoration or Repression

Depending on the conditions of BCG delivery and the immune status of the host, at least 2 different extremes in outcome may result. Once an adequate series of BCG stimuli is given, the host may ultimately clear the BCG infection, disperse/eliminate activated WBCs and repopulate the urothelium from a normal basal layer. Some resident T cells and macrophages persist in BCG granulomas in the bladder commonly seen even months to years after BCG therapy. In the event of excessive BCG infection, a self-protective down-modulatory anergy may occur that resembles the Th2 state in leprosy or anergic tuberculosis *(176)*. Such an anergic state has been observed in approximately 15% of bladder cancer patients, mostly in those receiving retreatment with BCG during the maintenance or reinduction phases. However, since most patients show increasing levels of immunosuppressive IL-10 following the peak IFN-γ urinary cytokine production, a general pattern of down-modulation probably occurs to some extent in all patients. Importantly, experiments in IL-10 knock-out mice have revealed that higher cancer successes can be obtained if this down-modulatory process is interrupted (Ratliff, personal communication).

Step 8: Rechallenge

During maintenance or reinduction therapy, usually started months after finishing the induction cycle, the entire process is accelerated likely due to reactivation and recruitment of resident and systemic memory T cells. Clinical responses in terms of symptoms and urinary Th1 cytokines are more rapid and stronger but down-regulation is also more likely *(176,177)*.

NEW PROSPECTS
AND CONTINUED CONTROVERSIES

Regimen Modifications

The conventional BCG treatment regimen has come under increased scrutiny with the emerging knowledge about BCG's effect on the human immune system during clinical therapy. Realizing that the original 6 weekly induction therapy by Morales from close to 25 yr ago was completely arbitrary (but nonetheless clearly successful), several rational modifications are likely to be explored in the near future (Table 7). Additionally, if a good surrogate marker of the appropriate immune response in the bladder can be found, it may be possible to eventually individualize therapy on a real-time basis.

Intravesical Combination Therapy Strategies

There have been several recent investigations into the use of combined intravesical chemotherapy plus BCG therapy for superficial bladder cancer using various regimens of sequential or alternating treatments (178–188) (Table 8). The results are difficult to interpret with confidence but suggest that peri-operative initiation with chemotherapy followed by an adequate course of BCG stimulation is superior to chemotherapy alone. There is already strong clinical evidence that a single peri-operative dose of chemotherapy is comparable to a longer course initiated 2–3 wk later, possibly as a consequence of reducing tumor seeding during TURB (189–191). There is also good experimental evidence that chemotherapy can increase fibronectin expression on the bladder surface, facilitating BCG adherence (178). However, a randomized control trial to test this specific hypothesis has not yet been performed.

The possibility of combining BCG plus interferon-alpha has also received much attention. In vitro studies have revealed that BCG and IFN-α are potentially synergistic via direct anti-proliferative effects against bladder cancer cell lines (107,192). IFN-α will also cooperate with BCG-induced cytokines IFN-α and TNF-α to induce potentially important phenotypic changes in bladder cancer cells (193,194). Most importantly, IFN-α has been shown to clearly potentiate and polarize in vitro human PBMC Th1 responses to BCG by at least an order of magnitude, predominantly by reducing IL-10 production (176). By itself, intravesical IFN-α has been shown to have moderate clinical activity as a single agent against bladder cancer, inducing a durable 15% complete response against patients with CIS failing BCG (195). Physical mixtures of BCG plus IFN-α are pharmacological biocompatible (196). Already 2 published trials using reduced dose BCG plus IFN-γ have demonstrated improved

Table 7

Immunological Observations and Clinical Implications for Future Study

Observation	Implication
Presensitized patients make earlier (usually within 1–2 weeks) and stronger PBMC and urinary cytokine responses when rechallenged or retreated while BCG naïve patients begin to respond usually after 3–4 weeks.	1) Inoculate patients with single intradermal BCG dose at time of TURB then treat 3 weeks later in bladder. 2) Extend induction treatment for BCG naïve patients by 2 weeks.
Once sensitized, patients continue to make strong recall local responses to BCG even 1,2,3 weeks later but may diminish thereafter.	Delays of 1 or 2 weeks off weekly BCG schedule are likely all right especially to increase tolerance.
Maximum immune activity occurs with the 2nd dose in a BCG retreatment or maintenance series (priming effect).	At least 2 sequential doses are preferable to monthly therapy.
Higher BCG doses and extended therapy can actually induce BCG unresponsiveness in previously treated patients.	1) Lower BCG dose during retreatment and maintenance. 2) Reduce re-induction from 6 to 3 or 4 treatments.
Local moderate symptoms generally correlate with the local cytokine immune responses in the bladder; exaggerated local symptoms often proceed onset of reduced immune responsiveness and prolonged local toxicity (BCG cystitis).	1) Titrate regimen intensity and duration to maintain moderate and acceptable toxicity. 2) Do not give next sequential treatment on schedule if symptoms from prior treatment have not resolved.
Patients without any local bladder symptoms often fail to make significant immune responses in the bladder.	Consider more intense regimens or alternatives especially if planning retreatment with BCG.
Maximum PBMC responses and local immunological changes in bladder subside between 3–6 months.	Optimal time for maintenance is likely q 3–6 months.

Table 8
Combined Chemotherapy-BCG Clinical Trials

Author	Year	Number	Tumor type	Chemo type	Regimen	Results single	Results chemo+BCG	Followup	Statistics	Remarks
Coplen	1990	14	Mixed	ADR	ADR qWk ×4 then BCG qWK ×6 alt BCG		11/14 (79%) NED	7 Mo	N/A	3 Patients removed for toxicity
Gelabert-Mas	1993	66	pTCC	MMC	MMC vs MMC alt BCG	Equal recurrence		NA	NS	Progression lower in combo but NS
Erol	1994	14	pTCC	Epirubicin	Epi x 2 h then BCG ×2 h qWk ×6 then qMo ×6		8/9 (89%) NED	14 Mo	N/A	7 Delayed and 5 unable to tolerate due to severe local toxicity
Uekado	1994	29	pTCC	Epirubicin	Periop Epi × 1 then BCG qWk ×6 beginning week 1		28/29 (97%) NED	20 Mo	N/A	1 Early failure @ 3 mo's w/ progression; well tolerated; 1 withdrawal for cystitis
Rintala	1995	68	CIS	MMC	Periop MMC then qWk ×4 then MMC vs BCG/alt MMC qMo ×1yr; q 3Mo ×1yr	47% NED @ 24 Mo	74% NED @ 24 Mo	33 Mo	p = 0.04	~25% Differential at all evaluation points progression 10% vs 7% (NS) well tolerated
Rintala	1996	182	Recurrent pTCC	MMC	Same as above	36% NED @ 24 Mo	38% NED @ 24 Mo	34 Mo	NS	Low progression rate 3% for both 6% termination in both for toxicity
Van der Meijden	1996	35	pTCC Marker lesion	MMC	MMC qWk ×4 then BCG qWk ×6		54% CR Ablation marker	3 Mo	N/A	Tolerable toxicity
Witjes	1998	182	MF or recurrent pTCC, CIS	MMC	MMC qWk ×10 vs MMC qWk ×4 then BCG qWk ×6	54% NED @ med f/u	61% NED @ med f/u	32 Mo	NS	Possible advantage to combo w/longer f/u progression 4% vs 6% (NS) toxicity similar; no worse than BCG alone
Wijkstrom	1999	291	CIS	MMC	BCG qWk ×6; qMo ×11 vs MMC qWk ×6; BCG/alt MMC qMo ×11	BCG: 65% NED	45% NED @ 18 Mo	18 Mo	p = 0.05	Preliminary results only toxicity higher in BCG monotherapy
Kaasinen	1999	202	pTCC Gr 1–2	MMC IFN-α	Periop MMC then qWk ×4 then BCG qMo ×10 vs BCG/alt IFN-α qMo ×10	MMC/BCG 75% NED @ 24 Mo	MMC/BCG IFN 34% NED @ 24 Mo	29 Mo	p < 0.001	Minimal toxicity Most Ta low grade tumors
Ali-el-dein	1999	124	MF or recurrent or T1 Gr2–3 or > 3 cm or CIS	Epirubicin	BCG/alt Epi qWk ×6; qMo ×10 vs BCG qWk ×6; qMo ×10	BCG: 68% NED	83% NED @ 36 Mo	30 Mo	p = 0.05	Toxicity 2× as great w/ BCG alone progression 8.6% vs 4.6%–combo (NS)

tolerability and at least equivalent efficacy to BCG alone *(197,198)*. Preliminary results from small pilot trials in two different centers further suggest improved efficacy over BCG monotherapy *(195)*. Even more provocative is the use of combination low-dose BCG plus interferon-alpha for BCG failures which has yielded a >55% disease free rate at 2 yr in a 37 patient single institution study *(199)*. However, until these results are confirmed in larger studies, combination immunotherapy must still be regarded as investigational.

Use of Megadose Vitamins Following BCG Therapy

Deficiency of vitamin A produces increased susceptibility to chemical carcinogenesis *(200)*. The vitamin A analog, etritinate, has reduced tumor occurrence in superficial bladder cancer but is associated with moderate toxicity *(201,202)*. Pyridoxine (vitamin B6) was found to be as effective as thiotepa in reducing superficial bladder cancer recurrence *(203)*. The antioxidant vitamins C and E have not been specifically studied in bladder cancer but have been shown to reduce colon cancer and prostate cancer, respectively *(204,205)*. Vitamin E has also been shown to increase the skin test responsiveness to the BCG derivative PPD and protect against potential vitamin A toxicity *(206)*. With this in mind, a 65 patient randomized, double blind study comparing standard recommended daily allowance (RDA) vitamins to a megadose antioxidant formulation (primarily A, B6, C, E) for papillary superficial bladder cancer recurrence after BCG was performed *(20)*. Overall recurrence was 80% for RDA vs 40% ($p = 0.001$) for megavitamins with benefits first apparent after 1 yr of therapy but which persisted throughout the study period. These potentially exciting results also await independent verification.

Treating the High-Risk
Superficial Bladder Cancer Patient with BCG

The worst thing that can happen to a patient with bladder cancer is that he or she progresses to an unresectable stage during the time in which intravesical therapy or observation is underway. Given the very aggressive nature of stage T1 grade 3 bladder cancer which progresses to muscle invasive disease or metastatic disease at a rate of up to 50% in 3–5 yr *(207,207)*, it has been argued that immediate cystectomy is the most appropriate option *(209,210)*. However, multiple retrospective and prospective studies with BCG therapy have indicated that over two-thirds may achieve long progression-free survival with their bladders intact *(70,211–214)*. One key stipulation is that accurate staging be performed from the onset as several investigators have reported unrecognized residual T1 disease or even muscle invasive disease in 30–40% of cases *(215, 216)*. Unfortunately, there does not appear to be any clinical or genetic feature that predicts pre-treatment, the likelihood of response to BCG *(64)*. Even positive p53 immunostaining, which has been associated with more aggressive disease, has not proven to be a reliable discriminator prior to the initiation of BCG *(217–220)*. A frontline trial of BCG immunotherapy thus appears justified in most cases of high grade superficial bladder cancer without putting the patient at excess risk.

What to Do When BCG Fails

Many if not most patients eventually fail BCG *(48)*. The decision of how to handle these patients must be individualized based on the intrinsic tumor risk, pattern of failure, co-morbidity, and patient preference. For patients at high risk for disease progression such as those with stage T1 grade 3 tumors with CIS that fail immediately after one cycle of BCG, the radical treatment option must be considered early since up to one third have unsuspected muscle invasive disease for which topical therapy is not effective *(64,221)*. Conversely, a patient with recurrences of stage Ta, grade 1–2 tumors may explore many other conservative options without great fear of jeopardizing his/her survival. An analysis of the type of BCG failure is also important. Patients that never achieve a disease free state of greater than 6 months duration or who fail on active maintenance are unlikely to benefit from additional BCG alone while those that relapse a few years later can be retreated with a reasonably high expectation of success *(222)*. Similarly, relapsers with tumors that have increased in stage, grade, positive cytology, or are p53 positive deserve more aggressive action *(48,64,217)*. A positive cytology in the absence of a bladder lesion should additionally prompt a search for disease in the upper tract or prostate that occurs in up to 20% of patients if followed long enough *(221, 223)*. Unfortunately, some patients with locally advanced superficial disease are not candidates for radical surgery due to co-morbid medical illnesses. Others frankly refuse to consider losing their bladders even after extended discussions of risk. For all these circumstances, alternative conservative measures may be appropriate.

The utility of chemotherapy or alternative immunotherapy to salvage BCG failures is limited. In one small study of 21 patients, only 4 (19%) were disease free at 3 yr with Mitomycin *(58)*. In the pivotal trial leading to FDA approval for Valrubicin, an anthracycline derivative with higher lipid solubility, of 90 high risk patients treated once weekly for 6 wk only 16 (18%) were disease free at 6 mo. With successive follow-up less than half have remained disease free at 2 yr. Interferon-alpha monotherapy has also been used for BCG failures with limited success. In small series, the rough 1 yr disease free rate is approximately 18% for CIS and papillary disease *(195)*. All BCG refractory patients with CIS relapsed within 6 months while half of nonrefractory BCG failures were disease free at 1 yr. Moreover, 4 of these 5 responders have maintained no evidence of disease status for 33+ mo. Anecdotal reports on Keyhole Limpet Hemocyanin (KLH) immunotherapy have been encouraging but the agent is generally only available in the research setting *(224,225)*. A more provocative protocol that awaits confirmation of efficacy is the use of combination low-dose BCG plus interferon-alpha *(199)*.

External beam radiation therapy is rarely appropriate for the treatment of superficial bladder cancer because it may cause significant local morbidity while displaying limited efficacy. CIS is particularly resistant and low grade disease responds more poorly than higher grade disease. Some benefit may be derived for patients with stage T1 grade 3 tumors especially if combined with aggressive TURB and chemotherapy *(226,227)*. Photodynamic therapy using hematoporphyrin derivatives can achieve a high initial complete response rate especially against CIS but generalized cutaneous photosensitivity remains limiting *(228)*. Moreover, severe local irritative symptoms persisting for months are not uncommon as well as occasional bladder contractures. Such therapy is also only available at select centers.

CONCLUSION

BCG remains the most powerful weapon in the arsenal of topical therapeutics against superficial bladder cancer, especially for aggressive cases. While it may not ultimately prevent progression in the majority of patients, the early use of BCG can provide a long term state free of meaningful disease worsening. With newer refinements in regimen optimization there is reasonable hope even better results can be obtained in the future. However, in all cases, constant vigilance is required since progression to more advanced disease can occur insidiously. Superficial bladder cancer is often a lifelong disease but it must not necessarily be a life-shortening one so long as a rational approach is taken, accepting and appreciating the practical limitations that exist.

REFERENCES

1. Pawinski A, Sylvester R, Kurth KH, Bouffioux C, van der Meijden A, Parmar MK and Bijnens L. A combined analysis of European Organization for Research and Treatment of Cancer, and Medical Research Council randomized clinical trials for the prophylactic treatment of stage TaT1 bladder cancer. European Organization for Research and Treatment of Cancer Genitourinary Tract Cancer Cooperative Group and the Medical Research Council Working Party on Superficial Bladder Cancer. J Urol 1996; 156: 1934–1940, discussion 1940–1941.

2. Lamm DL, Riggs DR, Traynelis CL, Nseyo UO. Apparent failure of current intravesical chemotherapy prophylaxis to influence the long-term course of superficial transitional cell carcinoma of the bladder. J Urol 1995; 153: 1444–1450.

3. Crispen R. History of BCG and its substrains. Prog Clin Biol Res 1989; 310: 35–50.

4. Luelmo F. BCG vaccination. Am Rev Respir Dis 1982; 125: 70–72.

5. Behr MA, Wilson MA, Gill WP, Salamon H, Schoolnik GK, Rane S, Small PM. Comparative genomics of BCG vaccines by whole-genome DNA microarray. Science 1999; 284: 1520–1523.

6. van der Meijden AP, Debruyne FM, Steerenberg PA, de Jong WH. Aspects of non-specific immunotherapy with BCG in superficial bladder cancer: an overview. Prog Clin Biol Res 1989; 310: 11–33.

7. Mathe G, Amiel JL, Schwarzenberg L, Schneider M, Cattan A, Schlumberger JR, et al. Active immunotherapy for acute lymphoblastic leukaemia. Lancet 1969; 1: 697–699.

8. Hadziev S, Kavaklieva-Dimitrova J. [Use of BCG in human cancer]. Folia Med (Plovdiv) 1969; 11: 8–14.

9. Morton D, Eilber FR, Malmgren RA, Wood WC. Immunological factors which influence response to immunotherapy in malignant melanoma. Surgery 1970; 68: 158–163; discussion 163–164.

10. Coe JE, Feldman JD. Extracutaneous delayed hypersensitivity, particularly in the guinea- pig bladder. Immunology 1966; 10: 127–136.

11. Zbar B, Bernstein ID, Bartlett GL, Hanna MG Jr, Rapp HJ. Immunotherapy of cancer: regression of intradermal tumors and prevention of growth of lymph node metastases after intralesional injection of living Mycobacterium bovis. J Natl Cancer Inst 1972; 49: 119–130.

12. Morales A, Eidinger D, Bruce AW. Intracavitary Bacillus Calmette-Guerin in the treatment of superficial bladder tumors. J Urol 1976; 116: 180–183.

13. Martinez-Pineiro JA, Muntanola P. Nonspecific immunotherapy with BCG vaccine in bladder tumors: a preliminary report. Eur Urol 1977; 3: 11–22.

14. Lamm DL, Sarodosy MS, DeHaven JI. Percutaneous, oral, or intravesical BCG administration: what is the optimal route? Prog Clin Biol Res 1989; 310: 301–310.

15. Cymes M, Fleishmann J, Smith E. Invasive bladder cancer treated with intravesical BCG. J Urol 1992; 147(Suppl): 273A.

16. Brenner DW, Yore LM, Schellhammer PF. Squamous cell carcinoma of bladder after successful intravesical therapy with Bacillus Calmette-Guerin. Urology 1989; 34: 93–95.

17. Lamm DL, Thor DE, Harris SC, Reyna JA, Stogdill VD, Radwin HM. Bacillus Calmette-Guerin immunotherapy of superficial bladder cancer. J Urol 1980; 124: 38–40.

18. Pinsky CM, Camacho FJ, Kerr D, Geller NL, Klein FA, Herr HA, et al. Intravesical administration of bacillus Calmette-Guerin in patients with recurrent superficial carcinoma of the urinary bladder: report of a prospective, randomized trial. Cancer Treat Rep 1985; 69: 47–53.

19. Herr HW, Pinsky CM, Whitmore WF Jr, Sogani PC, Oettgen HF, Melamed MR. Long-term effect of intravesical bacillus Calmette-Guerin on flat carcinoma in situ of the bladder. J Urol 1986; 135: 265–267.

20. Lamm DL, Riggs DR, Shriver JS, vanGilder PF, Rach JF, DeHaven JI. Megadose vitamins in bladder cancer: a double-blind clinical trial. J Urol 1994; 151: 21–26.

21. Luftenegger W, Ackermann DK, Futterlieb A, Kraft R, Minder CE, Nadelhaft P, Studer UE. Intravesical versus intravesical plus intradermal bacillus Calmette-Guerin: a prospective randomized study in patients with recurrent superficial bladder tumors. J Urol 1996; 155: 483–487.

22. Witjes JA, Fransen MP, van der Meijden AP, Doesburg WH, Debruyne FM. Use of maintenance intravesical bacillus Calmette-Guerin (BCG), with or without intradermal BCG, in patients with recurrent superficial bladder cancer. Long-term follow-up of a randomized phase 2 study. Urol Int 1993; 51: 67–72.

23. Blumenstein BA. Clinical trial design and analysis. Monograph: update on diagnosis and treatment of superficial bladder cancer. MPE Communications, Inc. 1998, pp. 23–25.

24. Lamm DL, Blumenstein B, Sarosdy M, Grossman B, Crawford ED. Significant long-term patient benefit with BCG maintenance therapy. J Urol 1997; 157(Suppl): 213.

25. Lamm DL. Bacillus Calmette-Guerin immunotherapy for bladder cancer. J Urol 1985; 134: 40–47.

26. Pagano F, Bassi P, Milani C, Meneghini A, Maruzzi D, Garbeglio A. A low dose bacillus Calmette-Guerin regimen in superficial bladder cancer therapy: is it effective? J Urol 1991; 146: 32–35.

27. Melekos MD, Chionis H, Pantazakos A, Fokaefs E, Paranychianakis G, Dauaher H. Intravesical bacillus Calmette-Guerin immunoprophylaxis of superficial bladder cancer: results of a controlled prospective trial with modified treatment schedule. J Urol 1993; 149: 744–748.

28. Yang DA, Li SQ, Li XT. [Prophylactic effects of zhuling and BCG on postoperative recurrence of bladder cancer]. Chung Hua Wai Ko Tsa Chih 1994; 32: 433–434.

29. Zhang S, Li H, Cheng H. [The preventive recurrent results of postoperative intravesical instillation therapy in bladder cancer]. Chung Hua Wai Ko Tsa Chih 1995; 33: 304–306.

30. Krege S, Giani G, Meyer R, Otto T, Rubben H. A randomized multicenter trial of adjuvant therapy in superficial bladder cancer: transurethral resection only versus transurethral resection plus mitomycin C versus transurethral resection plus bacillus Calmette-Guerin. Participating Clinics. J Urol 1996; 156: 962–966.

31. Tkachuk VN, al-Shukri A, al-Khani F. [The use of BCG vaccine for preventing recurrences of superficial bladder cancer]. Urol Nefrol (Mosk) 1996; 2: 23–25.

32. Iantorno R, Nicolai M, Mastroprimiano G, Ballone E, Passamonti M, Cipollone G, Tenaglia R. Randomized prospective study comparing long-term intravesical instillation of BCG after transurethral resection alone in patients with superficial bladder cancer. J Urol 1999; 161(Suppl): 284.

33. Douville Y, Pelouze G, Roy R, Charrois R, Kibrite A, Martin M, et al. Recurrent bladder papillomata treated with bacillus Calmette-Guerin: a preliminary report (phase I trial). Cancer Treat Rep 1978; 62: 551–552.

34. Morales A, Ottenhof P, Emerson L. Treatment of residual, non-infiltrating bladder cancer with bacillus Calmette-Guerin. J Urol 1981; 125: 649–651.

35. Brosman SA. BCG in the management of superficial bladder cancer. Urology 1984; 23: 82–87.

36. deKernion JB, Huang MY, Lindner A, Smith RB, Kaufman JJ. The management of superficial bladder tumors and carcinoma in situ with intravesical bacillus Calmette-Guerin. J Urol 1985; 133: 598–601.

37. Heney NM, Koontz WW, Weinstein R, Barton B. BCG in superficial bladder cancer. J Urol 1986; 135(Suppl): 184A.

38. Schellhammer PF, Ladaga LE, Fillion MB. Bacillus Calmette-Guerin for superficial transitional cell carcinoma of the bladder. J Urol 1986; 135: 261–264.

39. Pansadoro V, De Paula F. Intravesical bacillus Calmette-Guerin in the treatment of superficial transitional cell carcinoma of the bladder. J Urol 1987; 138: 299–301.

40. Kavoussi LR, Torrence RJ, Gillen DP, Hudson MA, Haaff EO, Dresner SM, et al. Results of 6 weekly intravesical bacillus Calmette-Guerin instillations on the treatment of superficial bladder tumors. J Urol 1988; 139: 935–940.

41. Khanna OP, Son DL, Mazer H, Read J, Nugent D, Cottone R, et al. Multicenter study of superficial bladder cancer treated with intravesical bacillus Calmette-Guerin or adriamycin. Urology 1990; 35: 101–108.

42. Akaza H. BCG treatment of existing Ta, T1 tumours or carcinoma in situ of the bladder. Eur Urol 1995; 27(Suppl 1): 9–12.

43. Witjes JA, Oosterhof GO, DeBruyne FM. Management of superficial bladder cancer Ta/T1/TIS: intravesical chemotherapy. In: *Comprehensive Textbook of Genitourinary Oncology* (Vogelzang NJ, Scardino PT, Shipley WU, Coffey DS, eds.). Williams & Wilkins, Baltimore, MD, 1996, pp. 416–427.

44. Hudson MA. Carcinoma in situ of the bladder. J Urol 1995; 153: 564–572.

45. Lamm DL. Carcinoma in situ. Urol Clin North Am 1992; 19: 499–508.

46. Jakse G. Intravesical instillation of BCG in carcinoma in situ of the urinary bladder. EORTC protocol 30861. EORTC-GU Group. Prog Clin Biol Res 1989; 310: 187–192.

47. Herr HW, Wartinger DD, Fair WR, Oettgen HF. Bacillus Calmette-Guerin therapy for superficial bladder cancer: a 10- year followup. J Urol 1992; 147: 1020–1023.

48. Nadler RB, Catalona WJ, Hudson MA, Ratliff TL. Durability of the tumor-free response for intravesical bacillus Calmette-Guerin therapy. J Urol 1994; 152: 367–373.

49. Lamm DL, Blumenstein BA, Crawford ED, Montie JE, Scardino P, Grossman HB, et al. A randomized trial of intravesical doxorubicin and immunotherapy with bacille Calmette-Guerin for transitional-cell carcinoma of the bladder. N Engl J Med 1991; 325: 1205–1209.

50. Brosman SA. Experience with bacillus Calmette-Guerin in patients with superficial bladder carcinoma. J Urol 1982; 128: 27–30.

51. Tachibana M, Jitsukawa S, Iigaya T, Shibayama T, Baba S, Deguchi N, et al. [Comparative study on prophylactic intravesical instillation of bacillus Calmette-Guerin (BCG) and adriamycin for superficial bladder cancers]. Nippon Hinyokika Gakkai Zasshi 1989; 80: 1459–1465.

52. Martinez-Pineiro JA, Jimenez Leon J, Martinez-Pineiro L Jr, Fiter L, Mosteiro JA, Navarro J, et al. Bacillus Calmette-Guerin versus doxorubicin versus thiotepa: a randomized prospective study in 202 patients with superficial bladder cancer. J Urol 1990; 143: 502–506.

53. Rintala E, Jauhiainen K, Alfthan O, Hansson E, Juusela H, Kanerva K, et al. Intravesical chemotherapy (mitomycin C) versus immunotherapy (bacillus Calmette-Guerin) in superficial bladder cancer. Eur Urol 1991; 20: 19–25.

54. Lamm DL, Blumenstein B, Crawford ED, Crissman J, deVere White R, Wolf M, et al. Randomized intergroup comparison of bacillus Calmette Guerin immunotherapy and mitomycin C chemotherapy prophylaxis in superficial transitional cell carcinoma of the bladder. Urol Oncol 1995; 1: 119–126.

55. Melekos MD, Zarakovitis I, Dandinis K, Fokaefs E, Chionis H, Dauaher H, Barbalias G. BCG versus epirubicin in the prophylaxis of multiple superficial bladder tumours: results of a prospective randomized study using modified treatment schemes. Int Urol Nephrol 1996; 28: 499–509.

56. Vegt PD, Witjes JA, Witjes WP, Doesburg WH, Debruyne FM, van der Meijden AP. A randomized study of intravesical mitomycin C, bacillus Calmette-Guerin Tice and bacillus Calmette-Guerin RIVM treatment in pTa-pT1 papillary carcinoma and carcinoma in situ of the bladder. J Urol 1995; 153: 929–933.

57. Witjes JA, van der Meijden AP, Sylvester LC, Debruyne FM, van Aubel A, Witjes WP. Long-term follow-up of an EORTC randomized prospective trial comparing intravesical bacille Calmette-Guerin-RIVM and mitomycin C in superficial bladder cancer. EORTC GU Group and the Dutch South East Cooperative Urological Group. European Organisation for Research and Treatment of Cancer Genito-Urinary Tract Cancer Collaborative Group. Urology 1998; 52: 403–410.

58. Malmstrom PU, Wijkstrom H, Lundholm C, Wester K, Busch C, Norlen BJ. 5-year followup of a randomized prospective study comparing mitomycin C and bacillus Calmette-Guerin in patients with superficial bladder carcinoma. Swedish-Norwegian Bladder Cancer Study Group. J Urol 1999; 161: 1124–1127.

59. DeJager R, Guinan P, Lamm D, Khanna O, DeKernion J, Williams R, et al. Long-term complete remission in bladder carcinoma in situ with intravesical Tice bacillus Calmette Guerin. Urology 1991; 38: 507–513.

60. Coplen DE, Marcus MD, Myers JA, Ratliff TL, Catalona WJ. Long-term followup of patients treated with 1 or 2, 6-week courses of intravesical bacillus Calmette-Guerin: analysis of possible predictors of response free of tumor. J Urol 1990; 144: 652–657.

61. Herr HW, Laudone VP, Badalament RA, Oettgen HF, Sogani PC, Freedman BD, et al. Bacillus Calmette-Guerin therapy alters the progression of superficial bladder cancer. J Clin Oncol 1988; 6: 1450–1455.

62. Herr HW, Schwalb DM, Zhang ZF, Sogani PC, Fair WR, Whitmore WF Jr, Oettgen HF. Intravesical bacillus Calmette-Guerin therapy prevents tumor progression and death from superficial bladder cancer: ten-year follow-up of a prospective randomized trial. J Clin Oncol 1995; 13: 1404–1408.

63. Cookson MS, Herr HW, Zhang ZF, Soloway S, Sogani PC, Fair WR. The treated natural history of high risk superficial bladder cancer: 15-year outcome. J Urol 1997; 158: 62–67.

64. Herr HW, Badalament RA, Amato DA, Laudone VP, Fair WR, Whitmore WF Jr. Superficial bladder cancer treated with bacillus Calmette-Guerin: a multivariate analysis of factors affecting tumor progression. J Urol 1989; 141: 22–29.

65. Okamura T, Tozawa K, Yamada Y, Sakagami H, Ueda K, Kohri K. Clinicopathological evaluation of repeated courses of intravesical bacillus Calmette-Guerin instillation for preventing recurrence of initially resistant superficial bladder cancer. J Urol 1996; 156: 967–971.

66. Hudson MA, Ratliff TL, Gillen DP, Haaff EO, Dresner SM, Catalona WJ. Single course versus maintenance bacillus Calmette-Guerin therapy for superficial bladder tumors: a prospective, randomized trial. J Urol 1987; 138: 295–298.

67. Badalament RA, Herr HW, Wong GY, Gnecco C, Pinsky CM, Whitmore WF Jr, et al. A prospective randomized trial of maintenance versus nonmaintenance intravesical bacillus Calmette-Guerin therapy of superficial bladder cancer. J Clin Oncol 1987; 5: 441–449.

68. Palou J, Laguna P, Algaba F, Salvador J, Hall RR, Vincente J. High grade superficial transitional cell carcinoma of the bladder and/or CIS treated with BCG: control vs. maintenance treatment. Br J Urol 1997; 80(Suppl): 32.

69. Lamm DL, Blumenstein BA, Crissman JD, Montie JE, Gottesman JE, Lowe BA, et al. Maintenance BCG immunotherapy for recurrent Ta, T1 and carcinoma in situ transitional cell carcinoma: a randomized Southwest Oncology Group study. J Urol 2000; 163: 1124–1129.

70. Lebret T, Gaudez F, Herve JM, Barre P, Lugagne PM, Botto H. Low-dose BCG instillations in the treatment of stage T1 grade 3 bladder tumours: recurrence, progression and success. Eur Urol 1998; 34: 67–72.

71. Rintala E, Jauhiainen K, Alfthan O. Mitomycin-C and BCG in intravesical chemo-therapy and immunotherapy of superficial bladder cancer. Finnbladder Research Group. Prog Clin Biol Res 1989; 310: 271–274.

72. Blumenstein BA, Lamm D, Jewett MA. Effect of colony-forming unit dose of Connaught BCG on outcome to immunotherapy in superficial bladder cancer. J Urol 1990; 143(Suppl): 340A.

73. Rivera P, Caffarena E, Cornejo H, Del Pino M, Foneron A, Haemmersli J, et al. [Microdoses of BCG vaccine for prophylaxis in bladder cancer stage T1]. Actas Urol Esp 1993; 17: 243–246.

74. Mack D, Frick J. Low-dose bacille Calmette-Guerin (BCG) therapy in superficial high- risk bladder cancer: a phase II study with the BCG strain Connaught Canada. Br J Urol 1995; 75: 185–187.

75. Hurle R, Losa A, Ranieri A, Graziotti P, Lembo A. Low dose Pasteur bacillus Cal-mette-Guerin regimen in stage T1, grade 3 bladder cancer therapy. J Urol 1996; 156: 1602–1605.

76. Morales A, Nickel JC, Wilson JW. Dose-response of bacillus Calmette-Guerin in the treatment of superficial bladder cancer. J Urol 1992; 147: 1256–1258.

77. Takashi M, Wakai K, Ohno Y, Murase T, Miyake K. Evaluation of a low-dose intravesical bacillus Calmette-Guerin (Tokyo strain) therapy for superficial blad-der cancer. Int Urol Nephrol 1995; 27: 723–733.

78. Martinez-Pineiro JA, Solsona E, Flores N, Isorna S. Improving the safety of BCG immunotherapy by dose reduction. Cooperative Group CUETO. Eur Urol 1995; 27(Suppl 1): 13–18.

79. Pagano F, Bassi P, Piazza N, Abatangelo G, Drago Ferrante GL, Milani C. Improv-ing the efficacy of BCG immunotherapy by dose reduction. Eur Urol 1995; 27 (Suppl 1): 19–22.

80. Bassi P, Pappagallo GL, Piazza N, Spinadin R, Carando R, Mazzariol C, et al. Low dose vs. standard dose BCG therapy of superficial bladder cancer: final results of a phase III randomized trial. J Urol 1999; 161(Suppl): 285.

81. Bassi P. 1999, (personal communication).

82. Orihuela E, Herr HW, Pinsky CM, Whitmore WF Jr. Toxicity of intravesical BCG and its management in patients with superficial bladder tumors. Cancer 1987; 60: 326–333.

83. van der Meijden AP. Practical approaches to the prevention and treatment of adverse reactions to BCG. Eur Urol 1995; 27(Suppl 1): 23–28.

84. Steg A, Adjiman S, Debre B. BCG therapy in superficial bladder tumours—complications and precautions. Eur Urol 1992; 21(Suppl 2): 35–40.

85. Berry DL, Blumenstein BA, Magyary DL, Lamm DL, Crawford ED. Local tox-icity patterns associated with intravesical bacillus Calmette-Guerin: a Southwest Oncology Group Study. Int J Urol 1996; 3: 98–100; discussion 101.

86. van der Meijden PM, van Klingeren B, Steerenberg PA, de Boer LC, de Jong WH, Debruyne FM. The possible influence of antibiotics on results of bacillus Calmette-Guerin intravesical therapy for superficial bladder cancer. J Urol 1991; 146: 444–446.

87. Durek C, Rusch-Gerdes S, Joacham D, Bohle A. Interference of modern antibi-otics with bacillus Calmette-Guerin (BCG) viability. J Urol 1999; 161(Suppl): 285.

88. Vegt PD, van der Meijden AP, Sylvester R, Brausi M, Holtl W, de Balincourt C. Does isoniazid reduce side effects of intravesical bacillus Calmette- Guerin therapy in superficial bladder cancer? Interim results of European Organization for Research and Treatment of Cancer Protocol 30911. J Urol 1997; 157: 1246–1249.

89. Bohle A, Balck F, von Weitersheim J, Jocham D. The quality of life during intraves-ical bacillus Calmette-Guerin therapy. J Urol 1996; 155: 1221–1226.

90. Mack D, Frick J. Quality of life in patients undergoing bacille Calmette-Guerin therapy for superficial bladder cancer. Br J Urol 1996; 78: 369–371.

91. Lamm DL, Steg A, Boccon-Gibod L, Morales A, Hanna MG Jr, Pagano F, et al. Complications of Bacillus Calmette-Guerin immunotherapy: review of 2602 patients and comparison of chemotherapy complications. Prog Clin Biol Res 1989; 310: 335–355.

92. Steg A, Leleu C, Debre B, Boccon-Gibod L, Sicard D. Systemic bacillus Calmette-Guerin infection in patients treated by intravesical BCG therapy for superficial bladder cancer. Prog Clin Biol Res 1989; 310: 325–334.

93. DeHaven JI, Traynellis C, Riggs DR, Ting E, Lamm DL. Antibiotic and steroid therapy of massive systemic bacillus Calmette-Guerin toxicity. J Urol 1992; 147: 738–742.

94. Lamm DL, van der Meijden PM, Morales A, Brosman SA, Catalona WJ, Herr HW, et al. Incidence and treatment of complications of bacillus Calmette-Guerin intravesical therapy in superficial bladder cancer. J Urol 1992; 147: 596–600.

95. Anonymous. Case records of the Massachusetts General Hospital. Weekly clinicopathological exercises. Case 29-1998. A 57-year-old man with fever and jaundice after intravesical instillation of bacille Calmette-Guerin for bladder cancer [clinical conference]. N Engl J Med 1998; 339: 831–837.

96. Wittes R, Klotz L, Kosecka U. Severe bacillus Calmette-Guerin cystitis responds to systemic steroids when antituberculous drugs and local steroids fail. J Urol 1999; 161: 1568–1569.

97. Saporta L, Gumus E, Karadag H, Kuran B, Miroglu C. Reiter syndrome following intracavitary BCG administration. Scand J Urol Nephrol 1997; 31: 211–212.

98. Hansen CP, Mortensen S. Epididymo-orchitis and Reiter's disease. Two infrequent complications after intravesical bacillus Calmette-Guerin therapy. Scand J Urol Nephrol 1997; 31: 317–318.

99. Wang MH, Chen YQ, Gercken J, Ernst M, Bohle A, Flad HD, Vlmer AJ. Specific activation of human peripheral blood gamma/delta$^+$ T lymphocytes by sonicated antigens of mycobacterium tuberculosis: role in vitro in killing human bladder carcinoma cell lines. Scand J Immunol 1993; 38: 239–246.

100. Thanhauser A, Bohle A, Flad HD, Ernst M, Mattern T, Vlmer AJ. Induction of bacillus Calmette-Guerin activated killer cells from human peripheral blood mononuclear cells against human bladder carcinoma cell lines in vitro. Cancer Immunol Immunother 1993; 37: 105–111.

101. Peuchmaur M, Benoit G, Vieillefond A, Chevelier A, Lemaigre G, Martin ED, Jardin A. Analysis of mucosal bladder leucocyte subpopulations in patients treated with intravesical bacillus Calmette-Guerin. Urol Res 1989; 17: 299–303.

102. Prescott S, James K, Hargreave TB, Chisholm GD, Smith JF. Intravesical Evans strain BCG therapy: quantitative immunohistochemical analysis of the immune response within the bladder wall. J Urol 1992; 147: 1636–1642.

103. Inoue T, Yoshikai Y, Matsuzaki G, Nomoto K. Early appearing gamma/delta T cells during infection with Calmette-Guerin bacillus. J Immunol 1991; 146: 2754–2762.

104. DeBoer EC, DeJong WH, Van der Meijden AP, Steerenberg PA, Witjes JA, Vegt PD, et al. Presence of activated lymphocytes in the urine of patients with superficial bladder cancer after intravesical immunotherapy with bacillus Calmette-Guerin. Cancer Immunol Immunother 1991; 33: 411–416.

105. Bruno S, Machi AM, Semino C, Meta M, Ponte M, Varaldo M, et al. Phenotypic, functional and molecular analysis of lymphocytes associated with bladder cancer. Cancer Immunol Immunother 1996; 42: 47–54.

106. Adams DO, Marino PA. Evidence for a multistep mechanism of cytolysis by BCG-activated macrophages: the interrelationship between the capacity for cytolysis, target binding, and secretion of cytolytic factor. J Immunol 1981; 126: 981–987.
107. Pryor K, Stricker P, Russell P, Golovsky D, Penny R. Antiproliferative effects of bacillus Calmette-Guerin and interferon alpha 2b on human bladder cancer cells in vitro. Cancer Immunol Immunother 1995; 41: 309–316.
108. Wolfe SA, Tracey DE, Henney CS. Induction of "natural killer" cells by BCG. Nature 1976; 262: 584–586.
109. Uyemura K, Wang XH, Ohmen J. Cytokine patterns of immunologically mediated tissue damage. J Immunol 1992; 149: 1470–1475.
110. Orme IM. Immunity to mycobacteria. Curr Opin Immunol 1993; 5: 497–502.
111. Fleischmann JD, Toossi Z, Ellner JJ, Wentworth DB, Ratliff TL, Imbembo AL. Urinary interleukins in patients receiving intravesical Bacillus Calmette-Guerin therapy for superficial bladder cancer. Cancer 1989; 64: 1447–1454.
112. Schamhart DHJ, Kurth KH, deReijke TM, Vleeming R. BCG treatment and the importance of inflammatory response. Urol Res 1992; 20: 199–203.
113. Prescott S, James K, Hargreave TB, Chisholm GD, Smyth JF. Radio-immunoassay detection of interferon-gamma in urine after intravesical Evans BCG therapy. J Urol 1990; 144: 1248–1251.
114. Huygen K, Abramowicz D, Vandenbussche P, Jacobs F, DeBruyn J, Kentos A, et al. Spleen cell cytokine secretion in Mycobacterium bovis BCG-infected mice. Infection and Immunity 1992; 60: 2880–2886.
115. DeBoer EC, DeJong WH, Steerenberg PA, Aarden LA, Tetteroo E, DeGroot ER, et al. Induction of urinary interleukin-1 (IL-1), IL-2, IL-6 and tumor necrosis factor during intravesical immunotherapy with bacillus Calmette-Guerin in superficial bladder cancer. Cancer Immunol Immunother 1992; 34: 306–312.
116. Bohle A, Nowc C, Ulmer AJ, Musehold J, Gerdes J, Hofstetter AG, Flad HD. Detection of urinary TNF, IL-1, and IL-2 after local BCG immunotherapy for bladder carcinoma. Cytokine 1990; 2: 175–181.
117. Murray PJ, Aldovini A, Young RA. Manipulation and potentiation of antimycobacterial immunity using recombinant bacille Calmette-Guerin strains that secrete cytokines. Proc Natl Acad Sci USA 1996; 93: 934.
118. Shin JS, Park JH, Kim JD, Lee JM, Kim SJ. Induction of tumour necrosis factor-alpha (TNF-alpha) mRNA in bladders and spleens of mice after intravesical administration of bacillus Calmette-Guerin. Clin Exp Immunol 1995; 100: 26–31.
119. O'Donnell MA, Chen X, DeWolf WC. Maturation of the cytokine immune response to BCG in the bladder: implications for treatment schedules. J Urol 1996; 155: 1030A.
120. DeReijke TM, DeBoer EC, Kurth KH, Schamhart DH. Urinary cytokines during intravesical bacillus Calmette-Guerin therapy for superficial bladder cancer: processing, stability and prognostic value. J Urol 1996; 155: 477–482.
121. Thalmann GN, Dewald B, Baggiolini M, Studer UE. Interleukin-8 expression in the urine after BCG therapy: a potential predictor of tumor recurrence and progression. J Urol 1996; 155: 34A.
122. Wallis RS, Amir-Tahmasseb M, Ellner JJ. Induction of interleukin 1 and tumor necrosis factor by mycobacterial proteins: the monocyte Western blot. Proc Natl Acad Sci USA 1990; 87: 3348–3352.
123. O'Donnell MA, Aldovini A, Duda RB, Yang H, Szilvasi A, Young RA, DeWolf WC. Recombinant Mycobacterium bovis BCG secreting functional interleukin-2 enhances gamma interferon production by splenocytes. Infect Immun 1994; 62: 2508–2514.

124. DeJong WH, DeBoer EC, Van Der Meijden APM. Presence of interleukin-2 in urine of superficial bladder cancer patients after intravesical treatment with bacillus Calmette-Guerin. Cancer Immunol Immunother 1990; 31: 182–186.

125. Poppas DP, Folkman J, Pavlovich CP, Voest EE, Chen X, Luster AD, O'Donnell MA. Intravesical bacillus Calmette-Guerin (BCG) induces the anti-angiogenic chemokine IP-10. Urology 1998; 52: 268–276.

126. Ikemoto S, Kishimoto T, Wada S. Clinical studies on cell-mediated immunity in patients with bladder carcinoma: blastogenic response, interleukin-2 production and interferon-γ production of lymphocytes. Br J Urol 1990; 65: 333–338.

127. Jackson AM, Ivshina AV, Senko O, Kuznetsova A, Sundan A, O'Donnell MA, et al. Prognosis of intravesical bacillus Calmette-Guerin therapy for superficial bladder cancer by immunological urinary measurements: statistically weighted syndromes analysis. J Urol 1998; 159: 1054–1063.

128. Flynn JL, Chan J, Triebold KJ, Dalton DK, Stewart TA, Bloom BR. An essential role for interferon-γ in resistance to Mycobacterium tuberculosis infection. J Exp Med 1993; 178: 2249–2254.

129. Newport MJ, Kuxley CM, Huston S, Hawrylowicz CM, Oostra BA, Williamson R, Levin M. A mutation in the interferon-γ-receptor gene and susceptibility to mycobacterial infections. N Engl J Med 1996; 335: 1941–1949.

130. Shapiro A, Lijovetzky G, Pode D. Changes of the mucosal architecture and of urine cytology during BCG treatment. World J Urol 1988; 6: 61–64.

131. Pagano F, Bassi P, Milani C. Pathologic and structural changes in the bladder after BCG intravesical therapy in men. Prog Clin Biol Res 1989; 310: 81–91.

132. Ratliff TL, Ritchey JK, Yuan JJ, Andriole GL, Catalona WJ. T-cell subsets required for intravesical BCG immunotherapy for bladder cancer. J Urol 1993; 150: 1018–1023.

133. Bohle A, Gerdes J, Ulmer AJ, Hofstetter AG, Flad HD. Effects of local BCG therapy in patients with bladder carcinoma on immunocompetent cells of the bladder wall. J Urol 1990; 144: 53–58.

134. Cornel EB, Van Moorselaar RJ, Van Stratum P, Debruyne FM, Schalken JA. Antitumor effects of bacillus Calmette-Guerin in a syngeneic rat bladder tumor model system, RBT323. J Urol 1993; 149: 179–182.

135. Boccafoschi C, Montefiore F, Pavesi M. Immunophenotypic characterization of the bladder mucosa infiltrating lymphocytes after intravesical BCG treatment for superficial bladder carcinoma. Eur Urol 1992; 21: 304–308.

136. Stefanini GF, Bercovich E, Mazzeo V, Grigioni WF, Emili E, D'errico A, et al. Class I and Class II HLA antigen expression by transitional cell carcinoma of the bladder: correlation with T cell infiltration and BCG treatment. J Urol 1989; 141: 1449–1453.

137. Drowart A, Zlotta AR, Van Vooren JP, Simon J, Schulman CC, Huygen K. What is the optimal regimen for intravesical BCG therapy: are six weekly instillations necessary? J Urol 1999; 161(Suppl): 285.

138. Haaff EO, Catalona WJ, Ratliff TL. Detection of interleukin-2 in the urine of patients with superficial bladder tumors after treatment with intravesical BCG. J Urol 1986; 136: 970–974.

139. Kaempfer R, Gerez L, Farbstein H, Madar L, Hirschman O, Nussinovich R, Shapiro A. Prediction of response to treatment in superficial bladder carcinoma through pattern of interleukin-2 gene expression. J Clin Oncol 1996; 14: 1778–1786.

140. Patard JJ, Guille F, Lobel B, Abbou CC, Chopin D. [Current state of knowledge concerning the mechanisms of action of BCG]. Prog Urol 1998; 8: 415–421.

141. Patard J-J, Muscatelli-Groux F, Saint Z, Popov P, Maille C, Chopin D. Evaluation of local immune response after intravesical bacille Calmette-Guerin treatment for superficial bladder cancer. Br J Urol 1996; 78: 709–714.

142. Esuvaranathan K, Alexandroff AB, McIntyre M, Jackson AM, Prescott S, Chisholm GD, James K. Interleukin-6 production by bladder tumors is upregulated by BCG immunotherapy. J Urol 1995; 154: 572–575.

143. Zlotta AR, Drowart A, Huygen K, De Bruyn J, Shekarsarai H, Decock M, et al. Humoral response against heat shock proteins and other mycobacterial antigens after intravesical treatment with bacille Calmette-Guerin in patients with superficial bladder cancer. Clin Exp Immunol 1997; 109: 157–165.

144. O'Donnell MA, Luo Y, Chen X, Szilvasi A, Hunter SE, Clinton SK. Role of IL-12 in the induction and potentiation of IFN-γ in response to Bacillus Calmette-Guerin. J Immunol 1999; 163: 4246–4252.

145. Kurisu H, Matsuyama H, Ohmoto Y, Shimabukuro T, Naito K. Cytokine-mediated antitumor effect of bacillus Calmette-Guerin on tumor cells in vitro. Cancer Immunol Immunother 1994; 39: 249–253.

146. Campbell SC, Tanabe K, Alexander JP, Edinger M, Tubbs RR, Klein EA. Intercellular adhesion molecule-1 expression by bladder cancer cells: functional effects. J Urol 1994; 151: 1385–1390.

147. Hawkyard SJ, Jackson AM, James K, Prescott S, Smyth JF, Chisholm GD. The inhibitory effects of interferon gamma on the growth of bladder cancer cells. J Urol 1992; 147: 1399–1403.

148. Jackson AM, Alexandrov AB, Prescott S, James K, Chisholm GD. Expression of adhesion molecules by bladder cancer cells: modulation by interferon-gamma and tumour necrosis factor-alpha. J Urol 1996; 148: 1583–1586.

149. Pryor K, Goddard J, Goldstein D, Stricker P, Russell P, Golovsky D, Penny R. Bacillus Calmette-Guerin (BCG) enhances monocyte- and lymphocyte-mediated bladder tumor cell killing. Br J Cancer 1995; 71: 801–807.

150. Lattime EC, Gomella LG, McCue PA. Murine bladder carcinoma cells present antigen to BCG specific CD4+ T-cells. Cancer Res 1992; 52: 4286–4290.

151. Ratliff TL. Role of the immune response in BCG for bladder cancer. Eur Urol 1992; 21: 17–21.

152. Ratliff TL. Mechanisms of action of intravesical BCG for bladder cancer. Prog Clin Biol Res 1989; 310: 107–122.

153. Paul WE, Seder RA. Lymphocyte responses and cytokines. Cell 1994; 76: 241–251.

154. Luo Y, Szilvasi A, Chen X, DeWolf WC, O'Donnell MA. A novel method for monitoring Mycobacterium bovis BCG trafficking using recombinant BCG expressing green fluorescent protein. Clin Diag Lab Immunol 1996; 3: 761–768.

155. O'Donnell MA, Szilvasi A, Luo Y, DeWolf WC. Fas mediated killing of transitional cell carcinoma (TCC). J Urol 1996; 155: 567A.

156. Klein LT, Miller MI, Ikeguchi E, Buttyan R, Connor JP, Katz A, et al. Anti-fas antibody mediated apoptosis in bladder tumor cells: a potential intravesical therapeutic agent. Proc Annu Meet Amer Assoc Cancer Res 1996; 37: A103.

157. Bohle A, Thanhauser A, Ulmer A, Ernst M, Flad HD, Jocham D. Dissecting the immunobiological effects of bacillus Calmette-Guerin (BCG) in vitro: evidence of a distinct BCG-activated killer (BAK) cell phenomenon. J Urol 1993; 150: 1932–1937.

158. Bohle A, Thanhauser A, Ulmer AJ, Mattern T, Ernst M, Flad HD, Jocham D. On the mode of action of intravesical bacillus Calmette-Guerin: in vitro characterization of BCG-activated killer cells. Urol Res 1994; 22: 185–190.

159. Ratliff TL, Shapiro A, Catalona WJ. Inhibition of murine bladder tumor growth by bacillus Calmette-Guerin: lack of a role of natural keller cells. Clin Immunol Immunopathol 1986; 41: 108–115.

160. Ratliff TL, Gillen D, Catalona WJ. Requirement of a thymus dependent immune response for BCG-mediated antitumor activity. J Urol 1987; 137: 155–158.

161. Nadler RB, Ritchey JK, Day ML, Ratliff TL. Cytokine patterns in BCG treated mouse bladders. J Urol 1994; 151: 515A.

162. Halak BK, Maguire HC Jr, Lattime EC. Tumor-induced interleukin-10 inhibits type 1 immune responses directed at a tumor antigen as well as a non-tumor antigen present at the tumor site. Cancer Res 1999; 59: 911–917.

163. Kavoussi LR, Brown EJ, Ritchey JK, Ratliff TL. Fibronectin-mediated Calmette-Guerin bacillus attachment to murine bladder mucosa. Requirement for the expression of an antitumor response. J Clin Invest 1990; 85: 62–67.

164. Zhao W, Schorey JS, Groger R, Allen PM, Brown EJ, Ratliff TL. Characterization of the fibronectin binding motif for a unique mycobacterial fibronectin attachment protein, FAP. J Biol Chem 1999; 274: 4521–4526.

165. Becich MJ, Carroll S, Ratliff TL. Internalization of bacille Calmette-Guerin by bladder tumor cells. J Urol 1991; 145: 1316–1324.

166. Matzinger P. Tolerance, danger, and the extended family. Annu Rev Immunol 1994; 12: 991–1045.

167. Iantorno R, Nicolai M, Cipollone G, Di Federico G, Tenaglia R. [Role of MCP-1 chemokine in the response of monocytes of patients with superficial tumors of the bladder treated with BCG immunotherapy]. Arch Ital Urol Androl 1997; 69(Suppl 1): 71–72.

168. DiTirro J, Rhoades ER, Roberts AD, Burke JM, Mukasa A, Cooper AM, et al. Disruption of the cellular inflammatory response to Listeria monocytogenes infection in mice with disruptions in targeted genes. Infect Immun 1998; 66: 2284–2289.

169. Troy AJ, Davidson JT, Atkinson CH, Hart DNJ. C1A dendritic cells predominate in transitional cell carcinoma of bladder and kidney but are minimally activated. J Urol 1999; 161: 1962–1967.

170. Stoll S, Jonuleit H, Schmitt E, Muller G, Yamauchi H, Kurimoto M, et al. Production of functional IL-18 by different subtypes of murine and human dendritic cells (DC): DC-derived IL-18 enhances IL-12-dependent Th1 development. Eur J Immunol 1998; 28: 3231–3239.

171. Kuniyoshi JS, Kuniyoshi CJ, Lim AM, Wang FY, Bade ER, Lau R, et al. Dendritic cell secretion of IL-15 is induced by recombinant huCD40LT and augments the stimulation of antigen-specific cytolytic T cells. Cell Immunol 1999; 193: 48–58.

172. Cruickshank S, Southgate J, Selby P, Trejdosiewicz L. Lymphoepithelial interactions in the normal and malignant bladder. Eur Urol 1999; 36: 468 (Abstr).

173. Glazier DB, Bahnson RR, McLeod DG, von Roemeling RW, Messing EM, Ernstoff MS. Intravesical recombinant tumor necrosis factor in the treatment of superficial bladder cancer: an Eastern Cooperative Oncology Group Study. J Urol 1995; 154: 66–68.

174. Geboers AD, van Bergen TN, Oosterlinck W. Gamma-interferon in the therapeutic and prophylactic management of superficial bladder cancer. J Urol (Pt 2) 1987; 137: 276A.

175. Alexandroff AB, Jackson AM, O'Donnell MA, James K. BCG immunotherapy of bladder cancer: 20 years on. Lancet 1999; 353: 1689–1694.

176. Luo Y, Chen X, Downs TM, DeWolf WC, O'Donnell MA. IFN-alpha 2B enhances Th1 cytokine responses in bladder cancer patients receiving Mycobacterium bovis bacillus Calmette-Guerin immunotherapy. J Immunol 1999; 162: 2399–2405.

177. DeReijke TM, DeBoer EC, Kurth KH, Schamhart DH. Urinary interleukin-2 monitoring during prolonged bacillus Calmette- Guerin treatment: can it predict the optimal number of instillations? J Urol 1999; 161: 67–71.

178. Coplen DE, Ratliff TL, Kavoussi LR, Marcus MD, Myers J, Yuan JJ, et al. Combination of adriamycin and BCG in the treatment of superficial bladder cancer. J Urol 1990; 143(Suppl): 341A.

179. Gelabert-Mas A, Arango Toro O, Bielsa Gali O, Llado Carbonell C. [A prospective and randomized study of the complete response, index of recurrences and progression in superficial bladder carcinoma treated with mitomycin C alone versus mitomycin C and BCG alternatively]. Arch Esp Urol 1993; 46: 379–382.

180. Erol A, Ozgur S, Basar M, Cetin S. Trial with bacillus Calmette-Guerin and epirubicin combination in the prophylaxis of superficial bladder cancer. Urol Int 1994; 52: 69–72.

181. Uekado Y, Hirano A, Shinka T, Ohkawa T. The effects of intravesical chemoimmunotherapy with epirubicin and bacillus Calmette-Guerin for prophylaxis of recurrence of superficial bladder cancer: a preliminary report. Cancer Chemother Pharmacol 1994; 35(Suppl): 65–68.

182. Rintala E, Jauhiainen K, Rajala P, Ruutu M, Kaasinen E, Alfthan O. Alternating mitomycin C and bacillus Calmette-Guerin instillation therapy for carcinoma in situ of the bladder. The Finnbladder Group. J Urol 1995; 154: 2050–2053.

183. Rintala E, Jauhiainen K, Kaasinen E, Nurmi M, Alfthan O. Alternating mitomycin C and bacillus Calmette-Guerin instillation prophylaxis for recurrent papillary (stages Ta to T1) superficial bladder cancer. Finnbladder Group. J Urol 1996; 156: 56–59; discussion 59–60.

184. Van der Meijden AP, Hall RR, Macaluso MP, Pawinsky A, Sylvester R, Van Glabbeke M. Marker tumour responses to the sequential combination of intravesical therapy with mitomycin-C and BCG-RIVM in multiple superficial bladder tumours. Report from the European Organisation for Research and Treatment on Cancer-Genitourinary Group (EORTC 30897). Eur Urol 1996; 29: 199–203.

185. Witjes JA, Caris CT, Mungan NA, Debruyne FM, Witjes WP. Results of a randomized phase III trial of sequential intravesical therapy with mitomycin C and bacillus Calmette-Guerin versus mitomycin C alone in patients with superficial bladder cancer. J Urol 1998; 160: 1668–1671; discussion 1671–1672.

186. Wijkstrom H, Kassinen E, Malmstrom P, Hellsten S, Duchek M, Wahlvist R, Rintala E. A nordic study comparing intravesical instillations of alternating mitomycin C and BCG with BCG alone in carcinoma in situ of the urinary bladder. J Urol 1999; 161(Suppl): 286.

187. Kassinen E, Rintala E, Anna-Kaisa P, Kallio J, Veli-Matti P, Jauhiainen K, Tuhkanen K. Monthly BCG preceded by five weekly mitomycin C instillations gives an excellent tumor control in the prophylaxis of recurrent papillary superficial bladder carcinoma (pTa to pT1) - no use of alternating interferon-a2b monthly with BCG. J Urol 1999; 161(Suppl): 286.

188. Ali-El-Dein B, Nabeeh A, Ismail EH, Ghoneim MA. Sequential bacillus Calmette-Guerin and epirubicin versus bacillus Calmette-Guerin alone for superficial bladder tumors: a randomized prospective study. J Urol 1999; 162: 339–342.

189. Oosterlinck W, Kurth KH, Schroder F, Bultinck J, Hammond B, Sylvester R. A prospective European Organization for Research and Treatment of Cancer Genitourinary Group randomized trial comparing transurethral resection followed by a single intravesical instillation of epirubicin or water in single stage Ta, T1 papillary carcinoma of the bladder. J Urol 1993; 149: 749–752.

190. Tolley DA, Parmar MK, Grigor KM, Lallemand G, Benyon LL, Fellows J, et al. The effect of intravesical mitomycin C on recurrence of newly diagnosed super-

ficial blad-der cancer: a further report with 7 years of follow up. J Urol 1996; 155: 1233–1238.

191. Solsona E, Iborra I, Ricos JV, Monros JL, Casanova J, Dumont R. Effectiveness of a single immediate mitomycin C instillation in patients with low risk superficial bladder cancer: short and long-term followup. J Urol 1999; 161: 1120–1123.

192. Zhang Y, Khoo HE, Esuvaranathan K. Effects of bacillus Calmette-Guerin and interferon alpha-2B on cytokine production in human bladder cancer cell lines. J Urol 1999; 161: 977–983.

193. Hawkyard SJ, Jackson AM, Prescott S, James K, Chisholm GD. The effect of recombinant cytokines on bladder cancer cells in vitro. J Urol 1993; 150: 514–518.

194. Bandyopadhyay S, Fazeli-Matin S, Rackley R, Chandra P, Novick A. Interferon-resistant transitional cell carcinomas (TCC) have defective signal transduction factors: a clinical basis for interferon combination therapy. J Urol 1999; 161(Suppl): 113.

195. Belldegrun AS, Franklin JR, O'Donnell MA, Gomella LG, Klein E, Neri R, et al. Superficial bladder cancer: the role of interferon-alpha [published erratum appears in J Urol 1998; 160(4): 1444]. J Urol 1998; 159: 1793–1801.

196. Downs TM, Szilvasi A, O'Donnell MA. Pharmacological biocompatibility between intravesical preparations of BCG and interferon-alpha 2B. J Urol 1997; 158: 2311–2315.

197. Stricker P, Pryor K, Nicolson T, Goldstein D, Golovsky D, Fersuson R, et al. Bacillus Calmette-Guerin plus intravesical interferon alpha-2b in patients with superficial bladder cancer. Urology 1996; 48: 957–962.

198. Bercovich E, Deriu M, Manferrari F, Irianni G. BCG vs. BCG plus recombinant alpha-interferon 2b in superficial tumors of the bladder. Arch Ital Urol Androl 1995; 67: 257–260.

199. O'Donnell MA, Downs TM, DeWolf WC. Co-administration of interferon-alpha 2B with BCG is effective in patients with superficial bladder cancer previously failing BCG alone. J Immunother 1999; 22: 463.

200. Harris CC, Kaufman DG, Sporn MB, Staffiotti U. Histogenesis of squamous metaplasia and squamous cell carcinoma of the respiratory epithelium in an animal model. Cancer Chemother Rep [3] 1973; 4: 43–47.

201. Alfthan O, Tarkkanen J, Grohn P, Heinonen E, Pyrhonen S, Saila K. Tigason (etretinate) in prevention of recurrence of superficial bladder tumors. A double-blind clinical trial. Eur Urol 1983; 9: 6–9.

202. Studer UE, Biedermann C, Chollet D, Karrer P, Kraft R, Toggenburg H, Vonbank F. Prevention of recurrent superficial bladder tumors by oral etretinate: preliminary results of a randomized, double blind multicenter trial in Switzerland. J Urol 1984; 131: 47–49.

203. Byar D, Blackard C. Comparisons of placebo, pyridoxine, and topical thiotepa in preventing recurrence of stage I bladder cancer. Urology 1977; 10: 556–561.

204. Bussey HJ, DeCosse JJ, Deschner EE, Eyers AA, Lesser ML, Morson BC, et al. A randomized trial of ascorbic acid in polyposis coli. Cancer 1982; 50: 1434–1439.

205. Heinonen OP, Albanes D, Virtamo J, Taylor PR, Huttunen JK, Hartman AM, et al. Prostate cancer and supplementation with alpha-tocopherol and beta-carotene: incidence and mortality in a controlled trial. J Natl Cancer Inst 1998; 90: 440–446.

206. Meydani SN, Meydani M, Blumberg JB, Leka LS, Siber G, Loszewski R, et al. Vitamin E supplementation and in vivo immune response in healthy elderly subjects. A randomized controlled trial. JAMA 1997; 277: 1380–1386.

207. Heney NM, Ahmed S, Flanagan MJ, Frable W, Corder MP, Hafermann MD, Hawkins IR. Superficial bladder cancer: progression and recurrence. J Urol 1983; 130: 1083–1086.

208. Kaubisch S, Lum BL, Reese J, Freiha F, Torti FM. Stage T1 bladder cancer: grade is the primary determinant for risk of muscle invasion. J Urol 1991; 146: 28–31.

209. Stockle M, Alken P, Engelmann U, Jacobi GH, Riedmiller H, Hohenfellner R. Radical cystectomy—often too late? Eur Urol 1987; 13: 361–367.

210. Esrig D, Freeman JA, Stein JP, Skinner DG. Early cystectomy for clinical stage T1 transitional cell carcinoma of the bladder. Semin Urol Oncol 1997; 15: 154–160.

211. Pansadoro V, Emiliozzi P, Defidio L, Donadio D, Florio A, Maurelli S, et al. Bacillus Calmette-Guerin in the treatment of stage T1 grade 3 transitional cell carcinoma of the bladder: long-term results. J Urol 1995; 154: 2054–2058.

212. Cookson MS, Sarosdy MF. Management of stage T1 superficial bladder cancer with intravesical bacillus Calmette-Guerin therapy. J Urol 1992; 148: 797–801.

213. Baniel J, Grauss D, Engelstein D, Sella A. Intravesical bacillus Calmette-Guerin treatment for Stage T1 grade 3 transitional cell carcinoma of the bladder. Urology 1998; 52: 785–789.

214. Hurle R, Losa A, Manzetti A, Lembo A. Intravesical bacille Calmette-Guerin in Stage T1 grade 3 bladder cancer therapy: a 7-year follow-up. Urology 1999; 54: 258–263.

215. Klan R, Loy V, Huland H. Residual tumor discovered in routine second transurethral resection in patients with stage T1 transitional cell carcinoma of the bladder. J Urol 1991; 146: 316–318.

216. Herr HW. The value of a second transurethral resection in evaluating patients with bladder tumors. J Urol 1999; 162: 74–76.

217. Lacombe L, Dalbagni G, Zhang ZF, Cordon-Cardo C, Fair WR, Herr HW, Reuter VE. Overexpression of p53 protein in a high-risk population of patients with superficial bladder cancer before and after bacillus Calmette-Guerin therapy: correlation to clinical outcome. J Clin Oncol 1996; 14: 2646–2652.

218. Zlotta AR, Noel JC, Fayt I, Drowart A, Van Vooren JP, Huygen K, et al. Correlation and prognostic significance of p53, p21WAF1/CIP1 and Ki- 67 expression in patients with superficial bladder tumors treated with bacillus Calmette-Guerin intravesical therapy. J Urol 1999; 161: 792–798.

219. Lebret T, Becette V, Barbagelatta M, Herve JM, Gaudez F, Barre P, et al. Correlation between p53 over expression and response to bacillus Calmette-Guerin therapy in a high risk select population of patients with T1G3 bladder cancer. J Urol 1998; 159: 788–791.

220. Pages F, Flam TA, Vieillefond A, Molinie V, Abeille X, Lazar V, et al. p53 status does not predict initial clinical response to bacillus Calmette-Guerin intravesical therapy in T1 bladder tumors. J Urol 1998; 159: 1079–1084.

221. Merz VW, Marth D, Kraft R, Ackermann DK, Zingg EJ, Studer UE. Analysis of early failures after intravesical instillation therapy with bacille Calmette-Guerin for carcinoma in situ of the bladder. Br J Urol 1995; 75: 180–184.

222. Bui TT, Schellhammer PF. Additional bacillus Calmette-Guerin therapy for recurrent transitional cell carcinoma after an initial complete response. Urology 1997; 49: 687–690; discussion 690–691.

223. Schwalb MD, Herr HW, Sogani PC, Russo P, Sheinfeld J, Fair WR. Positive urinary cytology following a complete response to intravesical bacillus Calmette-Guerin therapy: pattern of recurrence. J Urol 1994; 152: 382–387.

224. Jurincic-Winkler C, Metz KA, Beuth J, Sippel J, Klippel KF. Effect of keyhole limpet hemocyanin (KLH) and bacillus Calmette- Guerin (BCG) instillation on carcinoma in situ of the urinary bladder. Anticancer Res 1995; 15: 2771–2776.

225. Wishahi MM, Ismail MH, Ruebben H, Otto T. Keyhole-limpet hemocyanin immunotherapy in the bilharzial bladder: a new treatment modality? phase II trial: superficial bladder cancer. J Urol 1995; 153: 926–928.

226. Quilty PM, Duncan W. Treatment of superficial (T1) tumours of the bladder by radical radiotherapy. Br J Urol 1986; 58: 147–152.

227. Shipley WU, Kaufman DS, Heney NM, Althausen AF, Zietman AL. An update of combined modality therapy for patients with muscle invading bladder cancer using selective bladder preservation or cystectomy. J Urol 1999; 162: 445–450; discussion 450–451.

228. Nseyo UO, Shumaker B, Klein EA, Sutherland K. Photodynamic therapy using porfimer sodium as an alternative to cystectomy in patients with refractory transitional cell carcinoma in situ of the bladder. Bladder Photofrin Study Group. J Urol 1998;160: 39–44.

10 Radical Cystectomy and Pelvic Lymphadenectomy in the Treatment of Infiltrative Bladder Cancer

John P. Stein, MD, Donald G. Skinner, MD, and James E. Montie, MD

INTRODUCTION

Transitional cell carcinoma of the bladder is the second most common malignancy of the genitourinary tract, and the second most common cause of death of all genitourinary tumors. In 1999, it is estimated that 54,200 new patients will be diagnosed with bladder cancer, and 12,100 projected deaths from the disease *(1)*. Approximately 75% to

From: *Current Clinical Urology: Bladder Cancer: Current Diagnosis and Treatment*
Edited by: M. J. Droller © Humana Press Inc., Totowa, NJ

85% of patients with primary transitional cell carcinoma of the bladder present with low grade tumors confined to the superficial mucosa. The risk of superficial recurrence in patients with bladder tumors confined to the mucosa is 75%, with the majority of these cancers amenable to initial transurethral resection and selected administration of intravesical immunotherapy or chemotherapy *(2–4)*. However, 20% to 40% of all patients with transitional cell carcinoma of the bladder will either present with, or develop an invasive tumor of the bladder. Furthermore, in the past it has been reported that nearly 50% of patients treated locally for invasive bladder tumors present with metastatic disease within 2 yr of therapy *(3)*. This clearly underscores a malignant subset of invasive bladder tumors which may be most effectively treated by early, and aggressive radical therapy. Radical cystectomy has traditionally been considered the standard of therapy for high grade, invasive bladder cancer with the best survival results and lowest local recurrence rates reported to date *(5)*.

Invasive bladder cancer includes a spectrum of tumors ranging from infiltration of the superficial lamina propria, to extension into and through the muscularis propria. Traditionally, tumor invasion of the bladder muscularis has been the indication for aggressive radical therapy. In addition, there is sufficient evidence to suggest that high grade tumors that invade the lamina propria (T1) are at high risk for muscularis propria invasion, and tumor progression *(6–12)*, and may warrant an early aggressive management scheme. Furthermore, superficial bladder tumors with lymphovascular invasion *(8,13)*, those with prostatic urethral involvement *(14)*, or those which are associated with carcinoma in situ *(15,16)*, in conjunction with a poor response to repeated transurethral resection and intravesical therapy *(12)*; may also adversely affect the natural history of a superficial bladder tumor, and require similar aggressive therapy.

Currently, radical cystectomy provides the optimal result with regards to accurate pathologic staging, prevention of local recurrence, and overall survival *(5,17,18)*. In addition, radical cystectomy may influence the decision for adjuvant chemotherapy based upon clear pathologic criteria. In contemporary series, the best long-term survival rates for invasive bladder cancer have been achieved with radical cystectomy *(5,17–21)*. This may be a result of the natural history of high grade, invasive bladder cancer. Invasive bladder tumors tend to progressively invade from their superficial origin in the mucosa, to the lamina propria, and sequentially into the muscularis propria, perivesical fat and contiguous pelvic organs; with an increasing incidence of lymph node involvement at each site *(18,21–23)*. Furthermore, despite recent advances in radiographic imaging techniques, error in clinical staging of the primary bladder tumor is very common *(18,24,25)*. Radical cystectomy however, provides accurate pathologic staging of the primary bladder tumor and regional lymph nodes, which may serve to influence the decision of adjuvant treatment strategies.

With improvements over the past several decades in medical, surgical and anesthetic techniques, the morbidity and mortality associated with radical cystectomy has dramatically decreased. Prior to 1970, the perioperative complication rate of radical cystectomy was reportedly close to 35%, with a mortality rate of nearly 20%. This has dramatically diminished to less than a 10% perioperative complication rate and 2% mortality rate reported in contemporary series *(3,5–7,21)*. In addition, radical cystectomy with en bloc pelvic lymphadenectomy, provides optimal local control of the tumor. Pelvic recurrence rates in patient undergoing radical cystectomy are less than 10% for patients with node-negative bladder tumors, and 10%–20% for patients with resected pelvic nodal metastases *(5,23,26–28)*. Furthermore, transitional cell carcinoma is generally resistant to radiation therapy even at high doses, and chemotherapy alone or as adjuvant therapy, coupled with bladder sparing surgery, has yet to demonstrate equivalent recurrence and long-term survival rates compared to radical cystectomy alone *(17,29)*.

With a better understanding of the anatomic innervation to the corpora cavernosa, coupled with the evolution of orthotopic lower urinary tract reconstruction; the social, sexual and psychological implications following radical cystectomy have dramatically improved. In 1982, Walsh and Donker demonstrated that impotence following radical prostatectomy involved injury to the nerve supply to the corpora cavernosa *(30)*. This important anatomical discovery has subsequently been carefully applied to the technique of cystoprostatectomy in order to improve potency results in well-selected patients following surgery *(31)*. In addition, improvements in urinary diversion now provide most men and women the opportunity to safely undergo orthotopic lower urinary tract reconstruction to the native intact urethra following cystectomy *(32–36)*. Clearly, orthotopic reconstruction most closely resembles the original bladder in both location and function, and provides a continent means to store urine, and allows volitional voiding per urethra. In addition, the orthotopic neobladder eliminates the need for a cutaneous stoma, urostomy appliance, and the need for intermittent catheterization in most cases. A dedicated effort has been made to improve the technique of radical cystectomy, and provide an acceptable form of urinary diversion without compromise of a sound cancer operation, in a hope that patients may undergo earlier aggressive therapy when the potential for cure is highest.

Definition

Radical cystectomy implies the removal of the pelvic-iliac lymph nodes with the pelvic organs anterior to the rectum: the bladder, urachus, prostate, seminal vesicles, and visceral peritoneum in men; the bladder, urachus ovaries, Fallopian tubes, uterus, cervix, vaginal cuff, and the anterior pelvic peritoneum in women. The perivesical fat, pelvic and iliac lymph nodes are also removed en bloc with the specimen by the University of Southern California (USC) group, but as a separate specimen by the University of Michigan (UM) group. Certain technical issues regarding the surgical technique of a radical cystectomy are critical in order to minimizes local recurrence and positive surgical margins, and maximizes cancer-specific survival. In addition, attention to surgical detail is important to the successful application of orthotopic diversion, in order to maintain the rhabdosphincter mechanism and optimize urinary continence in these patients.

PREOPERATIVE EVALUATION

The majority of patients with bladder cancer present with hematuria and/or irritative voiding symptoms. After excluding a urinary tract infection, an excretory urogram (IVP) is usually performed to evaluate the upper urinary tract. Cystoscopy and urine cytology are then performed. Any filling defect identified on the IVP can be further assessed at the time of cystoscopy with retrograde ureteropyelography. When a bladder wall filling defect is seen on IVP, associated with ipsilateral hydronephrosis, it is highly suggestive of an invasive lesion and can be further evaluated with a computerized tomography (CT) prior to transurethral resection.

When a bladder tumor is identified cystoscopically, or abnormal cells reported on urine cytology, a careful bimanual examination and transurethral resection (or deep biopsy of the tumor) is performed under general anesthesia to establish a pathologic diagnosis with determination of depth of tumor invasion. This should include directed bladder biopsies of adjacent and normal appearing bladder mucosa remote from the primary tumor. In order to avoid an inadvertent bladder perforation with potential tumor spill, caution should be taken when completely resecting an obvious invasive bladder tumor; particularly when radical cystectomy is anticipated should be avoided. In women, particular attention should be directed toward the anterior vaginal wall on bimanual pelvic examination. If the primary bladder tumor is a deeply invasive posterior lesion with involvement of the anterior vaginal wall, the bladder should be removed *en bloc* with the anterior vaginal wall. This may require vaginal reconstruction if sexual function is desired postoperatively. In addition, women with anterior vaginal wall involvement with tumor are at increased risk of urethral tumor involvement which may preclude orthotopic urinary diversion *(35–37)*. Furthermore, all women should undergo cystoscopic evaluation of the bladder neck (vesico-urethral junction) to evaluate for a bladder neck tumor involvement; a well known significant risk factor for concomitant urethral tumor involvement which would thus preclude orthotopic reconstruction in a female patient *(37,38)*.

Complete clinical staging for bladder cancer should evaluate the most common metastatic sites including the lungs, liver and bone. A chest X-ray, liver function tests, and serum alkaline phosphatase should be obtained routinely. Patients with an elevated serum alkaline phosphatase or with complaints of bone pain should undergo a bone scan. A CT scan of the chest is obtained when pulmonary metastases are suspected by history, or because of an abnormal chest X-ray. A CT scan of the abdomen/pelvis is not routinely performed as it is neither sensitive nor specific enough to evaluate the degree of bladder wall tumor invasion, or to accurately determine pelvic lymph node involvement with tumor *(24, 39)*. However, a CT scan of the abdomen/pelvis may be performed in patients with suspected metastases, elevated liver function tests, a bladder tumor associated with ipsilateral hydronephrosis, or in patients with a T4 primary bladder tumor, the results of which may impact upon the decision for neoadjuvant therapy.

Bladder tumors associated with ipsilateral hydronephrosis, generally suggest an invasive lesion of the bladder *(40,41)*. In fact, Hatch and Barry found ureteral obstruction to be associated with muscle invasion in over 90% of patients with transitional cell carcinoma and hydronephrosis *(40)*. Recently, a retrospective analysis of 415 consecutive patients who underwent radical cystectomy for invasive bladder cancer was reported evaluating the specific variable of hydronephrosis (unilateral and bilateral), as determined by preoperative radiographic imaging studies with regard to pathologic stage and clinical outcome *(41)*. Of these patients, 299 patients (72%) demonstrated no preoperative evidence of hydronephrosis, 94 patients (23%) had unilateral hydronephrosis, and 22 patients (5%) had bilateral hydronephrosis. All patients were uniformly treated and pathologically staged. A significant correlation between hydronephrosis and advanced bladder cancer stage, and decreased patient survival was identified. Of the 116 patients with either unilateral or bilateral hydronephrosis, 85% had muscle invasive tumors or greater ($\geq$P2). Of the 94 patients with unilateral hydronephrosis, 83% demonstrated bladder tumors with pathologic evidence of muscle invasion of the bladder ($\geq$P2). This confirms previous reports that patients presenting with unilateral hydronephrosis and bladder cancer generally have muscle invasive tumors. Furthermore, when evaluating patients with bladder cancer who present with bilateral hydronephrosis, over 90% of patients demonstrated advanced disease pathologically, with extension outside the bladder (> P3b, or lymph node positive disease). Moreover, the 5-yr survival for patients with no hydronephrosis was 62%, compared to 45% and 30% for those with unilateral and bilateral hydronephrosis respectively.

These data suggest that patients with unilateral hydronephrosis have muscle invasive tumors, while those patients presenting with bilateral hydronephrosis may have a more ominous prognosis (41). Obviously, the presence of hydronephrosis (unilateral or bilateral) as determined by preoperative radiographic imaging is an important piece of clinical information which may help dictate therapy and provide prognostic information.

PREOPERATIVE RADIATION THERAPY

The rationale for preoperative radiation therapy for invasive bladder cancer has been based upon 3 assumptions:

1. Preoperative radiation may reduce the primary bladder tumor burden, potentially impacting systemic metastases and improving survival rates.
2. Preoperative radiation may improve local control by decreasing microscopic or macroscopic tumor extension and reduce the positive surgical margin rate.
3. Preoperative radiation may make radical cystectomy technically easier by reducing the overall primary tumor burden.

However, these presumptions do not appear to be supported by data from contemporary series. Preoperative radiation is not an effective adjuvant therapy to cystectomy with regards to survival, compared to surgery alone for the treatment of invasive urothelial cancer (19,29,42–44). In addition, preoperative radiation therapy has not been found to improve local recurrence rates compared to cystectomy alone (19,42). Although preoperative radiation of less then 5000 rads has little significant impact on the operation in terms of complications or the ability to perform a successful procedure, this dose is generally ineffective against bladder cancer. However, radiation doses in excess of 6000 rads is definitely associated with increased surgical morbidity and mortality (45). Currently, the only sound indication for preoperative radiation therapy in the management of invasive bladder cancer is in the event of an inadvertent tumor spill. Wound implantation with tumor may occur in 10%–20% of these patients (46), and can be prevented by a high dose, short course of preoperative radiation (47).

EN BLOC RADICAL CYSTECTOMY AND PELVIC-ILIAC LYMPHADENECTOMY: SURGICAL TECHNIQUE IN THE MALE AND FEMALE PATIENT

Preoperative Preparation

Patients undergoing radical cystectomy are generally admitted the morning prior to surgery at USC and on the day of surgery at UM unless medical conditions dictate otherwise. All patients receive a mechanical and antibacterial bowel preparation the day prior to surgery. Intravenous hydration must be considered in these patients to prevent dehydration upon arrival to the operating room. In addition, all patients should be evaluated and counseled by the enterostomal therapy nurse prior to surgery. A clear liquid diet may be consumed until midnight, at which time the patient takes nothing per mouth. A standard modified Nichols bowel prep *(48)* is initiated the morning of admission: 120 mL of Neoloid per mouth at 9:00 AM; 1 g of neomycin per mouth at 10:00 AM, 11:00 AM, 12:00 PM, 1:00 PM, 4:00 PM, 8:00 PM, and 12:00 AM; and 1 g of erythromycin base per mouth at 12:00 PM, 4:00 PM, 8:00 PM, and 12:00 AM. This regimen is well tolerated, obviates the need for enemas, and maintains nutritional and hydrational support. Intravenous crystalloid fluid hydration is begun in the evening prior to surgery in those patients admitted to the hospital the day prior to surgery, and maintained to ensure an adequate circulating volume as the patient enters the operating room. This may be particularly important in the elderly, frail patient with associated co-morbidities.

Patients over 50 yr of age at the USC routinely undergo prophylactic digitalization prior to cystectomy unless there is a specific contraindication. Patients younger than 50 yr of age are not routinely digitalized at USC. Digoxin is given orally; 0.5 mg at 12:00 PM, 0.25 mg at 4:00 PM, and 0.125 mg at 8:00 PM. Evidence suggests that preoperative digitalization may decrease the risk of perioperative dysrhythmias and congestive heart failure in the elderly patient undergoing an extensive operative procedure *(49,50)*. At UM digoxin is not employed based on the judgment that congestive heart failure after surgery is almost exclusively related to fluid overload rather than poor cardiac function. Attention to fluid management is important in these elderly patients particularly on postoperative day three and four when mobilization of third-space fluid is highest, subsequently necessitating liberal use of diuretics. In addition, intravenous broad spectrum antibiotics are administered en route to the operating room, providing adequate tissue and circulating levels at the time of incision.

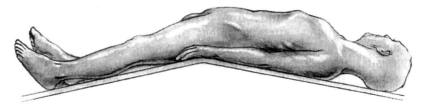

Fig. 1. Proper patient positioning for cystectomy. Note that the iliac crest is located at the break of the table. (Reproduced with permission from Skinner DG, Lieskovsky G (eds): *Diagnosis and Management of Genitourinary Cancer*. WB Saunders, Philadelphia, PA, 1988) (Skinner, Fig. 42-1).

Preoperative evaluation and counseling by the enterostomal therapy nurse is a critical component to the successful care of all patients undergoing cystectomy and urinary diversion. Currently, at USC approximately 90% of male and female patients requiring cystectomy for bladder cancer are appropriate candidates for orthotopic diversion *(33,36)*. At UM nearly 60% of men and 80% of women undergo orthotopic diversion. Patients determined to be appropriate candidates for orthotopic reconstruction are instructed how to catheterize per urethra should it be necessary postoperatively. All patients are site marked for a cutaneous stoma, instructed in the care of a cutaneous diversion (continent or incontinent form), and instructed in proper catheterization techniques should medical or technical factors preclude orthotopic reconstruction. The ideal cutaneous stoma site is determined only after the patient is examined in the supine, sitting and standing position. Proper stoma site selection is important to patient acceptance, and to the technical success of lower urinary tract reconstruction should a cutaneous form of diversion be necessary. In general, incontinent stoma sites are best located higher on the abdominal wall, while stoma sites for continent diversions can be positioned lower on the abdomen (hidden below the belt line) since they do not require an external collecting device. In addition, the use of the umbilicus as the site for catheterization may be employed with excellent functional and cosmetic results.

Patient Positioning

The patient is placed in the hyperextended supine position with the iliac crest located just below the fulcrum of the operating table (Fig. 1). The legs are slightly abducted so that the heels are positioned near the corners of the foot of the table. In the female patient considering orthotopic diversion, the modified frogleg or lithotomy position is employed, allowing easy access to the vagina. Care should be taken to ensure that all pressure points are well padded. Reverse Trendelenburg position levels the abdomen parallel with the floor and helps to keep the small bowel contents in the epigastrium. A nasogastric tube is placed, and the patient is prepped from nipples to mid-thigh. In the female patient the vagina is fully prepped. After the patient is draped, a 20F Foley catheter is placed in the bladder, and left open to gravity. A right handed surgeon stands on the patient's left hand side of the operating table.

Incision

A vertical midline incision is made extending from the pubic symphysis to the cephalad aspect of the epigastrium. The incision should be carried lateral to the umbilicus on the contralateral side of the marked cutaneous stoma site. When considering the umbilicus as the site for a catheterizable stoma, the incision should be directed 2–3 cm lateral to the umbilicus at this location. The anterior rectus fascia is incised, the rectus muscles retracted laterally, and the posterior rectus sheath and peritoneum entered in the superior aspect of the incision. As the peritoneum and posterior fascia are incised inferiorly to the level of the umbilicus, the urachal remnant (median umbilical ligament) is identified, circumscribed, and removed *en bloc* with the cystectomy specimen (Fig. 2). This maneuver prevents early entry into a high-riding bladder, and ensures complete removal of all bladder remnant tissue. Care is taken to remain medial and avoid injury to the inferior epigastric vessels (lateral umbilical ligaments) which course posterior to the rectus muscles. If the patient has had a previous cystotomy or segmental cystectomy, the cystotomy tract and cutaneous incision should be circumscribed full-thickness and excised *en bloc* with the bladder specimen. The medial insertion of the rectus muscles attached to the pubic symphysis are slightly incised, maximizing pelvic exposure throughout the operation.

Abdominal Exploration

A careful systematic intra-abdominal exploration is performed to determine the extent of disease, and to evaluate for any hepatic metastases, or gross retroperitoneal lymphadenopathy. The abdominal viscera are palpated to detect any concomitant unrelated disease. If no contraindication exists at this time, all adhesions should be incised and freed.

Bowel Mobilization

The bowel is mobilized starting with the right colon. A large right angle Richardson retractor elevates the right abdominal wall. The cecum

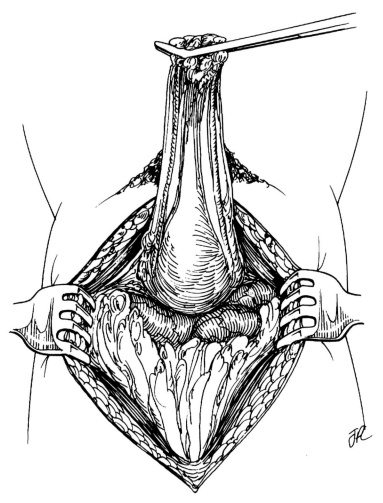

Fig. 2. Wide excision of the urachal remnant en bloc with the cystectomy speci-
men. (Reproduced with permission from Walsh PC, Retik AB, Stamey TA,
Vaughan ED (eds): *Cambell's Urology*, 6th edition. WB Saunders, Philadelphia,
PA, 1992) (Walsh, Fig. 74-3).

and ascending colon are reflected medially to allow incision of the lateral peritoneal reflection along the avascular/white line of Toldt. At USC
the mesentery to the small bowel is then mobilized off its retroperitoneal
attachments cephalad (toward the ligament of Treitz) until the retroperitoneal portion of the duodenum is exposed. This mobilization will facilitate a tension free urethroenteric anastomosis if orthotopic diversion is
performed. Combined sharp and blunt dissection facilitates mobilization of this mesentery along a characteristic avascular fibroareolar plane.

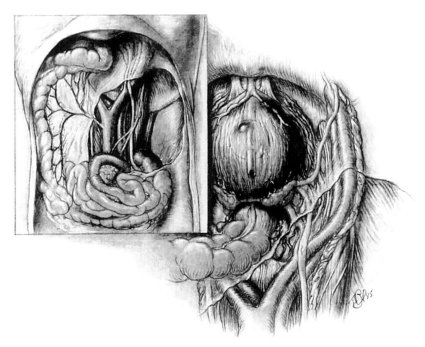

Fig. 3. View of the pelvis from overhead; after the ascending colon and peritoneal attachments of the small bowel mesentery have been mobilized up to the level of the duodenum. This mobilization allows the bowel to be properly packed in the epigastrium and exposes the area of the aortic bifurcation which is the starting point of the lymph node dissection. (Skinner, Fig. 42-2).

Conceptually, the mobilized mesentery forms an inverted right triangle; the base formed by the third and fourth portions of the duodenum, the right edge represented by the white line of Toldt along the ascending colon, the left edge represented by the medial portion of the sigmoid and descending colonic mesentery, and the apex represented by the ileocecal region (Fig. 3). This mobilization is critical in setting up the operative field, and facilitates proper packing of the intra-abdominal contents into the epigastrium. At UM, mobilization of the right-sided pelvic viscera is more limited, and only the region of the cecum is mobilized immediately to provide exposure to the common iliac vessels.

The left colon and sigmoid mesentery are then mobilized to the region of the lower pole of the left kidney by incising the peritoneum lateral to the colon along the avascular/white line of Toldt. The sigmoid mesentery is then elevated off the sacrum, iliac vessels, and distal aorta cephalad to the origin of the inferior mesenteric artery. This maneuver provides a mesenteric window through which the left ureter will pass (without angulation or tension) for the ureteroenteric anastomosis to the urinary

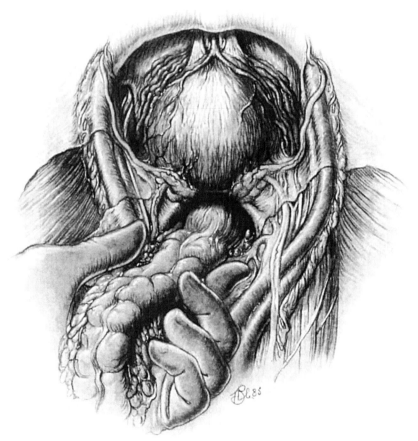

Fig. 4. View of the pelvis from overhead; after the ascending colon and small bowel have been packed in the epigastrium. Note that the sigmoid mesentery is mobilized off the sacral promontory and distal aorta up to the origin of the inferior mesenteric artery. (Skinner, Fig. 42-3).

reservoir at the terminal portions of the operation, and also facilitates retraction of the sigmoid mesentery while performing the lymph node dissection (Fig. 4). Care should be taken to dissect along the base of the mesentery which prevents injury to the inferior mesenteric artery and blood supply to the sigmoid colon.

Following mobilization of the bowel, a self-retaining retractor is placed (Finochietto retractor at USC, Bookwalter retractor at UM). The right colon and small intestine are carefully packed into the epigastrium with three moist lap pads, followed by a moistened towel rolled to the width of the abdomen. The descending and sigmoid colon are not packed, and left as free as possible, providing the necessary mobility required for the ureteral and pelvic lymph node dissection.

Successful packing of the intestinal contents is an art and prevents their annoying spillage into the operative field. Packing begins by sweeping the right colon and small bowel under the surgeon's left hand along the right sidewall gutter. A moist open lap pad is then swept with the right hand along the palm of the left hand, under the viscera along the retroperitoneum and sidewall gutter. In similar fashion, the left sidewall gutter is packed ensuring not to incorporate the descending or sigmoid colon. The central portion of the small bowel is packed with a third lap pad. A moist rolled towel is then positioned horizontally below the lap pads, but cephalad to the bifurcation of the aorta. Occasionally, prior to placement of the first moist lap pad, a mobile greater omental apron can be used to facilitate packing of the intestinal viscera in a similar fashion to the lap pad. After the bowel has been packed, a wide Deaver retractor or self-retaining right angle Bookwalter blade is placed with gentle traction on the previously packing to provide cephalad exposure.

Ureteral Dissection

The ureters are most easily identified in the retroperitoneum just cephalad to the common iliac vessels. They are dissected into the deep pelvis (several cm beyond the iliac vessels) and divided between two large hemoclips. A section of the proximal cut ureteral segment (distal to the proximal hemoclip) is then sent for frozen section analysis to ensure the absence of carcinoma in situ or overt tumor. The ureter is then mobilized cephalad and tucked under the rolled towel to prevent inadvertent injury. Frequently, an arterial branch from the common iliac artery or the aorta needs to be divided to provide adequate ureteral mobilization. In addition, the rich vascular supply emanating from the gonadal vessels should remain intact and undisturbed. These attachments are an important blood supply to the ureter which ensure an adequate vascular supply for the ureteroenteric anastomosis at the time of diversion. This is particularly important in irradiated patients. Leaving the proximal hemoclip on the divided ureter during the exenteration allows for hydrostatic ureteral dilation, and facilitates the ureteroenteric anastomosis.

Pelvic Lymphadenectomy

A meticulous pelvic lymph node dissection is routinely performed *en bloc* by the USC group and separately by the UM group with radical cystectomy. The extent of the lymphadenectomy may vary depending on the patient and surgeon preference. When performing a salvage procedure following definitive radiation treatment (greater then 5000 rads), a pelvic lymphadenectomy is usually not performed because of the significant risk of iliac vessel and obturator nerve injury *(39)*.

For a combined common and pelvic iliac lymphadenectomy the group at USC initiate the lymph node dissection 2 cm above the aortic bifurcation (superior limits of dissection), and extends laterally over the inferior vena cava to the genitofemoral nerve, representing the lateral limits of dissection. Distally, the lymph node dissection extends to the lymph node of Cloquet medially (on Cooper's ligament) and the circumflex iliac vein laterally.

The cephalad portion (2 cm above the aortic bifurcation) of the lymphatics are ligated with hemoclips to prevent lymphatic leak, while the caudal (specimen) side is ligated only when a blood vessel is encountered. Frequently, small anterior tributary veins originate from the vena cava just above the bifurcation, which should be clipped and divided. In men, the spermatic vessels are retracted laterally and spared. However, in women the infundibulopelvic ligament along with the corresponding ovarian vessels are ligated and divided at the pelvic brim.

All fibroareolar and lymphatic tissues are dissected caudally off the aorta, vena cava, and common iliac vessels over the sacral promontory into the deep pelvis. The initial dissection along the common iliac vessels is performed over the arteries, skeletonizing them. As the common iliac veins are dissected medially, care is taken to control small arterial and venous branches coursing along the anterior surface of the sacrum. Electrocautery is helpful at this location which allows the adherent fibroareolar tissue to be swept off the sacral promontory down into the deep pelvis with the use of a small gauze sponge. Significant bleeding from these presacral vessels can occur if not properly controlled. Hemoclips are discouraged in this location as they can be easily dislodged from the anterior surface of the sacrum, resulting in troublesome bleeding.

Once the proximal portion of the lymph node dissection is completed, a finger is passed from the proximal aspect of dissection under the pelvic peritoneum (anterior to the iliac vessels), distally toward the femoral canal. The opposite hand can be used to strip the peritoneum from the undersurface of the transversalis fascia, and connects with the proximal dissection from above. This maneuver elevates the peritoneum and helps define the lateral limit of peritoneum to be incised and removed with the specimen. In male patients, the peritoneum is divided medial to the spermatic vessels, and lateral to the infundibulopelvic ligament in female patients. The only structure encountered is the vas deferens in the male or round ligament in the female; these structures are clipped and divided.

A large right-angled rake retractor (e.g., Israel) is used to elevate the lower abdominal wall, including the spermatic cord or remnant of the round ligament, to provide distal exposure in the area of the femoral canal. Tension on the retractor is directed vertically toward the ceiling,

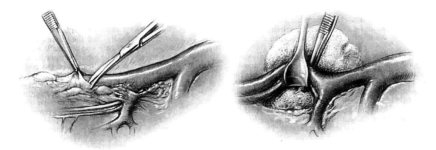

Fig. 5. (Left) Technique of skeletonizing the external iliac artery and vein. (Skinner, Fig. 42-4A.). **Fig. 6.** (Right) Technique of passing a small gauze sponge lateral to the external iliac vessels and medial to the psoas muscle. (Skinner, Fig. 42-4B).

with care taken to avoid injury to the inferior epigastric vessels. This provides excellent exposure to the distal external iliac vessels. The distal limits of the dissection are then identified: the circumflex iliac vein crossing anterior to the external iliac artery distally, the genitofemoral nerve laterally, and Cooper's ligament medially. The lymphatics draining the ipsilateral leg, particularly medial to the external iliac vein, are carefully clipped and divided to prevent lymphatic leakage. This includes the lymph node of Cloquet (also known as Rosenmuller) which represents the distal limit of the lymphatic dissection at this location. The distal external iliac artery and vein are then circumferentially dissected and skeletonized with care taken to ligate an accessory obturator vein (present in 40% of patients) originating from the inferiomedial aspect of the external iliac vein.

Following completion of the distal limits of dissection, the proximal and distal dissections are joined. The proximal external iliac artery and vein are skeletonized circumferentially to the origin of the hypogastric artery (Fig. 5). Care should be taken to clip and divide a commonly encountered vessel arising from the lateral aspect of the proximal external iliac vessels coursing to the psoas muscle. The external iliac vessels are then retracted medially, and the fascia overlying the psoas muscle is incised medial to the genitofemoral nerve. On the left side, branches of the genitofemoral nerve often pursue a more medial course and may be intimately related to the iliac vessels, in which case they are excised.

At this point, the lymphatic tissue surrounding the iliac vessels are composed of a medial and lateral component attached only at the base within the obturator fossa. The lateral lymphatic compartment (freed medially from the vessels and laterally from the psoas) is bluntly swept into the obturator fossa by retracting the iliac vessels medially, and passing a small gauze sponge lateral to the vessels along the psoas and

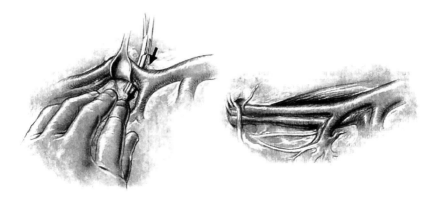

Fig. 7. (Left) Technique of withdrawing the gauze sponge with the left hand. This aids in dissecting the obturator fossa, sweeping all fibroareolar and lymphatic tissue toward the bladder. (Skinner, Fig. 42-4C). **Fig. 8.** (Right) Obturator fossa cleaned. This allows proper identification of the obturator nerve passing deep to the external iliac vein. (Skinner, Fig. 42-4D).

pelvic sidewall (Fig. 6). This sponge should be passed anterior and distal to the hypogastric vein, directed caudally into the obturator fossa. The external iliac vessels are then elevated and retracted laterally while the gauze sponge is carefully withdrawn from the obturator fossa with gentle traction using the left hand (Fig. 7). This maneuver effectively sweeps all lymphatic tissue into the obturator fossa, and facilitates identification of the obturator nerve deep to the external iliac vein. The obturator nerve is best identified proximally and carefully dissected free from all lymphatics. The obturator nerve is then retracted laterally along with the iliac vessels (Fig. 8). At this point, the obturator artery and vein are entrapped between the index finger laterally (medial to the obturator nerve) and the middle finger medially of the left hand. This isolates the obturator vessels exiting the obturator canal along the pelvic floor. These vessels are then carefully clipped and divided ensuring to stay medial to the obturator nerve. The obturator lymph node packet is then swept medially toward the sidewall of the bladder, ligating small tributary vessels and lymphatics from the pelvic sidewall, and removed en bloc with the cystectomy specimen.

Ligation of the Lateral Vascular Pedicle to the Bladder

Following dissection of the obturator fossa and dividing the obturator vessels, the lateral vascular pedicle to the bladder is isolated and divided. Developing this plane isolates the lateral vascular pedicle to the bladder; a critical maneuver in performing a safe cystectomy with proper vascular control. Isolation of the lateral vascular pedicle is performed with the

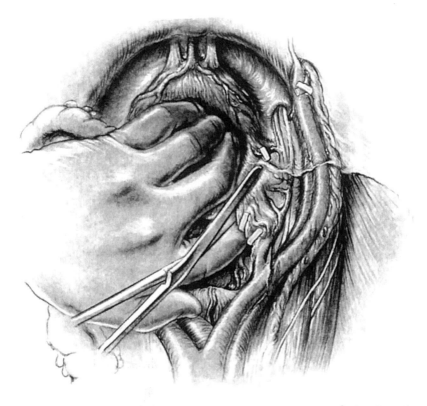

Fig. 9. The left hand is used to define the right lateral pedicle, extending from the bladder to the hypogastric artery. This plane is developed by the index finger (medial) and the middle finger (lateral), exposing the anterior branches of the hypogastric artery. This vascular pedicle is clipped and divided down to the endopelvic fascia. Traction with the left hand defines the pedicle, allows direct visualization, and protects the rectum from injury. (Skinner, Fig. 42-5).

left hand. The bladder is retracted toward the pelvis, placing traction on the anterior branches of the hypogastric artery. The left index finger is passed medial to the hypogastric artery, posterior to the anterior visceral branches, and lateral to the previously transected ureter. The index finger is directed caudally toward the endopelvic fascia, parallel to the sweep of the sacrum. This maneuver defines the two major vascular pedicles to the anterior pelvic organs: the lateral pedicle; anterior to the index finger, composed of the visceral branches of the anterior hypogastric vessel, and the posterior pedicle; posterior to the index finger, composed of the visceral branches between the bladder and rectum.

With the lateral pedicle entrapped between the left index and middle fingers, firm traction is applied vertically and caudally. This facilitates skeletonization of the anterior branches off the hypogastric artery (Fig. 9). The posterior division of the hypogastric artery including the superior gluteal, ilio-lumbar, and lateral sacral arteries are preserved to avoid gluteal claudication. Distal to this posterior division, the hypogastric artery may be ligated for vascular control, but should not be divided since the lateral pedicle is easier to dissect if left in continuity. The largest and most consistent anterior branch to the bladder, the superior vesical artery, can usually be isolated and individually ligated and divided. The remaining anterior branches of the lateral pedicle are then divided between large hemoclips down to the endopelvic fascia, or as far as is technically possible. With blunt dissection the index finger of the left hand helps identify this lateral pedicle, and protects the rectum as it is pushed medially. Large right angle hemoclip appliers are ideally suited for proper placement of the clips. Each pair of hemoclips are positioned as far apart as possible to ensure that 0.5–1 cm of tissue projects beyond each clip when the pedicle is divided. This prevents the hemoclips from being dislodged resulting in unnecessary bleeding. Occasionally, in patients with an abundance of pelvic fat, the lateral pedicle may be thick and require division into two manageable pedicles. The inferior vesicle vein serves as an excellent landmark as the endopelvic fascia is just distal to this structure. The endopelvic fascia just lateral to the prostate may then be incised which helps identify the distal limit of the lateral pedicle.

Ligation of the Posterior Pedicle to the Bladder

Following division of the lateral pedicles, the bladder specimen is retracted anteriorly exposing the cul-de-sac (pouch of Douglas). The surgeon elevates the bladder with a small gauze sponge under the left hand, while the assistant retracts on the peritoneum of the rectosigmoid colon in a cephalad direction. This provides excellent exposure to the recess of the cul-de-sac, and places the peritoneal reflection on traction which facilitates proper division. The peritoneum lateral to the rectum is incised, and extended anteriorly across the cul-de-sac to join the incision on the contralateral side (Fig. 10). It should be emphasized that the anterior and posterior peritoneal reflections converge in the cul-de-sac to form Denonvilliers' fascia, which extends caudally to the urogenital diaphragm (Fig. 11, *large arrow*). This important anatomic boundary in the male separates the prostate and seminal vesicles anterior to the rectum posterior. The plane between the prostate and seminal vesicles, and the anterior sheath of Denonvilliers' will not develop easily. However, the plane between the rectum and the posterior sheath of Denonvilliers' (Denonvilliers' space) should develop easily with blunt dissection. Therefore, the peritoneal incision in the cul-de-sac must be made on the rectal

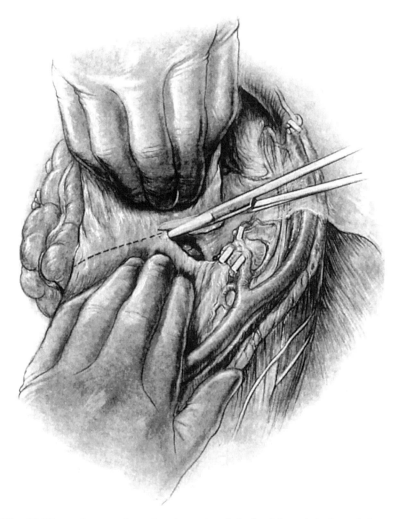

Fig. 10. The peritoneum lateral to the rectum is incised down into the cul-de-sac, and carried anteriorly over the rectum to join the opposite side. Note that the incision should be made precisely so the proper plane behind Denonvilliers' fascia can be developed safely. (Skinner, Fig. 42-7).

side rather than the bladder side (Fig. 11, *small arrow*). This allows proper and safe development of Denonvilliers' space between the anterior rectal wall and the posterior sheath of Denonvilliers' fascia (Fig. 12). Employing a posterior sweeping motion of the fingers, the rectum can be carefully swept off the seminal vesicles, prostate, and bladder in men, and off the posterior vaginal wall in women. This sweeping motion, when extended laterally, helps to thin and develop the posterior pedicle which appears like a collar emanating from the lateral aspect of the rectum.

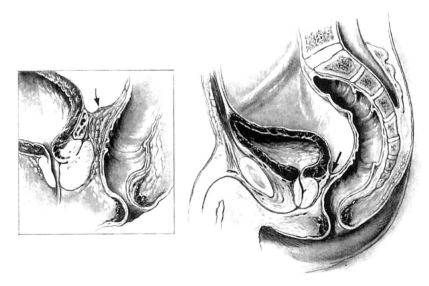

Fig. 11. Illustration of the formation of Denonvilliers' fascia. Note that it is derived from a fusion of the anterior and posterior peritoneal reflections. Denonvilliers' space lies behind the fascia. To successfully enter this space and facilitate mobilization of the anterior rectal wall off Denonvilliers' fascia, the incision in the cul-de-sac is made close to the peritoneal fusion on the anterior rectal wall side, and not on the bladder side. (Skinner, Fig. 42-6).

Care should be taken as one develops this posterior plane more caudally as the anterior rectal fibers often are adherent to the specimen, and can be difficult to bluntly dissect. In the region just cephalad (proximal) to the urogenital diaphragm, sharp dissection may be required to dissect the anterior rectal fibers off the apex of the prostate in order to prevent rectal injury at this location.

Particular mention should be made concerning several situations which may impede the proper development of this posterior plane. Most commonly, when the incision in the cul-de-sac is made too far anteriorly, proper entry into Denonvilliers' space is prevented. Improper entry can occur in between the two layers of Denonvilliers' fascia, or even anterior to this, making the posterior dissection difficult, increasing the risk of rectal injury. Furthermore, posterior tumor infiltration, or previous high dose pelvic irradiation can obliterate this plane making the posterior dissection difficult. To prevent injury to the rectum in these situations, dissection of this plane can be facilitated by combining an initial perineal approach (*see* salvage cystectomy) from below with sharp dissection from above or by relying on a retrograde dissection of the prostate under direct vision similar to that employed during a radical

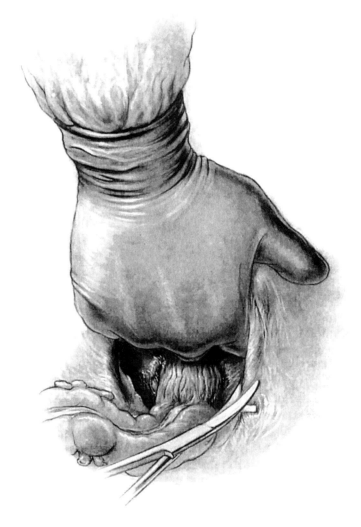

Fig. 12. After the peritoneum of the cul-de-sac has been incised, the anterior rectal wall can be swept off the posterior surface of the Denonvilliers' fascia. This effectively defines the posterior pedicle that extends from the bladder to the lateral aspect of the rectum on either side. (Skinner, Fig. 42-8).

prostatectomy. The key to prevent a rectal injury is to avoid blunt dissection with the finger in areas where normal tissue planes have been obliterated by previous surgery or radiation. Sharp dissection under direct vision will dramatically reduce the potential for rectal injury. If a rectotomy occurs, a two or three layer closure is recommended. A diverting proximal colostomy is not routinely required unless gross contamination occurs, or if the patient has received previous pelvic radiation therapy. If orthotopic diversion or vaginal reconstruction is planned, an omental interposition is recommended to prevent fistulization between suture lines.

Once the posterior pedicles have been defined, they are clipped and divided to the endopelvic fascia in the male patient. The endopelvic fascia is then incised adjacent to the prostate, medial to the levator ani muscles (if not done previously), to facilitate the apical dissection. In the female patient, the posterior pedicles including the cardinal ligaments are divided 4 to 5 cm beyond the cervix. With cephalad pressure on a previously placed vaginal sponge stick, the apex of the vagina can be identified, and opened posteriorly just distal to the cervix. The vagina is then circumscribed anteriorly with the cervix attached to the cystectomy specimen. If there is concern about an adequate surgical margin at the posterior or base of the bladder, then the anterior vaginal wall should be removed en bloc with the bladder specimen; subsequently requiring vaginal reconstruction postoperatively if sexual function is desired. It is preferable to spare the anterior vaginal wall if orthotopic diversion is planned. This eliminates the need for vaginal reconstruction, and helps maintain the complex musculofascial support system and helps prevent injury to the pudendal innervation to the rhabdosphincter proximal urethra, both important components to the continence mechanism in women. The anterior vaginal wall is then sharply dissected off the posterior bladder down to the region of the bladder neck (vesicourethral junction) which is identified by palpating the Foley catheter balloon. At this point, the specimen is attached only at the apex in men and vesicourethral junction in women.

Anterior Apical Dissection in the Male Patient

Attention is now directed anteriorly. All fibroareolar connections between the anterior bladder wall, prostate, and undersurface of the pubic symphysis are divided. The superficial dorsal vein is identified, ligated and divided. With tension placed posteriorly on the prostate, the puboprostatic ligaments are identified, and divided just beneath the pubis, and lateral to the dorsal venous complex which courses in between these ligaments. Following transection of the puboprostatic ligaments, the levator muscle fibers are mobilized laterally off the prostate. The apex of the prostate and membranous urethra now becomes palpable. Several methods can be performed to control the dorsal venous plexus. One may carefully pass an angled clamp beneath the dorsal vein complex, anterior to the urethra. The venous complex is then ligated with a 2-0 absorbable suture, and divided close to the apex of the prostate. Any bleeding from the transected venous complex can then be oversewn with an absorbable (2-0 polyglycolic acid) suture. In similar fashion, the dorsal venous complex may be gathered anterior to the urethra, distal to the apex of the prostate with a long Allis clamp, and a figure of eight 2-0 absorbable suture placed under direct vision anterior to the urethra around the venous complex. This maneuver avoids passage of any instruments between the dorsal venous complex and rhabdosphincter which could potentially disrupt or injure these structures and compromise the continence mechanism. After the complex has been ligated it can be sharply divided with excellent exposure to the anterior surface of the urethra. The urethra is then incised just beyond the apex of the prostate, and a series of 2-0 Monocryl (at USC) or 3-0 Monocryl (at UM) sutures placed in the urethra circumferentially. To provide better purchase to the sutures they may be carefully placed, incorporating the edge of the dorsal venous complex anteriorly and recto-urethralis muscle posteriorly, or the caudal extent of Denonvilliers' fascia. The Foley catheter is then clamped with a curved Kocher clamp and transected distal to the specimen removed.

Alternatively, the dorsal venous complex can be sharply transected without dividing the puboprostatic ligaments, with or without securing vascular control. Cephalad traction on the prostate elongates the proximal and membranous urethra, and allows the urethra to be skeletonized laterally by dividing the so-called "lateral pillars" which are extensions of the rhabdosphincter. The anterior two-thirds of the urethra is divided, exposing the urethral catheter. The urethral sutures can then be placed under direct vision. Six 2-0 Monocryl (at USC), or four 3-0 Monocryl (at UM) sutures are placed equally spaced into the urethral mucosa and lumen anteriorly. At USC the rhabdosphincter, the edge of which acts as a hood overlying the dorsal vein complex, is included in these sutures if the venous complex was sharply incised. This maneuver serves to maintain urinary continence, and compresses the dorsal vein complex against the urethra for hemostatic purposes. At UM, efforts are made to place small, 3–4 mm bites into the urethra to minimize an "accordion" effect on the urethra by the sutures. These maneuvers serve to enhance urinary continence. The urethral catheter is then drawn through the urethrotomy, clamped on the bladder side and divided. Cephalad traction on the bladder side with the clamped catheter occludes the bladder neck, prevents tumor spill from the bladder, and provides exposure excellent to the posterior urethra. One or two additional sutures can then be placed in the posterior urethra incorporating the recto-urethralis muscle or distal Denonvilliers' fascia. The posterior urethra is then divided and the specimen removed. The urethral sutures are appropriately tagged to identify their location and placed under a towel until the urethroenteric anastomosis is performed. Bleeding from the dorsal vein is usually minimal at this point. If additional hemostasis is required, 1 or 2 anterior urethral sutures can be tied to stop the bleeding. Frozen section analysis of the distal urethral margin of the cystectomy specimen is then performed to exclude tumor involvement.

These aforementioned technical modifications in the apical dissection in men undergoing orthotopic diversion are based on the excellent functional results observed in female patients undergoing the same form of diversion. Women retain their continence mechanism almost immediately following removal of the urethral catheter which may be attributed to the limited dissection performed anterior to the urethra along the pelvic floor. Based on the improved results of more rapid return of continence in women, it is likely that the continence mechanism in men may also be maximized if dissection in the region of the anterior urethra is minimized. These observations have recently led to modifications in the technique by many groups of the apical dissection in the male patient undergoing orthotopic reconstruction, all in an attempt to minimize the apical dissection along the pelvic floor and maximize the continence mechanism.

If a cutaneous form of urinary diversion is planned, urethral preparation is slightly modified. Once the dorsal venous complex is secured and divided, the anterior urethra is identified. The urethra is mobilized from above as far distally as possible into the pelvic diaphragm. With cephalad traction, the urethra is stretched above the urogenital diaphragm, a curved clamp is placed as distal on the urethra as feasible and divided distal to the clamp. Care must be taken avoid rectal injury with this clamp. This is prevented by placing gentle posterior traction with the left hand or index finger on the rectum and ensuring the clamp is passed anterior. The specimen is then removed. Mobilization of the urethra as distally as possible facilitates a late urethrectomy should it be necessary. The levator musculature can then be reapproximated along the pelvic floor to facilitate hemostasis.

Anterior Dissection in the Female

Female cystectomies are easier than in men in some ways and more difficult in others. Exposure is better in a woman, particularly at the vesicourethral junction. However, many urologists are less familiar with pelvic surgery in women than in men, paravaginal vascular control may be difficult in women, and the venous plexus anterior to the urethra is less well defined in women but may clearly bleed equally briskly. When considering orthotopic diversion in female patients undergoing cystectomy, several technical issues are critical to the procedure in order to maintain the continence mechanism in these women.

When developing the posterior pedicles in women, the posterior vagina is incised at the apex just distal to the cervix. This incision is carried anteriorly along the lateral and anterior vaginal wall forming a circumferential incision. The anteriorlateral vaginal wall is then grasped with a curved Kocher clamp. This provides counter traction, and facilitates dissection between the anterior vaginal wall and the bladder specimen. Careful dissection of the proper plane will prevent entry into the posterior bladder and also reduce the amount of bleeding in this vascular area. Development of this posterior plane and vascular pedicle is best performed sharply with the use of hemoclips, and carried just distal to the vesicourethral junction. Palpation of the Foley catheter balloon assists in identifying this region. This dissection effectively maintains a functional vagina. Furthermore, an intact anterior vaginal wall helps support the proximal urethra through a complex musculofascial support system that extends from the anterior vagina. The vagina is then closed at the apex and in the past was suspended to Cooper's ligament to prevent vaginal prolapse or the development of an enterocele postoperatively. Currently, the group at USC prefers a colposacralplexy incorporating Marlex mesh which fixates the vagina without angulation or undo tension. The need or effectiveness of this maneuver remains under study. At UM, women who have any element of preoperative stress incontinence are studied with fluorourodynamic studies with consideration given to a pubovaginal sling with extremely light tension. While this may lessen the risk of stress urinary incontinence, the degree to which this will increase the potential for urinary retention is uncertain. If indeterminate, one can consider postoperative paraurethral collagen injection or even a sling procedure if urinary incontinence remains postoperatively.

Alternatively, in the case of a deeply invasive posterior bladder tumor with concern of an adequate surgical margin, the anterior vaginal wall should be removed en bloc with the cystectomy specimen. After dividing the posterior vaginal apex, the lateral vaginal wall subsequently serves as the posterior pedicle and is divided distally. This leaves the anterior vaginal wall attached to the posterior bladder specimen. Again, the Foley catheter balloon facilitates identification of the vesicourethral junction. The surgical plane between the vesicourethral junction and the anterior vaginal wall is then developed distally at this location. A 1 cm length of proximal urethra is mobilized while the remaining distal urethra is left intact with the anterior vaginal wall. Vaginal reconstruction by a clam shell (horizontal), or side-to-side (vertical) technique is required.

Other means of vaginal reconstruction may include: a rectus myocutaneous flap, detubularized cylinder of ileum, a peritoneal flap, or an omental flap. Regardless, a well vascularized omental pedicle graft is placed between the reconstructed vagina and neobladder, and secured to the levator ani muscles to separate the suture lines and prevent fistulization.

It is important that no dissection be performed anterior to the urethra along the pelvic floor and that the endopelvic fascia is not opened in women considering orthotopic diversion. This prevents injury to the rhabdosphincter region and corresponding innervation which is critical in maintaining the continence mechanism. Anatomic studies have demonstrated that the innervation to this rhabdosphincter region in women arises from branches off the pudendal nerve that course along the pelvic floor posterior to the levator muscles (51). Any dissection performed anteriorly may injure these nerves and compromise the continence status. Some reports suggest that a sympathetic nerve sparing cystectomy is important in maintaining continence in these women. The USC and UM groups have routinely sacrificed the autonomic nerves coursing along the lateral aspect of uterus and vagina, and relied upon the pudendal innervation of the rhabdosphincter region for continence and have observed excellent continence in women undergoing orthotopic diversion with this technique. Flurourodynamic studies in women undergoing orthotopic diversion have also identified the rhabdosphincter region as the area which provides the continence mechanism in these women (52). It is possible that preservation of the sympathetic nerves may contribute to the high incidence of hypercontinence and urinary retention requiring continuous intermittent catheterization reported by Hautmann and associates (53). The precise mechanisms however, of incontinence or retention following neobladder formation in women, are poorly defined. In addition to neurogenic innervation as described above, an inability to adequately relax the external sphincter during Valsalva, development of "pouchocele" with descent of the anterior vaginal wall during Valsalva maneuver for voiding, and angulation of the junction between the urethra and neobladder have all been identified in individual patients (54–56).

When the posterior dissection is completed (ensuring to dissect just distal to the vesicourethral junction), a Statinski vascular clamp is placed across the bladder neck. With gentle traction the proximal urethra is divided anteriorly, distal to the bladder neck and clamp. The anterior urethral sutures are placed as described in the male patient. The distal portion of the catheter is then drawn into the wound through the urethrotomy and divided. The Statinski vascular clamp placed across the catheter at the bladder neck prevents any tumor spill from the bladder. Gentle cephalad tract on the clamped catheter allows placement of the posterior urethral sutures. The posterior urethra is then transected and the specimen is removed. Frozen section analysis is performed on the distal urethral margin of the cystectomy specimen to exclude tumor.

If a cutaneous diversion is planned in the female patient, the posterior pedicles are developed as previously mentioned. Attention is then directed anteriorly and the pubourethral ligaments are divided. A curved clamp is placed across the urethra, and the anterior vaginal wall is opened distally and incised circumferentially around the urethral meatus. The vaginal cuff is closed as previously described and suspended to Cooper's ligament. Alternatively, a perineal approach made be used for this dissection with complete removal of the entire urethra.

Following removal of the cystectomy specimen, the pelvis is irrigated with warm sterile water. The presacral nodal tissue previously swept off the common iliac vessels and sacral promontory into the deep pelvis is collected, and sent separately for pathologic evaluation. Nodal tissue in the presciatic notch, anterior to the sciatic nerve, is also sent for histologic analysis. Hemostasis is obtained and the pelvis is packed with a lap pad while attention is directed to the urinary diversion.

The use of various tubes and drains postoperatively are important but varies depending on surgeon and institutional preference. The USC group prefers to drain the pelvis for any urine or lymph leak with a 1-in Penrose drain for 3 wk, and a large suction hemovac drain for the evacuation of blood for 24 h. At UM, the pelvis is drained for 3–4 d with flat closed-suction Jackson Pratt drains. Although some groups prefer nasogastric decompression for a short period of time, at USC a gastrostomy tube 18 French Foley catheter is routinely placed utilizing a modified Stamm technique which incorporates a small portion of omentum (near the greater curvature of the stomach) interposed between the stomach and the abdominal wall. This provides a simple means to drain the stomach, and prevents the need for an uncomfortable nasogastric tube while the postoperative ileus resolves. Alternatively, at UM for the past 3 yr, most patients do not have either a nasogastric tube or gastrostomy tube; later insertion of a nasogastric tube secondary to abdominal distention is needed in only 15–20% of patients (57).

MANAGEMENT OF THE URETHRA IN PATIENTS WITH BLADDER CANCER

Indications for Urethrectomy in the Female Patient

In the past, urethrectomy was routinely performed in all women undergoing cystectomy. However, with a better understanding of the continence mechanism in women (51), coupled with sound pathologic criteria in which to safely select appropriate female candidates for orthotopic diversion *(37)*; urethrectomy is currently performed in those female patients not suitable candidates for an orthotopic reservoir, or who would prefer an alternative form of diversion. Currently, the vast majority of women undergoing cystectomy can undergo orthotopic diversion *(35, 36)*. The clinical and functional results in women undergoing orthotopic urinary diversion has been excellent.

Urethrectomy is performed at the time of cystectomy in women with a high risk for urethral tumor involvement, with known urethral tumor involvement, or in patients who prefer a cutaneous form of diversion. An extensive analysis of female cystectomy specimens removed for urothelial carcinoma of the bladder demonstrates that tumor involving the bladder neck is an important risk factor for urethral tumor involvement *(37)*. All cystectomy specimens with carcinoma involving the urethra had concomitant tumor involvement at the bladder neck. However, not all specimens with tumor involving the bladder neck demonstrated urethral tumor involvement. This is an important issue because, although bladder neck involvement with tumor is a risk factor for urethral tumor involvement, approximately 50% of patients with tumor at the bladder neck will have a urethra free of tumor. In this situation, the female patient may be considered an appropriate candidate for orthotopic diversion.

It has recently been demonstrated that intraoperative pathologic evaluation of the proximal urethra is the most critical determinant for orthotopic diversion in women *(36)*. Intraoperative frozen section analysis of the distal cystectomy margin (proximal urethra) is an accurate and reliable method to prospectively evaluate the proximal urethra for tumor involvement. Furthermore, because of the potential risk of injuring the continence mechanism with a preoperative biopsy of the bladder neck and urethra in women, coupled with a reliable method to evaluate the proximal urethra intraoperatively; one can rely primarily upon intraoperative frozen section analysis of the proximal urethra for proper patient selection in women considering orthotopic lower urinary tract reconstruction *(36)*.

Indications for Urethrectomy in the Male Patient

With the increasing familiarity and application of orthotopic diversion, the management of the urethra in the male patient undergoing cystectomy for bladder cancer is of particular importance. Urethral recurrences develop in approximately 10% of male patients following cystectomy for bladder cancer *(58)*. The greatest risk factor for urethral recurrence is tumor involvement of the prostate in the radical cystectomy specimen;

with prostatic stromal invasion more ominous then either ductal or mucosal involvement. Patients considering orthotopic diversion have traditionally undergone precystectomy screening of the prostate by means of a deep transurethral biopsy at the 5 and 7 o'clock position adjacent to the verumontanum, which has been suggested to be the most common sites of involvement of the prostatic urethra, ducts, and stroma with transitional cell carcinoma (59,60).

Recently, the incidence of urethral recurrence in male patients undergoing a cutaneous form of diversion was compared to the urethral recurrence rate in men undergoing an orthotopic diversion was reviewed (57). Interestingly, the estimated probability of a urethral recurrence at 5 yr following cystectomy was significantly increased in male patients with a cutaneous diversion, compared to those undergoing an orthotopic diversion (10% compared to 4%, respectively). Even those patients with high risk pathology (prostate involvement), diverted by means of an orthotopic diversion, had a lower probability of urethral recurrence compared to patients with similar pathology undergoing a non-orthotopic form of diversion. The 5-yr risk of recurrence in these patients with prostate involvement was only 5% in the orthotopic group compared to 24% for the non-orthotopic group. Although the exact etiology is unknown, it has been suggested that the orthotopic form of diversion may provide some protective effect, perhaps by the mucus or some other secretory product of the intestine, that prevents the development of cancer in the retained urethra (62). Alternatively, selection factors and stage migration with earlier cystectomy may also contribute to a lower recurrence rate in the retained urethra.

The current indications for urethrectomy (contraindication to orthotopic diversion) in male patients include those demonstrating carcinoma in situ or overt carcinoma of the urethral margin detected on intraoperative frozen section analysis. En bloc urethrectomy is performed at the time of cystectomy in those male patients with known tumor involving the urethra. A delayed urethrectomy is performed in patients with prostatic stromal tumor involvement demonstrated on final pathologic examination of the cystectomy specimen who have undergone a cutaneous form of urinary diversion. Those patients with prostatic stromal involvement of tumor demonstrated in the cystectomy specimen, who underwent an orthotopic diversion are closely monitored postoperatively with urethral wash cytology for recurrence purposes. Furthermore, it is no longer necessary to perform a preoperative biopsy of the prostate because orthotopic diversion is contraindicated in only those patients with overt tumor of the urethra diagnosed on intraoperative frozen section analysis.

POSTOPERATIVE CARE

A meticulous, team-oriented approach to the care of these generally elderly patients undergoing radical cystectomy helps reduce perioperative morbidity and mortality. At USC, all patients are monitored in the surgical intensive care unit (ICU) for at least 24 h or until stable. At UM, patients are not routinely sent to the ICU, and in a recent review of 137 consecutive cases, only 17.5% required an ICU stay. Regardless, careful attention to fluid management is imperative as third space fluid loss in these patients can be tremendous and deceiving. In patients with severely compromised cardiac or pulmonary function, it may be necessary for invasive cardiac monitoring with a pulmonary artery catheter placed prior to surgery to precisely ascertain the cardiac response to fluid shifts. A combination of crystalloid and colloid fluid replacement is given on the night of surgery, and converted to crystalloid on postoperative d 1. Prophylaxis against stress ulcer is initiated with an H_2 blocker. Intravenous broad spectrum antibiotics are continued in all patients at USC and in neobladder patients at UM, subsequently converting to orals antibiotics as the diet progresses. Pulmonary toilet is encouraged with incentive spirometry, deep breathing, and coughing.

Prophylaxis against deep vein thrombosis is important in these patients undergoing extensive pelvic operations for malignancies. The USC group prefers initiating the anticoagulation in the recovery room with 10 mg of sodium warfarin via the nasogastric or gastrostomy tube. The daily dose is adjusted to maintain a prothrombin time in the range of 18–22 s. If the prothrombin time exceeds 22 s, 2.5 mg of vitamin K is administered intramuscularly to prevent bleeding. At UM, only intermittent compression stockings are used with early aggressive ambulation. No systemic anticoagulation is used. Pain control is maintained with either an epidural catheter, or a patient controlled analgesic system, or a combination of the two at USC. At UM, an epidural catheter is avoided because of a possible propensity for a prolonged ileus; Ketoralac is used for 72 h at UM. Patient comfort enhances deep breathing, and early ambulation. At USC, if digoxin was given preoperatively, it is continued until discharge. If a tube gastrostomy is employed it is removed on postoperative d 7, or later if bowel function is delayed. At UM, if a nasogastric tube was omitted, the patient is fed slowly only after flatus is evident. Patients in whom there is evidence of abdominal distention or any vomiting require replacement of a nasogastric tube. The catheter and drain management is specific to the form of urinary diversion. Some patients may develop a prolonged ileus or some other complication which delays the quick return of oral intake. In such circumstances, total parenteral nutrition (TPN) is wisely instituted earlier rather than later, in which situation

Table 1
Operative Mortality and Early Complication Rates
in 1051 Patients Undergoing Cystectomy and Urinary Diversion:
Stratified by the Form of Urinary Diversion and Preoperative Therapy

		No. of patients	Perioperative mortality[a]	Early complication[b]
Form of	Conduit[c]	278 (27%)	8 (3%)	80 (29%)
urinary diversion	Continent[d]	773 (73%)	18 (2%)	205 (26%)
Preoperative	None	883 (84%)	25 (3%)	240 (27%)
adjuvant	Radiation only	111 (11%)	1 (1%)	31 (30%)
therapy	Chemotherapy only	48 (4%)	0	11 (26%)
	Radiation and	8 (1%)	0	3 (33%)
Totals	chemotherapy	1051	26 (2.5%)	285 (27%)

[a] Any death within 30 d of surgery or prior to discharge.
[b] Any complication within the first 4 mo postoperative.
[c] Including ileoconduit and colon conduits.
[d] Including continent cutaneous, orthotopic, and rectal reservoirs.

the patient may become farther behind nutritionally. In recent experience at UM, TPN is required in approximately 15–20% of patients for a variety of reasons.

RESULTS OF RADICAL CYSTECTOMY AND URINARY DIVERSION

The USC group recently reported on an extensive computerized cystectomy data base containing detailed, comprehensive clinical and pathological information on patients undergoing cystectomy from August 1971 through December 1997 (5). A total of 1051 patients underwent radical cystectomy for primary transitional cell carcinoma of the bladder with the intent to cure. Of the 1051 patients, 839 were male (80%) and 212 were female. The median age for this large group was 66 yr (range 22–93 yr), with a median followup of 7.9 yr (range 0–24 yr).

Perioperative mortality (any death within 30 d of surgery or prior to discharge) occurred in 26 of 1051 patients (2.5%). No significant difference in mortality was observed when evaluated by the form of urinary diversion or when stratified by the administration of preoperative therapy. A total of 285 patients (27%) suffered an early complication. No significant difference was observed in the early complication rate when evaluated by the form of urinary diversion or when stratified by the administration of preoperative therapy (Table 1).

At UM, a care pathway system has been in place for four years defining the daily milestones anticipated for patients during the recovery process. This is available and widely used by the attending physicians, residents, and nursing staff. Standardization of postoperative care has been shown to be beneficial after many surgical procedures and reduces variability and thus probably improves care and is cost effective. However, in spite of a standardized pathway, it has been difficult to substantially decrease the length of stay in cystectomy patients. The current median length of stay is approximately 9.5 d at UM. Many patients have substantial comorbidity that delays discharge, particularly evident when an aggressive strategy toward cystectomy is used for elderly patients over 75 yr of age as used at USC and UM. However, even as a more aggressive philosophy towards cystectomy in the elderly has evolved, mortality rates have fortunately remained very low. In a recent series of 147 consecutive cases at UM, in patients ranging from 36–100 yr of age, the perioperative mortality rate was only 0.5%.

Pathologic staging of the 1051 patients included 76% without evidence of lymph node involvement: 65 patients (6%) with P0, 99 patients (9%) with Pis, 41 patients (4%) with Pa, 195 patients (19%) with P1, 95 patients (9%) with P2 (superficial muscle invasion), 98 patients (9%) with P3a (deep muscle invasion), 135 patients (13%) with P3b (extravesical tumor extension), and 78 patients (7%) with P4 tumors. Pathologic subgroups include: 593 patients (56%) with organ confined lymph node negative tumors, and 213 patients (20%) with non-organ confined (extravesical) lymph node negative tumors (Table 2).

A total of 245 patients (24%) were found to have lymph node positive disease (Table 3). Increasing incidence of lymph node involvement was found with increasing p-stage of the primary bladder tumor. Lymph node positive disease was found in only 19 of 419 patients (5%) with superficial (P0, Pis, Pa, P1) primary bladder tumors (p-stage). The incidence of lymph node involvement increased with muscle invasive primary bladder tumors; 21 of 116 patients (18%) with P2, and 35 of 133 patients (27%) with P3a disease. Lymph node positive disease was highest in patients with non-organ confined primary bladder tumors; 112 of 247 patients (27%) with P3b, and 58 of 136 patients (43%) with P4 primary bladder tumors.

The recurrence-free and overall survival for the entire 1051 patients at 5 and 10 yr was 69% and 66%, and 62% and 46% respectively (Table 2). Recurrence-free and overall survival for the entire cohort was significantly related to the pathologic stage and lymph node status. Increasing pathologic stage and lymph node positive disease were associated with significantly higher recurrence rates and worse overall survival. The recurrence-free and overall survival for the 593 patients (56%) with organ confined, lymph node negative bladder tumors (P0, Pa, Pis, P1, P2, P3a) was not statistically different when stratified by each individual patho-

Table 2
Recurrence-free and Overall Survival in 1051 Patients Undergoing Radical
Cystectomy and Urinary Diversion for High Grade, Invasive Bladder Cancer:
Stratified by Pathologic Stage and Pathologic Subgroups

Variable		No. of patients	Recurrence-free survival (%) 5-Yr	10-Yr	Overall survival (%) 5-Yr	10-Yr
Pathologic	P0	65 (6%)	93	86	85	69
stage	Pis	99 (9%)	90	90	90	72
	Pa	41 (4%)	79	71	78	72
	P1	195 (19%)	82	79	77	54
	P2	95 (9%)	91	89	78	56
	P3a	98 (9%)	76	74	68	46
	P3b	135 (13%)	62	61	51	32
	P4	78 (7%)	50	47	43	30
Lymph node −	All patients	806 (76%)	78	75	71	51
Lymph node +	All patients	245 (24%)	35	34	33	26
	1–4 nodes	161	42	40	41	33
	≥5 nodes	84	23	23	27	23
	Organ confined (p-stage)	75	47	45	50	41
	Extravesical (p-stage)	170	30	30	24	19
Pathologic	Organ confined[a]	593 (56%)	85	82	79	58
subgroups	Extravesical[b]	213 (20%)	59	56	48	31
Entire group		1051	69	66	62	46

[a] Including P0, Pa, Pis, P1 P2, P3a (lymph node negative).
[b] Including P3b, P4 (lymph node negative).

Table 3
Incidence of Lymph Node Involvement Stratified
by p-stage in 1051 Patients Undergoing Radical Cystectomy
and Urinary Diversion for High Grade, Invasive Bladder Cancer

		No. of patients	Lymph node involvement Positive	Negative
Primary	P0, Pis, Pa, P1[a]	419 (40%)	19 (5%)	400 (95%)
bladder tumor	P2	116 (11%)	21 (18%)	95 (82%)
(p-stage)	P3a	133 (13%)	35 (27%)	98 (73%)
	P3b	247 (23%)	112 (45%)	135 (55%)
	P4	136 (13%)	58 (43%)	78 (57%)
Entire group		1051	245 (24%)	806 (76%)

[a] Superficial (nonmuscle) tumors.

logic stage. The 5 and 10-yr recurrence-free and overall survival for the pathologic subgroup of organ confined lymph node negative tumors, was 85% and 82%, and 79% and 58% respectively (Table 2).

Table 4
Incidence of Local (Pelvic) and Distant Recurrence
in 1051 Patients Undergoing Radical Cystectomy
and Urinary Diversion for High Grade, Invasive Bladder Cancer

Pathologic groups	Total No. of patients	Recurrence site Local	Distant
Organ confined	593 (56%)	25 (4%)	51 (5%)
Extravesical disease[a]	213 (20%)	20 (9%)	47 (22%)
Lymph node positive	245 (24%)	26 (11%)	93 (38%)
Totals	1051	71 (7%)	191 (18%)

[a]P0, Pa, Pia, P1, P2, P3a, P3b, P4.

The recurrence-free and overall survival for the 213 patients (20%) with non-organ confined (extravesical) lymph node negative bladder tumors (P3b, P4) was not a significant difference when stratified by each individual pathologic stage. The 5 and 10-yr recurrence-free and overall survival for the pathologic subgroup of extravesical, lymph node negative tumors was 59% and 56%, and 48% and 31% respectively (Table 2).

Patients with lymph node positive disease demonstrated significantly worse survival and higher recurrence rates compared to those without lymph node involvement. The recurrence-free and overall survival for all 245 patients (24%) with lymph node positive disease at 5 and 10 yr was 35% and 33%, and 32% and 26% respectively (Table 2). Survival rates in this group of patients with lymph node positive disease could be further stratified by the primary bladder tumor (p-stage), and by the total number of lymph nodes involved. Patients with less than 5 positive lymph nodes and organ confined primary bladder tumors had significantly lower recurrence rates and improved survival compared to those with 5 or more lymph nodes involved, or those with non-organ confined (extravesical) primary bladder tumors.

Recurrence-free and overall survival was significantly related to the pathologic subgroup. Patients with organ confined lymph node negative tumors had statistically the lowest recurrence and highest survival rates, compared to patients with lymph node positive disease who had the highest recurrence and worse survival rate. Patients with non-organ confined (extravesical) lymph node negative tumors demonstrated intermediate recurrence and survival rates.

A total of 262 patients (25%) developed a bladder cancer recurrence (Table 4). The median time to tumor recurrence was 12 mo (range 13 d to 11.1 yr). Of the 262 recurrences, 191 patients (18%) developed a distant recurrence, while 71 patients (7%) developed a local pelvic tumor recurrence. The median time for a distant, and local recurrence was 12 and 18 mo, respectively.

DISCUSSION

The authors at USC and UM have developed and employ an aggressive surgical approach to the treatment of high grade, invasive bladder cancer which is ideal. This rationale is based on the natural progression of bladder cancer with its inherent metastatic and lethal potential. Bladder tumors tend to progressively invade their superficial origin of the mucosa, to the lamina propria and sequentially into the muscularis propria, perivesical region, and contiguous pelvic structures, with increasing incidence of lymph node involvement with progression *(18,21–23)*.

Improvements in medical, surgical and anesthetic therapy have reduced the morbidity and mortality associated with radical cystectomy. Radical cystectomy currently provides the optimal results with regard to survival and prevention of local recurrence *(5,17)*. Unlike any other therapy, radical cystectomy also provides accurate pathologic staging, which may influence the need for adjuvant therapy based on clear histologic analysis of the primary bladder tumor and regional lymph nodes. Furthermore, the evolution of orthotopic lower urinary tract reconstruction to the native intact urethra has provided male and female patients more acceptable means to store and eliminate urine *(32–36)*; lessening the impact of removal of the bladder following cystectomy. Lastly, equally effective forms of therapy for high grade, invasive bladder cancer have yet to emerge.

The previous mentioned data, in a large group of patients with long-term followup, suggests that radical cystectomy with *en bloc* bilateral pelvic iliac lymphadenectomy and urinary diversion can be performed safely with excellent bladder cancer control. Survival results are exceptional, with a low incidence of local pelvic recurrence *(5)*. Lastly, no other form of therapy with similar outcomes for the treatment of high grade, invasive bladder cancer has emerged.

Furthermore, the results from this series provides strong evidence that radical cystectomy provides excellent survival results for the treatment of high grade, invasive bladder cancer. No other single or combined modality of treatment appear to have similar survival rates. Overall, 69% were alive without evidence of disease with an overall survival of 62% at 5 yr. Most deaths occurring in patients within the first 3 yr following cystectomy are primarily related to bladder cancer. Following this, deaths in this elderly group of patients are associated primarily with comorbid diseases, unrelated to bladder cancer. Although a bladder cancer recurrence can occur at any time, most occur within the first several years following surgery, and are responsible for the majority of deaths during this time period.

These data also confirm that pathologic stage is an important survival determinate in patients undergoing cystectomy for bladder cancer. In addition, pathologic subgroups can be identified that stratify patients into different prognostic categories, which may help dictate the need for adjuvant therapy. The recurrence-free survival in the pathologic subgroup of organ confined lymph node negative bladder tumors was remarkably 85% at 5 yr, and 82% at 10 yr. Similar results for superficial bladder tumors treated with cystectomy have been reported by others *(18)*. The recurrence-free survival in the pathologic subgroup of non-organ confined lymph node negative tumors was 59% at 5 yr, and 56% at 10 yr. Patients with non-organ confined tumors demonstrated significantly higher recurrence rates and worse survival compared to those with organ confined tumors. This suggests that patients with extravesical bladder tumors are at high risk and should be considered for adjuvant therapy following surgery.

A significant number of patients will have lymph node involvement at the time of cystectomy. This underscores the virulent and metastatic capabilities of high grade, invasive bladder cancer. Despite lymph node involvement, nearly 35% of patients were alive without evidence of disease at 10 yr. The prognosis in patients with lymph node positive disease could be further stratified by the number of lymph nodes involved, and by the stage of the primary bladder tumor (p-stage). Although patients with lymph node involvement have the highest recurrence rates, there remains a substantial number of patients who may benefit from a meticulous lymph node dissection. Similar results with lymph node positive disease following cystectomy have been previously reported *(18,23,63)*. Clearly, some patients with lymph node involvement are at high risk for recurrence and should be considered for adjuvant treatment strategies.

As a result of improved medical, surgical and anesthetic techniques, the mortality and morbidity from radical cystectomy has dramatically decreased. An anticipated perioperative mortality rate following cystectomy is 1–3% *(5,23,26–28)*. The administration of preoperative therapy (radiation and/or chemotherapy), and the form of urinary diversion performed (continent or incontinent) did not significantly alter the mortality rate or the perioperative complication rate. Strict attention to perioperative details, meticulous surgery, and a team-oriented surgical and postoperative approach is critical to minimize morbidity and mortality, and to ensure the best clinical outcomes following radical cystectomy.

Radical cystectomy unequivocally provides the best local control for the treatment of high grade, invasive bladder cancer, with an overall local pelvic recurrence rate of 7% in the USC series. Even those at highest risk of a local recurrence (lymph node positive disease) had only an 11% local recurrence rate following cystectomy. Other series have reported higher pelvic recurrence rates in patients with clinical T3b disease (a palpable pelvic mass) and in this adversely selected population, certainly additional adjuvant therapies are needed. Nevertheless, no other local therapy approaches the pelvic control rate of cystectomy *(64)*. These results are important as it is generally known that those who suffer a local pelvic recurrence have a poor prognosis despite all forms of therapy. This excellent local control following cystectomy also suggests that orthotopic forms of urinary diversion may be appropriate even in high-risk patients with extravesical tumor extension or lymph node positive disease. Currently, no other form of therapy for high grade, invasive bladder cancer provides comparable local control.

The development of orthotopic lower urinary tract reconstruction has dramatically lessened the impact of cystectomy on the quality of life of patients following removal of their bladder. Orthotopic diversion has eliminated the need for a cutaneous stoma, urostomy appliance, and the need for intermittent catheterization. Continence rates following orthotopic diversion are excellent, providing patients a more natural voiding pattern per urethra *(33,36)*. Currently orthotopic diversion should be considered the diversion of choice in all cystectomy patients and the urologist should have a specific reason why an orthotopic diversion is **not** performed. Patient factors such as frail general health, motivation, or comorbidity and the cancer factor of a positive urethral margin may disqualify some patients. Nevertheless, the option of lower urinary tract reconstruction to an intact urethra has been shown to decrease physician reluctance and increase patient acceptance to undergo earlier cystectomy when the disease may be at a more curable stage *(65)*.

Currently, no equally effective alternative form of therapy for high grade, invasive bladder cancer has evolved. Bladder cancer appears to be resistant to radiation therapy, even at high doses. Other bladder-sparing techniques employing chemotherapy alone, or in combination with radiation have substantially higher local recurrence rates, and do not appear to result in long-term survival or recurrence rates comparable to radical cystectomy *(66)*. Whether patients have a better quality of life following cystectomy or following bladder-sparing protocols, which require significant treatment to the bladder with the potential for tumor recurrence, has not been clarified. However, the argument for bladder-sparing protocols has diminished with the advent and successful application of orthotopic diversion following radical cystectomy.

Unlike any other therapy, radical cystectomy pathologically stages the primary bladder tumor and regional lymph nodes. This histologic evaluation will provide important prognostic information and may help identify high risk patients who could benefit from adjuvant therapy. Patients with extravesical tumor extension, or with lymph node positive disease are at risk for recurrence and should be considered for adjuvant treatment strategies. Additionally, the recent application of molecular markers based on pathologic staging and analysis, may also serve to identify patients at risk for tumor recurrence who may benefit from adjuvant forms of therapy *(67)*.

The clinical results reported from the large, contemporary group of patients, clearly demonstrate that radical cystectomy provides excellent survival, with the lowest reported local recurrence rates. Improvements in orthotopic urinary diversion have improved the quality of life in patients following cystectomy. These data may provide a standard to which other treatment modalities should be compared.

REFERENCES

1. Landis SH, Murray T, Bolden S, Wingo PA. Cancer statistics, 1999. CA Cancer J Clin 1999; 49: 8–31.
2. Crawford ED, Davis MA. Nontransitional cell carcinomas of the bladder. In: *Genitourinary Cancer Management* (de Kernian JB, Paulson DF, eds.). Lea & Febiger, Philadelphia, PA, 1987, pp. 95–105.
3. Skinner DG, Lieskovsky G. Management of invasive and high-grade bladder cancer. In: *Diagnose and Management of Genitorurinary Cancer* (Skinner DG, Lieskovsky G, eds.). WB Saunders, Philadelphia, PA, 1988, pp. 295–312.
4. Droller MJ. Individualizing the approach to invasive bladder cancer. Contemp Urol 1990; 7/8; 54–61.
5. Stein JP, Freeman JA, Boyd SD, Groshen S, Skinner EC, Lieskovsky G, Skinner DG. Radical cystectomy in the treatment of invasive bladder cancer: long-term results in a large group of patient. J Urol 1998; 159: 213 (abstract 823).
6. Thrasher JB, Crawford ED. Minimally invasive transitional cell carcinoma (T1 and T2). In: *Current Therapy in Genitourinary Surgery*, 2nd edition. (Resnick MI, Kursh E, eds.). BC Decker, St. Louis, MO, 1992, pp. 74–78.
7. Freeman JA, Esrig D, Stein JP, Simoneau AR, Skinner EC, Chen S-C, et al. Radical cystectomy for high risk patients with superficial bladder cancer in the era of orthotopic urinary reconstruction. Cancer 1995; 76: 833–839.
8. Anderstrom C, Johansson S, Nilsson S. The significance of lamina propria invasion on the prognosis of patients with bladder tumors. J Urol 1980; 124: 23–26.
9. Heney NM, Ahmed S, Flanagan MJ, Frable W, Corder MP, Hafermann MD, Hawkins IR. Superficial bladder cancer: progression and recurrence. J Urol 1983; 130: 1083–1086.
10. Dalesio O, Schulman CC, Sylvester R, DePauw M, Robinson M, Denis L, et al. Prognostic factors in superficial bladder tumors. A study of the European Organization for Research on Treatment of Cancer: Genitourinary Tract Cancer Cooperative Group. J Urol 1983; 129: 730–733.
11. Herr HW, Jakse G, Sheinfeld J. The T1 bladder tumor. Sem Urol 1990; 8: 254–261.
12. Fitzpatrick JM. The natural history of superficial bladder cancer. Sem Urol 1993; 11: 127–136.
13. Malkowicz SB, Nichols P, Lieskovsky G, Boyd SD, Huffman J, Skinner DG. The role of radical cystectomy in the management of high grade superifiial bladder cancer (PA, P1, PIS and P2). J Urol 1990; 144: 641–645.

14. Schellhammer PF, Bean MA, Whitmore WF Jr. Prostatic involvement by transitional cell carcinoma: pathogenesis, patterns, and prognosis. J Urol 1977; 118: 399–403.
15. Prout GR Jr, Griffin PP, Daly JJ, Henery NM. Carcinoma in situ of the urinary bladder with and without asssociated vesical neoplasms. Cancer 1983; 52: 524–532.
16. Utz DC, Farrow DM. Management of carcinoma in situ of the bladder: a case for surgical management. Urol Clin N Am 1980; 7: 533–540.
17. Montie JE. Against bladder sparing surgery. J Urol 1999; 162: 452–457.
18. Ghoneim MA, El-Mekresh MM, El-Baz MA. El-Attar IA, Ashamallah A. Radical cystectomy for carcinoma of the bladder: critical evaluation of the results in 1,026 cases. J Urol 1997; 158: 393–399;
19. Skinner DG, Lieskovsky G. Contemporary cystectomy with pelvic node dissection compared to preoperative radiation therapy plus cystectomy in management of invasive bladder cancer. J Urol 1984; 131: 1069–1072.
20. Montie JE, Strafton RA, Stewart BH. Radical cystectomy without radiation therapy for carcinoma of the bladder. J Urol 1984; 131: 477–482.
21. Frazier HA, Robertson JE, Dodge RK, Paulson DF. The value of pathologic factors in predicting cancer-specific survival among patients treated with radical cystectomy for transitional cell carcinoma of the bladder and prostate. Cancer 1993; 71: 3993–4001.
22. Skinner DG, Tift JP, Kaufman JJ. High dose, short course preoperative radiation therapy and immediate single stage radical cystectomy with pelvic node dissection in the management of bladder cancer. J Urol 1982; 127: 671–674.
23. Lerner SP, Skinner DG, Lieskovsky G, Boyd SD, Groshen SL, Ziogas A, et al. The rationale for en bloc pelvic lymph node dissection for bladder cancer patients with nodal metastases: long-term results. J Urol 1993; 149: 758–765.
24. Soloway MS, Lopez AE, Patel J, Lu Y. Result of radical cystectomy for transitional cell carcinoma of the bladder and the effect of chemotherapy. Cancer 1994; 73: 1926–1931.
25. Voges GE, Tauschke E, Stöckle M, Alken P, Hohenfellner R. Computerized tomography: an unreliable method for accurate staging of bladder tumors in patients who are candidates for radical cystectomy. J Urol 1989; 142: 972–974.
26. Wishnow KI, Dmochowski R. Pelvic recurrence after radical cystectomy without preoperative radiation. J Urol 1988; 140: 42–43.
27. Roehrborn CG, Sagalowsky AI, Peters PC. Long-term patient survival after cystectomy for regional metastatic transitional cell carcinoma of the bladder. J Urol 1991; 146: 36–39.
28. Mathur VK. Krahn HP, Ramsey EW. Total cystectomy for bladder cancinoma. J Urol 1981; 125: 784–786.
29. Thrasher JB, Crawford ED. Current management of invasive and metastatic transitional cell carcinoma of the bladder. J Urol 1993; 149: 957–972.
30. Walsh PC, Donker PJ. Impotence following radical prostatectomy: insight into etiology and prevention. J Urol 1982; 128: 492–497.
31. Schlegel PN, Walsh PC. Neuroanatomical approach to radical cystoprostatectomy with preservation of sexual function. J Urol 1987; 138: 1402–1406.
32. Elmajian DA, Stein JP, Skinner DG. Orthotopic urinary diversion: the Kock ileal neobladder. W J Urol 1996; 14: 40–46.
33. Elmajian DA, Stein JP, Esrig D, Freeman JA, Skinner EC, Boyd SD, et al. The Kock ileal neobladder: update experience in 295 male patients. J Urol (in press).
34. Stein JP, Stenzl A, Esrig D, Freeman JA, Boyd SD, Lieskovsky G, et al. Lower urinary tract reconstruction following cystectomy in women using the Kock ileal

reservoir with bilateral ureteroileal urethrostomy: initial clinical experience. J Urol 1994; 152: 1404–1408.

35. Stein JP, Grossfeld G, Freeman JA, Esrig D, Ginsberg DA, Cote RJ, et al. Orthotopic lower urinary tract reconstruction in women using the Kock ileal neobladder: updated experience in 27 patients. J Urol 1997; 158: 400–405.

36. Stein JP, Esrig D, Freeman JA, Grossfeld GD, Ginsberg DA, Cote RC, et al. Prospective pathologic analysis of female cystectomy specimens: risk factors for orthotopic diversion in women. Urology 1998; 51: 951–955.

37. Stein JP, Cote RJ, Freeman JA, Esrig D, Elmajian DA, Groshen S, et al. Indications for lower urinary tract reconstruction in women after cystectomy for bladder cancer: a pathological review of female cystectomy specimens. J Urol 1995; 154: 1329–1322.

38. Stenzl A, Draxl H, Posch B, Colleselli K, Falk M, Bartsch G. The risk of urethral tumors in female bladder cancer: can the urethra be used for orthotopic reconstruction of the lower urinary tract? J Urol 1995; 153: 950–955.

39. Pagano F, Bassi P, Galetti TP, Meneghini A, Milani C, Artibani W, Garbeglio A. Results of contemporary radical cystectomy for invasive bladder cancer: a clinicopathological study with an emphasis on the inadequacy of the tumor, nodes and metastases classification. J Urol 1991; 145: 45–50.

40. Hatch TR, Barry JM. The value of excretory radiography in staging bladder cancer. J Urol 1986; 135: 49.

41. Haleblian GE, Skinner EC, Dickinson MG, Lieskovsky G, Skinner DG. Hydroureteronephrosis as a prognostic indicator in bladder cancer patients. J Urol 1997; 160: 2011–2014.

42. Crawford ED, Das S, Smith JA Jr. Preoperative radiation therapy in the treatment of bladder cancer. Urol Clin N Am 1987; 14: 781–787.

43. Anderstrom C, Johansson S, Nilsson S, Unsgaard B. Wahlqvist LA. A prospective randomized study of preoperative irradiation with cystectomy or cystectomy alone for invasive bladder carcinoma. Eur Urol 1983; 9: 142–147.

44. Smith JA Jr, Crawford ED, Paradelo JC, Blumenstein B, Herschman BR, Grossman HB, Christie DW. Treatment of advanved bladder cancer with combined preoperative irradiation and radical cystectomy versus radical cystectomy alone: a phase III intergroup study. J Urol 1997; 157: 805–808.

45. Crawford ED, Skinner DG. Salvage cystectomy after radiation failure. J Urol 1980; 123: 32–34.

46. Magri J. Partial cystectomy: review of 104 cases. Br J Urol 1962; 34: 74–87.

47. van der Werf-Messing B. Carcinoma of the bladder treated by suprapubic radium implants: the value of additional external irradiation. Eur J Urol 1969; 5: 277–281.

48. Nichols RL, Broido P, Condon RE, Gorbach SL, Nyhus LM. Effect of preoperative neomycin-erythromycin intestinal preparation on the incidence of infectious complications following colon surgery. Ann Surg 1973; 178: 453–462.

49. Pinaud MLJ, Blanloeil YAG, Souron RJ. Preoperative prophylactic digitalization of patients with coronary artery disease-a randomized echocardiographic and hemodynamic study. Anesth Analg 1983; 62: 685–689.

50. Burman SO. The prophylactic use of digitalis before thoracotomy. Ann Thorac Surg 1972; 14: 359–368.

51. Colleselli K, Stenzl A, Eder R, Strasser H, Poisel S, Bartsch G. The female urethral sphincter: a morphological and topographical study. J Urol 1998; 160: 49–50.

52. Grossfeld GD, Stein JP, Bennett CJ, Ginsberg DA, Boyd SD, Lieskovsky G, Skinner DG. Lower urinary tract reconstruction in the female using the Kock ileal reservoir with bilateral ureteroileal urethrostomy: update of continence results and flurourodynamic findings. Urology 1996; 48: 383–388.

53. Hautmann RE, Paiss T. Does the option of the ileal neobladder stimulate patient and physician decision towards earlier cystectomy? J Urol 1998; 159: 1845–1850.
54. Park JM, Montie JE. Mechanism of incontinence and retention after orthotopic neobladder diversion. Urology 1998; 51: 601–609.
55. Arai Y, Okubo K, Konami T, Kin S, Kanba T, Okabe T, et al. Voiding function of orthotopic ileal neobladder in women. Urology 1999; 54: 44–49.
56. Ali-El-Dein B, El-Sobky E, Hohenfellner M, Ghoneim MA. Orthotopic bladder substitution in women: functional evaluation. J Urol 1999; 161: 1875–1880.
57. Donat SM, Slaton JW, Pisters LL, Swanson DA. Early nasogastric tube removal combined with metoclopramide after radical cystectomy and urinary diversion. J Urol 1999; 162: 1599–1602.
58. Freeman JA, Esrig D, Stein JP, Skinner DG. Management of the patient with bladder cancer. Urethral recurrence. Urol Clin N Am 1994; 21(4): 645–651.
59. Sakamoto N, Tsuneyoshi M, Naito S, Kumazawa J. An adequate sampling of the prostate to identify prostatic involvement by urothelial carcinoma in bladder cancer patients. J Urol 1993; 149: 318–321.
60. Wood DP Jr, Montie JE, Pontes JE, Levin HS. Identification of transitional cell carcinoma of the prostate in bladder cancer patients: a prospective study. J Urol 1989; 142: 83–85.
61. Freeman JA, Tarter AT, Esrig D, Stein JP, Elmajian DA, Chen S-C, et al. Urethral recurrence in patients with orthotopic ileal neobladders. J Urol 1996; 156: 1615–1619.
62. Crocitto LE, Simpson J, Wilson TG. Bladder augmentation in the prevention of cyclophosphamide induced hemorrhagic cystitis in the rat model. J Urol 1994; 151(2): 379A, abstract 608.
63. Vieweg J. Gschwend JE, Herr HW, Fair WR. Pelvic lymph node dissection can be curative in patients with node positive bladder cancer. J Urol 1999; 161: 449–454.
64. Hall CM, Dinney P.M. Radical cystectomy for stage T3b bladder cancer. Semin Urol Oncol 1996; 14: 73–80.
65. Hautmann RE, Paiss T. Does the option of the ileal neobladder stimulate patient and physician decision toward earlier cystectomy? J Urol 1998; 159: 1845–1850.
66. Shipley WU, Kaufman DS, Heney NM, Althausen AF, Zietman AL. An update of combined modality therapy for patients with muscle invading bladder cancer using selective bladder preservation or cystectomy. J Urol 1999; 162: 445–451.
67. Stein JP, Grossfeld GD, Ginsberg DA, Esrig D, Freeman JA, Figueroa AJ, et al. Prognostic markers in bladder cancer: a contemporary review of the literature. J Urol 1999; 160: 645–659.

11 Considerations in the Use of Neoadjuvant and Adjunctive Systemic Chemotherapy in Treatment of Invasive Bladder Cancer by Cystectomy

Seth P. Lerner, MD
and Derek Raghavan, MD, PHD

CONTENTS

INTRODUCTION
CHEMOTHERAPY
CONCLUSION
REFERENCES

INTRODUCTION

Approximately 10,000 cases of muscle invasive bladder cancer are diagnosed in the United States each year, representing about 20% of new cases of urinary tract malignancy *(1)*. Results from contemporary radical cystectomy and pelvic lymph node dissection for T2-4NXM0 transitional cell carcinoma (TCC) of the bladder indicate that this operation is safe with a surgical mortality rate of 0.5%–6%. Radical cystectomy accomplishes excellent, durable, local control of the primary tumor, provides accurate pathologic staging of the primary tumor and lymph nodes, and, due to increasing expertise with continent urinary diversion, affords preservation of quality of life *(2)*. Despite these advances, the 5-yr survival rate for all patients with pT2 tumors is 50%–80%, with patients with

From: *Current Clinical Urology: Bladder Cancer: Current Diagnosis and Treatment*
Edited by: M. J. Droller © Humana Press Inc., Totowa, NJ

negative lymph nodes having 64%–86% 5-yr survival. The 5-yr survival rates for regionally advanced cancers, pT3 and pT4, in contemporary series range from 22%–58%. Among patients with pathologically proven lymph node metastasis, the 5-yr survival probability following radical cystectomy is only 29% *(3)*. The 5-yr survival rate is 50% for patients with nodal metastases and tumors confined to the muscularis propria, whereas with more advanced primary tumors, the survival rate drops significantly to 18% or less.

CHEMOTHERAPY

The early clinical trials of chemotherapy for bladder cancer showed that several single agents have activity, including cyclophosphamide, the vinca alkaloids, methotrexate, mitomycin C, 5-fluorouracil, doxorubicin and cisplatin *(4)*. More recently, ifosfamide *(5)*, gallium nitrate *(6)*, paclitaxel *(7)*, docetaxel *(8)*, and gemcitabine *(9–11)* have been shown in a series of phase I–II clinical trials to have substantial antitumor effect against TCC of the urinary tract.

In the early development of chemotherapy for bladder cancer, combination chemotherapy regimens produced higher objective response rates than single agents, but did not improve survival *(12,13)*. The first randomized trial to demonstrate a survival benefit from combination chemotherapy was reported from an international group (USA, Canada, Australia), and showed that the combination of methotrexate, vinblastine, doxorubicin and cisplatin (MVAC regimen) yielded a significantly increased response rate, progression-free and total survival, compared to single agent cisplatin *(14)*. A randomized study from the MD Anderson Cancer Institute confirmed this result by demonstrating a statistically improved survival from the MVAC regimen compared to the combination of cyclophosphamide, doxorubicin and cisplatin *(15)*. This result was anticipated as randomized trials had already demonstrated equivalence between the cyclophosphamide-doxorubicin-cisplatin combination and the single agents, cisplatin *(16)* and cyclophosphamide *(10)*.

Saxman et al. have recently published a long-term follow-up of the international trial and reported only 2 of 122 patients alive at 6 yr after treatment with cisplatin alone, compared to 9 of 133 alive after MVAC *(17)*. Although MVAC constitutes the standard treatment in 1999 for patients with metastatic disease, it is clear that with such a low cure rate and a median survival of only one year, new treatments are urgently required *(18)*.

Several of the novel compounds listed above are currently under evaluation in combination chemotherapy regimens. Paclitaxel has been incorporated into combination regimens with carboplatin *(19,20)*, cisplatin *(21)*, ifosfamide plus cisplatin *(22)*, and methotrexate plus cisplatin *(23)*. Objective response rates in the range of 30–70% have been documented, but in many instances, the median survival has been shorter than would be expected from the MVAC regimen.

The combination of gemcitabine with cisplatin increases the objective response rate to nearly 70%, with a median survival greater than 12 mo *(24)*, and trials in progress are also assessing its use in association with carboplatin, paclitaxel and ifosfamide *(25,26)*.

These agents are particularly important, as they appear to be much less toxic than some of the earlier agents (e.g., the MVAC regimen), and hence may be more easily introduced into combined modality regimens. A randomized trial comparing the MVAC regimen against the cisplatin-gemcitabine combination has been completed and awaits statistical analysis. It should not be forgotten that paclitaxel and gemcitabine are radiosensitizers. Thus, they may have a role in improving local control in combination with radiotherapy and may potentially be important in the control of systemic disease.

Neoadjuvant Chemotherapy

Invasive bladder cancer is now considered to be a systemic disease. More than half of the presenting patients will eventually relapse with distant metastases *(27)*, presumably because micrometastases are present early in the course of the disease. Systemic chemotherapy has been added to locoregional treatment in an attempt to improve cure rates by downstaging the primary tumor, reducing micrometastases and, in some instances, by functioning as a radiosensitizer *(28)*.

Neoadjuvant chemotherapy implies treatment prior to definitive local therapy that is based upon the clinical stage of the cancer defined by TURBT and bimanual examination under anesthesia. The advantages are the presence of measurable disease to assess response, introduction of chemotherapy with the smallest potential volume of metastatic disease, and the opportunity for downstaging of "unresectable" tumors making them "resectable". In contrast, the possible drawbacks of this strategy include the risk of using an ineffective initial treatment, thus delaying potentially definitive treatment approaches (such as radiotherapy or surgery) and the use of systemic treatment to control a localized tumor that may have more side effects.

The initial, nonrandomized single agent trials were very promising as they demonstrated substantial tumor downstaging and apparently improved tumor resection rates *(29–33)*. However, randomized clinical trials that tested single agent chemotherapy plus local treatment versus local treatment alone did not show any benefit from this strategy *(34–36)*. Similarly, the use of combination chemotherapy regimens, such as cisplatin, methotrexate, and vinblastine (CMV) or MVAC, as neoadjuvant treatment initially appeared to be highly effective *(37–41)*, but late follow-up studies did not indicate any apparent long-term benefit *(42)*. Also of relevance, Kaye et al. *(43)* demonstrated an apparent absence of objective response when using the combination of cyclophosphamide, methotrexate and 5-fluoruracil. However, their recorded median survival figures were comparable to contemporary results with radiotherapy alone, suggesting that the noninvasive assessment of objective response within the bladder might be flawed.

By contrast, the Nordic Cooperative Bladder Cancer Study Group reported that two cycles of neoadjuvant cisplatin and doxorubicin conferred a reduced death rate in patients with T3 and T4a bladder cancer who were treated by cystectomy and pre-operative short course pelvic irradiation *(44)*. This study, however, had only a modest statistical power because of the patient numbers. A recent meta-analysis of all known randomized trials reviewed data from 479 cases and compared local treatment to neoadjuvant chemotherapy followed by local treatment. This study demonstrated an overall hazard ratio of 1.02 (favoring local treatment) and a 2% increase in relative risk of death from the use of neoadjuvant chemotherapy *(45)*. It should not be forgotten that this study was heavily dominated by single agent trials (4 out of 5 used single agent ciplatin).

An International Intergroup (MRC/EORTC) Trial, in which more than 950 patients were randomly allocated to neoadjuvant cisplatin/methotrexate/vinblastine plus local treatment or local treatment alone, was recently reported for the first time *(46)*. This study was well executed, with a high compliance to protocol design, but suffered from lack of central pathology review. The first report of this study failed to reveal a significant survival difference between the two arms, despite significant downstaging of tumors treated by neoadjuvant chemotherapy.

Similar results have been produced by the recent Radiation Therapy Oncology Group (RTOG) study, in which patients were randomly allocated to receive definitive chemoradiation (incorporating cisplatin and radical dose radiotherapy) or two cycles of neoadjuvant CMV chemotherapy, followed by an identical schedule of chemoradiation *(47)*. This study reported 5-yr survival rates of 48% and 49%, clearly showing an absence of survival benefit in comparison to neoadjuvant chemotherapy.

An important randomized trial carried out by the North American Intergroup has not been reported to date. In this study, patients were randomized to 3 cycles of MVAC followed by cystectomy or cystectomy alone.

Table 1
Results of Clinical Trials
of Neoadjuvant Chemotherapy for Invasive Bladder Cancer

Series	Regimen	Response rate after chemorx			Response rate after all Rx			Median survival (mo)	Actuarial long-term survival
		CR (%)	PR (%)	RR (%)	CR (%)	PR (%)	RR (%)		
Raghavan	C-RT/†	60		60	85		85	32	40% 5-yr 30% true 5-yr
Kaye	CyMF-RT	0	0	0	0	0	0	27	26% 3-yr,T4 26% 3-yr
Zincke	MVDC/†	50	19	69	0	0	92	?	?
Scher/ Schultz	MVDC/†	21	39	60	30	57	87	59.9	40% 8-yr
Shearer	M-RT	–	–	–	–	–	56	23	39% 3-yr
Shearer	RT only	–	–	–	–	–	50	20	37% 3-yr
Malmstrom	DC/†	–	–	–	–	–	–	Not reached	>50% 7-yr
Malmstrom	† only	–	–	–	–	–	–	72	50% 6-yr
Wallace	C	–	–	–	–	–	–	~24	39% 3-yr
Wallace	RT only	–	–	–	–	–	–	~22	39% 3-yr
Hall	RT/† only	–	–	–	–	–	–	Too early	62% 2-yr
Hall	CMV- RT/†	–	–	–	–	–	–	Too early	60% 2-yr

Abbreviations: Chemorx, chemotherapy; Rx, therapy; CR, complete remission; PR, partial remission; RR, total remission rate; RT, radiotherapy; C, cisplatin; M, methotrexate; F, fluorouracil; Cy, cyclophosphamide; D, doxorubicin.
†Cystectomy as definitive treatment.
Modified from Raghavan et al. (27).

The rigorous trial design and execution, accompanied by central pathological review, will be of particular importance in interpreting the significance of the study if the results differ from those of the larger MRC/ EORTC trial. However, until the results of this trial are available, the benefit of neoadjuvant chemotherapy remains unproven, as the majority of trials have failed to report improved median and 5-yr survival rates (Table 1).

Perioperative Chemotherapy

Chemotherapy has also been administered before and after definitive locoregional treatment for bladder cancer. Shearer et al. (1988) studied the role of methotrexate in this context in a randomized trial that predominantly assessed the impact of neoadjuvant chemotherapy, but also had a component of adjuvant therapy after completion of definitive treatment *(34)*. No survival gain was noted compared to standard treatment.

In a pilot study conducted by the Eastern Cooperative Oncology Group, two cycles of MVAC were administered before cystectomy, followed by another two cycles postoperatively *(48)*. Seventeen patients had T3 disease and one had a stage T2 tumor. Nearly half the cases showed downstaging in response to MVAC, but at a median follow-up time of 23 mo, 50% had died. Logothetis and colleagues *(49)* tested a similar strategy and reported an interim analysis of a trial in which 100 patients were randomized to receive either two cycles of MVAC followed by cystectomy and then 3 adjuvant cycles of MVAC, or initial cystectomy followed by 5 cycles of adjuvant MVAC. There was no statistically significant difference between the survival results in the two arms, despite the significant level of downstaging after neoadjuvant chemotherapy. The perioperative complication rates were similar for the two arms *(50)*. Both trials revealed an unexpectedly high rate of deaths from vascular complications, again demonstrating the importance of randomized trials in the assessment of these novel strategies of management *(51)*.

Neoadjuvant Chemotherapy: Conclusions

The conclusions from these randomized trials suggest that there is no clear rationale to support neoadjuvant chemotherapy outside a clinical trial for patients who are at high risk for relapse. Patients who have unresectable disease, either because of fixation to the pelvic side wall or pathologically proven pelvic lymph nodes above the bifurcation of the common iliac artery, may benefit with respect to disease-free survival from initial chemotherapy followed by cystectomy if there is a significant response to chemotherapy. This approach may reduce complications and morbidity from local progression of cancer, though this has not been formally evaluated in prospective studies. It should not be forgotten, however, that an overall survival benefit has not been demonstrated for neoadjuvant chemotherapy even in this context.

Adjuvant Chemotherapy

When cystectomy is performed as initial definitive therapy, complete pathologic staging becomes available, and patients are selected for adjuvant chemotherapy who are most likely to benefit from it. The chemotherapy is therefore given at a time of minimal disease burden. The disadvantages are the absence of measurable tumor to determine objective response to therapy, delay in treatment of micrometastatic disease, and that patients who are debilitated after cystectomy may eventually not receive chemotherapy at all. There are four published randomized trials of radical cystectomy with or without adjuvant chemotherapy. A fifth trial comparing combined neoadjuvant and adjuvant chemotherapy versus adjuvant therapy is discussed in the perioperative chemotherapy section earlier in this chapter.

The first contemporary randomized trial of adjuvant chemotherapy following cystectomy was performed at the University of Southern California (USC) *(52)*. This trial accrued 100 patients (91 evaluable) from a group of 160 that were eligible over 8.5 yr. Patients were randomized to four courses of adjuvant PAC (or CISCA–cisplatin 100 mg/M^2, doxorubicin 60 mg/M^2 and cyclophosphamide 600 mg/M^2) or observation following radical cystectomy and bilateral pelvic and iliac lymphadenectomy. Eligible patients had pathologic stage P3, P4, N0 or N+, M0 bladder TCC. Although the target accrual goal was to enroll 75 patients in each arm, only 100 patients total were enrolled. At 3 yr the probability of disease recurrence was 30 ± 8% for the chemotherapy arm and 54 ± 8% for the observation arm. The probability of cancer death at 3 yr was 29 ± 8% and 50 ± 8%, respectively. This benefit persisted with additional follow-up, but when analyzed for the subsets of node negative and node positive patients, it was significant only for patients with no or one positive node only *(52)*. This study has several methodological flaws common to many of the subsequent studies described in this chapter. Only 63% of the eligible patients were enrolled. Of the 44 patients randomized to chemotherapy, 11 refused treatment and several more were not treated with the protocol chemotherapy regimen. The initial statistical analysis used the Wilcoxan test, which emphasizes early differences in outcome measures. Subsequent analysis using the log rank test showed a statistically significant benefit for chemotherapy regarding the endpoint of time to recurrence but not survival *(53,54)*. Whether or not a prolongation of the time to recurrence is perceived as beneficial has not been formally addressed in quality of life studies.

A subsequent study from Mainz, Germany, randomized patients to three courses of MVAC/MVEC (substituting epirubicin for doxorubicin) in patients with pT3b, pT4, pN0 or pN1, pN2 TCC of the bladder *(55)*. Lymph node metastases were proven pathologically in 59% of patients. The trial design called for 100 randomized patients and was powered to detect an improvement in freedom from disease recurrence from 20% in the observation arm to 55% in the chemotherapy arm. Of the 60 eligible patients encountered over 3.5 yr, 49 patients were randomized: 26 to the chemotherapy arm and 23 to the observation arm. Eight patients randomized to chemotherapy were not treated with MVAC or MVEC. The trial did not permit chemotherapy at the time of relapse in the observation arm. Documented tumor progression occurred in 7 of

26 patients randomized to chemotherapy and in 18 of 23 patients in the observation arm ($p = 0.0015$). Chemotherapy ($p = 0.0007$) and the number of involved lymph nodes ($p = 0.0028$) were significant risk factors for recurrence in a Cox proportional hazards model that also included gender, age and pT stage.

The study was closed early because an interim analysis showed a significant advantage for the chemotherapy arm (55). No survival benefit could be determined due to the short followup (median followup for those alive was 21–24 mo). Furthermore, because of the lack of salvage chemotherapy being offered to patients who relapsed on the control arm, this study was effectively a trial that tested the role of chemotherapy at some time after cystectomy, rather than truly testing the role of planned adjuvant chemotherapy.

Subsequent to this the authors began offering adjuvant chemotherapy to patients with pathologically proven non organ-confined cancer and updated their experience in 1995 (56). With longer followup of the original patients in the randomized trial, there was a significant benefit attributed to adjuvant chemotherapy for both time to progression and event-free survival (defined as no progression and tumor unrelated death) ($p = 0.0005$ and $p = 0.0055$, respectively). Among patients with lymph node metastases treated with cystectomy and pelvic lymphadenectomy, adjuvant chemotherapy was associated with a decreased probability of tumor progression for patients with one positive node and for patients with two or more positive nodes (57). The potential for selection bias, given the small numbers of patients in this trial, and unplanned subset analysis clearly confound the results and make these data difficult to interpret in valid statistical terms. Non-randomized patients were then added to the randomized study and a survival benefit was reported, further confounding the statistical analysis of this study.

In 1994, these investigators initiated a new multi-center German trial with similar entry criteria to compare three cycles of MVAC and three cycles of cisplatin and methotrexate (57). The study design calls for enrolling 320 patients and will test for equivalence, which they define as lowering the progression rate by no more than 15%. As of March 1999, 230 patients have been enrolled and accrual may be complete by the end of the year 2000 (M. Stockle, personal communication).

A recent Swiss multicenter (SAKK) study evaluated three courses of adjuvant, single-agent cisplatin (90 mg/m^2), following cystectomy vs cystectomy alone (58). Patients with multifocal recurrent T1 cancer and patients with muscle-invasive cancers (T2–T4a) were eligible. A total of 80 patients were enrolled out of 168 who met the pathological entry criteria. Reasons for exclusion included ureteral obstruction, radiographic evidence of nodal metastases, impaired renal function or decreased performance status. Only 7/80 (9%) patients had pathologic nodal metastases and only 35/80 (44%) had P3b or P4 tumors *(59)*. Only 65% of patients received the 3 cycles of chemotherapy; 7 patients refused chemotherapy altogether and 6 had fewer than 3 courses. The study was closed early after a planned interim analysis on 80 patients failed to show a significant difference in 5-yr survival rates.

The Stanford trial evaluated total cystectomy and pelvic lymph node dissection plus adjuvant chemotherapy with four courses of CMV *(60)* vs cystectomy and node dissection alone *(61)*. All but one eligible patient evaluated at the institution was enrolled in the trial. A total of 55 patients with pT3b and pT4 cancers with or without nodal metastases were randomized with 88% of the 27 patients randomized to chemotherapy completing treatment (64% had positive nodes). At a median follow-up of 62 mo, the median time to progression was 12 mo vs 37 mo for the observation and chemotherapy arms, respectively, and the relapse rates were 80% and 52%, respectively. Despite this improvement in time to progression, there was no survival benefit with adjuvant chemotherapy. This may be due to the very small numbers of cases entered, or due to the fact that the study was designed prospectively to treat all patients in the observation arm with CMV chemotherapy at time of relapse. A total of 19 of 25 patients treated with cystectomy alone relapsed and 15 of 19 did receive chemotherapy (1–6 cycles of CMV). Three patients (16%) were without disease at 50, 75, and 77 mo after cystectomy. The toxicity was acceptable although one patient died of neutropenia and sepsis following cycle one of chemotherapy.

Despite the similar survival probabilities in the chemotherapy and observation arms, the authors argue that adjuvant chemotherapy in a high risk group of patients is preferable to chemotherapy at relapse which requires more chemotherapy in a frequently debilitated patient with 2-yr survival probabilities of 10–15% *(14)*. This study was criticized for small sample size, the long interval for accrual (7 yr), and early termination (*see* Table 2) which the authors state, occurred because the endpoint of freedom from progression had been reached with fewer than anticipated patients.

Adjuvant Chemotherapy: Conclusions

The data reported from randomized trials to date are insufficient to conclusively determine the efficacy of adjuvant chemotherapy following radical cystectomy for P3b,P4 node negative or node positive (any pT) TCC. The total number of patients (267) in the four studies discussed in this chapter is small and 70 of these patients were treated with sin-

Table 2
Results of Randomized Trials
of Adjuvant Chemotherapy and Radical Cystectomy

Series	Regimen	No. patients randomized	Progression Median	5-yr[a]	Survival Median	5-yr[a]	Survival benefit?
USC	CISCA	44	6.58 yr	51%	4.25 yr	39%	No
	Observation	47	1.92 yr	34%	2.41 yr	44%	
Mainz	M-VA(E)C[b]	26	not reached	63% 3 yr	–	–	Not
	Observation	23	16 mo	0% 3 yr	–	–	evaluated
Mainz	M-VA(E)C[c]	26	not reached	64% 3 yr	38 mo	54%[c]	Yes
	Observation	23	16 mo	14% 3 yr	17 mo	14%	
SAKK	Cisplatin	37	–	–	not reached	57%	No
	Observation	40	–	–	not reached	54%	
Stanford	CMV[d]	25	37 mo	50%	63 mo	55%	No
	Observation	25	12 mo	22%	36 mo	35%	

[a] Kaplan-Meier estimates.
[b] Survival data not reported.
[c] Followup report from original series; event-free survival (event defined as progression or tumor unrelated death) at 36 months estimated from Kaplan-Meier plots.
[d] Results estimated from Kaplan-Meier plots.

gle agent cisplatin which is inferior to combination chemotherapy for patients with measurable disease *(14)*. The percentage of patients randomized to chemotherapy who did not receive any chemotherapy ranges from 4–31%. These data should be accounted for when designing future studies as they will no doubt increase the sample size required to maintain the power of the study. In addition to pathologic tumor stage and nodal metastases, the use of histologic features (e.g., lymphatic or vascular invasion) and molecular markers (*see below*) to identify a high risk group that may benefit from adjuvant chemotherapy should be evaluated prospectively in clinical trials.

The limitations of published randomized trials of adjuvant chemotherapy suggest that there is no standard place for adjuvant chemotherapy in an unstructured setting. Entry into appropriate clinical trials is therefore our preferred approach. When no relevant trials are open, recommendations for adjuvant chemotherapy should be made in the context of a complete informed consent describing the risks of chemotherapy and the limitations of the studies conducted to date.

Molecular Staging

Molecular markers may provide a more accurate method to stratify patients into low-risk and high-risk categories for bladder cancer progression and survival following radical cystectomy. Mutations within the conserved region of the *p53* tumor suppressor gene are a common feature of CIS and high-grade TCC *(62)*. Immunohistochemical techniques take advantage of the prolonged half-life of the mutant *p53* protein, and *p53* nuclear immunoreactivity correlates highly with *p53* mutations identified by genomic sequencing *(63,64)*. For patients treated with radical cystectomy, *p53* nuclear immunoreactivity of the primary tumor has been associated with an increased risk of relapse and death for patients with P2 and P3a node-negative TCC of the bladder *(65)*. *P53* did not stratify patients with more advanced cancers (P3b, P4, or N+). At Baylor, we confirmed these observations in an analysis of 80 patients treated with radical cystectomy for TCC *(66)*.

Sarkis et al. found similar results for 90 patients undergoing neoadjuvant chemotherapy prior to planned radical cystectomy in a phase II study from the Memorial Sloan-Kettering Cancer Center *(67)*. The 5-yr survival probability was 62% for patients with tumors that were *p53* negative (wild type) and 40% for *p53* positive (mutated) ($p = 0.004$). As was observed in the USC study, the predictive value of *p53* was particularly evident for patients with tumors confined to the muscularis propria (77% vs 43.5%, $p = 0.007$).

Herr et al. recently analyzed long-term follow-up of 60 patients who achieved T0 status after neoadjuvant M-VAC chemotherapy *(68)*. Patients whose primary tumors were *p53* negative by immunohistochemistry had a survival probability of 87% at 10 yr compared to 51% for patients with *p53* positive tumors. This survival benefit was most significant for patients with T2 tumors where 100% of 19 patients with tumors that were *p53* negative survived compared to 9/19 (47%) patients with *p53* positive tumors. The survival of patients with T3 tumors was similar for patients with *p53* negative and *p53* positive tumors (67% and 60%, respectively). Based on these observations these authors have initiated a study to treat patients with T2 *p53* negative tumors with MVAC chemotherapy followed by transurethral resection alone *(68)*.

Investigators at USC and Baylor have initiated an NCI funded multicenter, multinational clinical trial to evaluate *p53* and other markers in patients treated with radical cystectomy for cancers pathologically confined to the muscularis propria or lamina propria. This study will test two hypotheses: 1) *P53* alterations in organ-confined bladder TCC significantly increase the risk of recurrence and death; and 2) Adjuvant chemotherapy may improve survival in patients with *p53* alterations. This study will also create a repository of archival tissue for the examination of other markers including *RB*, and cell cycle regulatory proteins including p16 and p21.

In the Memorial study the response to chemotherapy in the primary bladder tumor was similar for patients who were *p53* negative and those who were *p53* positive *(67)*. In an analysis of the USC adjuvant chemotherapy trial, cisplatin based chemotherapy was associated with a lower risk of recurrence and death in p53 positive tumors compared to *p53* negative tumors *(69)*. These observations contradict the prevailing opinion that mutations in the *p53* gene impart resistance to chemotherapy because tumor cells fail to undergo apoptosis despite DNA damage.

In an effort to understand these contradictory findings, it is important to consider some of the various pathways of induction of apoptosis as they relate to DNA damaging agents. Wild type *p53* regulates the transition between G1 and S phase. *P53* protein levels increase in response to DNA damage, inhibiting cell division by holding cells in G1 for repair or promoting cell death via the apoptotic pathway *(70)*. Defects in apoptosis caused by inactivation of *p53* may thus impart resistance to chemotherapy or irradiation *(71)*. In addition, some *p53* mutations may confer a selective gain of function that confers resistance to chemotherapy agents including etoposide or cisplatin, which may be overcome in vitro with high drug concentrations in the case of cisplatin *(72)*.

Waldman et al. have suggested, however, that alterations in *p53* might increase the sensitivity of tumors to chemotherapy by allowing multiple rounds of S phase leading to aneuploidy and apoptosis by alternate pathways *(73)*. In addition, apoptosis may occur via induction by tumor necrosis factor alpha (TNFα) *(74)*. Paclitaxel, an active agent in TCC, promotes microtubule assembly and induces apoptosis through both the TNFα and p53 pathways *(74)*. Thus in the case of *p53* alterations in bladder cancer, chemotherapy sensitivity may be retained via alternative apoptotic pathways and may depend on the particular chemotherapy agent and the spectrum of *p53* mutations in a particular tumor.

Inactivation of the retinoblastoma *(RB)* tumor suppressor gene is also a common event in bladder cancer and is seen more frequently in high-grade and invasive cancers *(75,76)*. Loss of *RB* expression has been associated with a higher probability of progression to invasive disease and decreased survival. It has recently been shown that patients whose bladder cancer demonstrates overexpression of *RB* protein by immunohistochemistry have an increased rate of progression and decreased survival probability similar to patients whose tumors demonstrate no RB expression *(77,78)*. Overexpression of *RB* protein, representing the hyperphosphorylated (inactivated) form of *RB*, is related to loss of function of *p16*, which is a cyclin-dependent kinase (CDK) inhibitor which acts upstream to *RB* *(79)*. While strong staining for *RB* is associated with absence of expression of p16 protein, absence of *RB* expression is associated with strong nuclear staining for p16. Loss of *p16* function may therefore have a similar deleterious effect as loss of *RB* function in bladder cancer.

Altered expression of the retinoblastoma tumor suppressor gene may add prognostic value to p53 immunohistochemistry *(66,77)*. Patients with p53 wild type/pRB wild type tumors have a significantly decreased probability of tumor recurrence and an increased probability of survival compared to patients with one or both altered. Both *p53* and the retinoblastoma tumor suppressor *(RB)* genes have been shown in multiple studies to define survival probabilities, particularly in patients with pT2 or pT3a node-negative tumors. P53 and RB immunostaining can be performed accurately in bladder biopsy samples prior to cystectomy *(66,79)*, and this will afford the opportunity to predict biologic behavior in advance of definitive therapy and provide additional selection criteria for neoadjuvant and adjuvant chemotherapy trials.

The data we have presented is selective and intended to demonstrate some potential uses for molecular markers. There is significant variability, however, regarding the predictive value of certain markers. Until prospective clinical trials are completed and techniques standardized, these markers should not be used in general clinical practice.

CONCLUSION

After more than 25 yr of research, the true role of combined modality treatment for locally advanced bladder cancer remains controversial. Neoadjuvant trials, while supporting a role for debulking and facilitation of surgical resection, have not shown an overall survival benefit. Adjuvant chemotherapy trials have been more intriguing, with at least the suggestion of improved disease-free survival and statistical trends that support a potential role for adjuvant chemotherapy in a series of statistically underpowered trials.

It is our belief that the improved tools of molecular prognostication will allow us to design randomized trials more precisely, and to identify the true utility of adjuvant chemotherapy strategies. In addition, with the advent of novel, less toxic chemotherapy regimens, it may be possible to introduce earlier, or more intensive, adjuvant regimens in an effort to improve outcome. One of the most important clinical trials currently in progress, initiated as a multicenter collaboration by investigators at USC and Baylor, will address these important issues. This and other well-designed clinical trials must be supported by the medical community if we are to improve the results of treatment for invasive bladder cancer.

REFERENCES

1. Landis SH, Murray T, Bolden S, Wingo PA. Cancer Statistics, 1999. CA Cancer J Clin 1999; 49: 8–31.

2. Lerner SP, Skinner DG. Radical cystectomy for bladder cancer. In: *Comprehensive Textbook of Genitourinary Oncology* (Vogelzang NJ, Shipley WU, Scardino PT, Coffey D, eds.). Williams and Wilkins, Philadelphia, PA, 1995, pp. 442–463.

3. Lerner SP, Skinner DG, Lieskovsky G, et al. The rationale for en bloc pelvic lymph node dissection for bladder cancer patients with nodal metastases: long-term results. J Urol 1993; 149: 758–765.

4. Loehrer PJS, DeMulder PP. Management of metastatic bladder cancer. In: *Principles and Practice of Genitourinary Oncology* (Raghavan D, Scher HI, Leibel SA, Lange PH, eds.). Lippincott-Raven, Philadelphia, PA, 1997, pp. 299–305.

5. Witte RS, Elson P, Bono B, et al. Eastern Cooperative Oncology Group phase II trial of ifosfamide in the treatment of previously treated advanced urothelial carcinoma. J Clin Oncol 1997; 15: 589–593.

6. Seligman PA, Crawford ED. Treatment of advanced transitional cell carcinoma of the bladder with continuous-infusion gallium nitrate. J Natl Cancer Inst 1991; 83: 1582–1584.

7. Roth BJ, Dreicer R, Einhorn LH, et al. Significant activity of paclitaxel in advanced transitional-cell carcinoma of the urothelium: a phase II trial of the Eastern Cooperative Oncology Group. J Clin Oncol 1994; 12: 2264–2270.

8. McCaffrey JA, Hilton S, Mazumdar M, et al. Phase II trial of docetaxel in patients with advanced or metastatic transitional-cell carcinoma. J Clin Oncol 1997; 15: 1853–1857.

9. Pollera CF, Ceribelli A, Crecco M, Calabresi F. Weekly gemcitabine in advanced bladder cancer: A preliminary report. Ann Oncol 1994; 5: 132–134.

10. Stadler W, Kuzel T, Roth B, Raghavan D, Dorr FA. Phase II study of single-agent gemcitabine in previously untreated patients with metastatic urothelial cancer. J Clin Oncol 1997; 15: 3394–3398.

11. Moore MJ, Tannock IF, Ernst DS, Huan S, Murray N. Gemcitabine: a promising new agent in the treatment of advanced urothelial cancer. J Clin Oncol 1997; 15: 3441–3445.

12. Soloway MS, Einstein A, Corder MP, Bonney W, Prout GR Jr, Coombs J. A comparison of cisplatin and the combination of cisplatin and cyclophosphamide in advanced urothelial cancer. A National Bladder Cancer Collaborative Group A study. Cancer 1983; 52: 767–772.

13. Hillcoat BL, Raghavan D, Matthews J, et al. A randomized trial of cisplatin versus cisplatin plus methotrexate in advanced cancer of the urothelial tract. J Clin Oncol 1989; 7: 706–709.

14. Loehrer PJ Sr, Einhorn LH, Elson PJ, et al. A randomized comparison of cisplatin alone or in combination with methotrexate, vinblastine, and doxorubicin in patients with metastatic urothelial carcinoma: a cooperative group study. J Clin Oncol 1992; 10: 1066–1073.

15. Logothetis CJ, Dexeus FH, Finn L, et al. A prospective randomized trial comparing MVAC and CISCA chemotherapy for patients with metastatic urothelial tumors. J Clin Oncol 1990; 8: 1050–1055.

16. Khandekar JD, Elson PJ, DeWys WD, Slayton RE, Harris DT. Comparative activity and toxicity of cis-diamminedichloroplatinum (DDP) and a combination of doxorubicin, cyclophosphamide, and DDP in disseminated transitional cell carcinomas of the urinary tract. J Clin Oncol 1985; 3: 539–545.

17. Saxman SB, Propert KJ, Einhorn LH, et al. Long-term follow-up of a phase III intergroup study of cisplatin alone or in combination with methotrexate, vinblastine, and doxorubicin in patients with metastatic urothelial carcinoma: a cooperative group study. J Clin Oncol 1997; 15: 2564–2569.

18. Levine EG, Raghavan D. MVAC for bladder cancer: time to move forward again. J Clin Oncol 1993; 11: 387–389.

19. Vaughn DJ, Malkowicz SB, Zoltick B, et al. Paclitaxel plus carboplatin in advanced carcinoma of the urothelium: an active and tolerable outpatient regimen. J Clin Oncol 1998; 16: 255–260.

20. Redman BG, Smith DC, Flaherty L, Du W, Hussain M. Phase II trial of paclitaxel and carboplatin in the treatment of advanced urothelial carcinoma. J Clin Oncol 1998; 16: 1844–1848.

21. Murphy BA, Johnson DR, Smith J, et al. Phase II trial of paclitaxel (P) and cisplatin (C) for metastatic or locally unresectable urothelial cancer. ASCO Program/Proc 1996; 15: 245 (Abstract 617).

22. McCaffrey J, Hilton S, Mazumdar M, et al. A phase II trial of ifosfamide, paclitaxel and cisplatin (ITP) in patients (pts) with advanced urothelial tract tumors. ASCO Program/Proc 1996; 15: 251 (Abstract 641).

23. Tu SM, Hossan E, Amato R, Kilbourn R, Logothetis CJ. Paclitaxel, cisplatin and methotrexate combination chemotherapy is active in the treatment of refractory urothelial malignancies. J Urol 1995; 154: 1719–1722.

24. Kaufman D, Stadler W, Carducci M, et al. Gemcitabine (GEM) plus cisplatin (CDDP) in metastatic transitional cell carcinoma (TCC): final results of a phase II study. ASCO Program/Proc 1998; 17: 320a (Abstract 1235).

25. Vaishampayan U, Smith D, Redman B, Kucuk O, Ensley J, Hussain M. Phase II evaluation of carboplatin, paclitaxel and gemcitabine in advanced urothelial carcinoma. ASCO Program/Proc 1999; 18: 333a (Abstract 1282).

26. Bellmunt J, Guillem V, Paz-Ares L, et al. A phase II trial of paclitaxel, cisplatin and gemcitabine (TCG) in patients (pts) with advanced transitional cell carcinoma (TCC) of the urothelium. ASCO Program/Proc 1999; 18: 332a (Abstract 1279).

27. Raghavan D, Shipley W, Garnick M, Russell PJ, Ritchie JP. Biology and management of bladder cancer. N Engl J Med 1990; 322: 1129–1138.

28. Raghavan D. Pre-emptive (neo-adjuvant) intravenous chemotherapy for invasive bladder cancer. Br J Urol 1988; 61: 1–8.

29. Herr HW. Preoperative irradiation with and without chemotherapy as adjunct to radical cystectomy. Urology 1985; 25: 127–134.

30. Soloway MS, Ikard M, Ford K. Cis-diamminedichloroplatinum (II) in locally advanced and metastatic urothelial cancer. Cancer 1981; 47: 476–480.

31. Fagg SL, Dawson-Edwards P, Hughes MA, Latief TN, Rolfe EB, Fielding JW. Cis-diamminedichloroplatinum (DDP) as initial treatment of invasive bladder cancer. Br J Urol 1984; 56: 296–300.

32. Raghavan D, Pearson B, Duval P, et al. Initial intravenous cis-platinum therapy: improved management for invasive high risk bladder cancer? J Urol 1985; 133: 399–402.

33. Pearson BS, Raghavan D. First-line intravenous cisplatin for deeply invasive bladder cancer: update on 70 cases. Br J Urol 1985; 57: 690–693.

34. Shearer RJ, Chilvers CF, Bloom HJ, Bliss JM, Horwich A, Babiker A. Adjuvant chemotherapy in T3 carcinoma of the bladder. A prospective trial: preliminary report. Br J Urol 1988; 62: 558–564.

35. Wallace DM, Raghavan D, Kelly KA, et al. Neo-adjuvant (pre-emptive) cisplatin therapy in invasive transitional cell carcinoma of the bladder. Br J Urol 1991; 67: 608–615.

36. Martinez-Pineiro JA, Gonzalez Martin M, Arocena F, et al. Neoadjuvant cisplatin chemotherapy before radical cystectomy in invasive transitional cell carcinoma of the bladder: a prospective randomized phase III study. J Urol 1995; 153: 964–973.

37. Meyers FJ, Palmer JM, Freiha FS, et al. The fate of the bladder in patients with metastatic bladder cancer treated with cisplatin, methotrexate and vinblastine: a Northern California Oncology Group study. J Urol 1985; 134: 1118–1121.

38. Vogelzang NJ, Moormeier JA, Awan AM, et al. Methotrexate, vinblastine, doxorubicin and cisplatin followed by radiotherapy or surgery for muscle invasive bladder cancer: the University of Chicago experience. J Urol 1993; 149: 753–757.

39. Scattoni V, Bolognesi A, Cozzarini C, et al. Neoadjuvant CMV chemotherapy plus radical cystectomy in locally advanced bladder cancer: the impact of pathologic response on long-term results. Tumori 1996; 82: 463–469.

40. Scher H, Herr H, Sternberg C, et al. Neo-adjuvant chemotherapy for invasive bladder cancer. Experience with the M-VAC regimen. Br J Urol 1989; 64: 250–256.

41. Zincke H, Sen SE, Hahn RG, Keating JP. Neoadjuvant chemotherapy for locally advanced transitional cell carcinoma of the bladder: do local findings suggest a potential for salvage of the bladder? Mayo Clin Proc 1988; 63: 16–22.

42. Schultz PK, Herr HW, Zhang ZF, et al. Neoadjuvant chemotherapy for invasive bladder cancer: prognostic factors for survival of patients treated with M-VAC with 5-year follow-up. J Clin Oncol 1994; 12: 1394–1401.

43. Kaye SB, MacFarlane JR, McHattie I, Hart AJ. Chemotherapy before radiotherapy for T3 bladder cancer. A pilot study. Br J Urol 1985; 57: 434–437.

44. Malmstrom PU, Rintala E, Wahlqvist R, Hellstrom P, Hellsten S, Hannisdal E. Five-year followup of a prospective trial of radical cystectomy and neoadjuvant chemotherapy: Nordic Cystectomy Trial I. The Nordic Cooperative Bladder Cancer Study Group (see comments). J Urol 1996; 155: 1903–1906.

45. Does neoadjuvant cisplatin-based chemotherapy improve the survival of patients with locally advanced bladder cancer: a meta-analysis of individual patient data from randomized clinical trials. Advanced Bladder Cancer Overview Collaboration. Br J Urol 1995; 75: 206–213.

46. Hall RR. Neo-adjuvant CMV chemotherapy and cystectomy or radiotherapy in muscle invasive bladder cancer. First analysis of MRC/EORTC Intercontinental trial. MRC Advanced Bladder Cancer Working Group, EORTC GU Group, NCI Canada, Norwegian Bladder Cancer Group, Australian Bladder Cancer Study Group, Club Urologica Espanol de Tratamiento and FinBladder. ASCO Program/ Proc 1996; 15: 244 (Abstract 612).

47. Shipley WU, Winter KA, Kaufman DS, et al. Phase III trial of neoadjuvant chemotherapy in patients with invasive bladder cancer treated with selective bladder preservation by combined radiation therapy and chemotherapy: initial results of Radiation Therapy Oncology Group 89-03. J Clin Oncol 1998; 16: 3576–3583.

48. Dreicer R, Messing EM, Loehrer PJ, Trump DL. Perioperative methotrexate, vinblastine, doxorubicin and cisplatin (M-VAC) for poor risk transitional cell carcinoma of the bladder: an Eastern Cooperative Oncology Group pilot study. J Urol 1990; 144: 1123–1126.

49. Logothetis C, Swanson D, Amato R, et al. Optimal delivery of perioperative chemotherapy: preliminary results of a randomized, prospective, comparative trial of pre-operative and postoperative chemotherapy for invasive bladder carcinoma. J Urol 1996; 155: 1241–1245.

50. Hall MC, Swanson DA, Dinney CP. Complications of radical cystectomy: impact of the timing of perioperative chemotherapy. Urology 1996; 47: 826–830.

51. Raghavan D. Perioperative chemotherapy for invasive bladder cancer—what should we tell our patients? (Editorial). J Urol 1996; 155: 1246–1247.

52. Skinner DG, Daniels JR, Russell CA, et al. The role of adjuvant chemotherapy following cystectomy for invasive bladder cancer: a prospective comparative trial. J Urol 1991; 145: 459–464.

53. Raghavan D. Editorial comment re: Skinner DG, Daniels JR, Russell CA, Lieskovsky G, Boyd SD, Nichols P, Kern W, Sakamoto J, Krailo M, Groshen S. The role

of adjuvant chemotherapy following cystectomy for invasive bladder cancer: a prospective comparative trial. J Urol 1991; 145: 465–466.

54. Droller MJ. Editorial comment re: Skinner DG, Daniels JR, Russell CA, Lieskovsky G, Boyd SD, Nichols P, Kern W, Sakamoto J, Krailo M, Groshen S. The role of adjuvant chemotherapy following cystectomy for invasive bladder cancer: a prospective comparative trial. J Urol 1991; 145: 465.

55. Stockle M, Meyenburg W, Wellek S, et al. Advanced bladder cancer (stages pT3b, pT4a, pN1 and pN2): improved survival after radical cystectomy and 3 adjuvant cycles of chemotherapy. Results of a controlled prospective study. J Urol 1992; 148: 302–306.

56. Stockle M, Meyenburg W, Wellek S, et al. Adjuvant polychemotherapy of nonorgan-confined bladder cancer after radical cystectomy revisited: long-term results of a controlled prospective study and further clinical experience. J Urol 1995; 153: 47–52.

57. Stockle M, Wellek S, Meyenburg W, et al. Radical cystectomy with or without adjuvant polychemotherapy for non- organ-confined transitional cell carcinoma of the urinary bladder: prognostic impact of lymph node involvement. Urology 1996; 48: 868–875.

58. Studer UE, Bacchi M, Biedermann C, et al. Adjuvant cisplatin chemotherapy following cystectomy for bladder cancer: results of a prospective randomized trial. J Urol 1994; 152: 81–84.

59. Anonymous. Manual for Staging of Cancer/American Joint Committee on Cancer. (Beahrs OH, Henson DE, Hutter RVP, Kennedy BJ, eds) 4th Edition. JB Lippincott, Philadelphia, PA, 1992, p. 280.

60. Harker GW, Meyers FJ, Freiha FS, et al. Cisplatin, methotrexate, and vinblastine (CMV): An effective chemotherapy regimen for metastatic transitonal cell carcinoma of the urinary tract—a Northern California Oncology Group Study. J Clin Oncol 1985; 3: 1463–1470.

61. Freiha F, Reese J, Torti FM. A randomized trial of radical cystectomy versus radical cystectomy plus cisplatin, vinblastine and methotrexate chemotherapy for muscle invasive bladder cancer (see comments). J Urol 1996; 155: 495–499.

62. Spruck CH, III, Ohneseit PF, Gonzalez-Zulueta M, et al. Two molecular pathways to transitional cell carcinoma of the bladder. Cancer Res 1994: 54: 784-788.

63. Esrig D, Spruck CH, III, Nichols PW, et al. p53 nuclear protein accumulation correlates with mutations in the p53 gene, tumor grade, and stage in bladder cancer. Am J Pathol 1993; 143: 1389–1397.

64. Cordon-Cardo C, Dalbagni G, Saez GT, et al. p53 mutations in human bladder cancer: genotypic versus phenotypic patterns. Int J Cancer 1994; 56: 347–353.

65. Esrig D, Elmajian D, Groshen S, et al. Accumulation of nuclear p53 and tumor progression in bladder cancer. N Engl J Med 1994; 331: 1259–1264.

66. Lerner SP, Benedict WF, Green A, et al. Molecular staging and prognosis following radical cystectomy using p53 and retinoblastoma protein expression. J Urol 1998; 159(Suppl): 165 (Abstract #630).

67. Sarkis AS. Prognostic value of p53 nuclear overexpression in patients with invasive bladder cancer treated with neoadjuvant M-VAC. J Clin Oncol 1995; 13: 1384–1390.

68. Herr HW, Bajorin DF, Scher HI, Cordon-Cardo C, Reuter VE. Can p53 help select patients with invasive bladder cancer for bladder preservation? J Urol 1999; 161: 20–23.

69. Cote RJ, Esrig D, Groshen S, Jones PA, Skinner DG. p53 and treatment of bladder cancer. Nature 1997; 385: 123–125.

70. Wu X, Levine AJ. p53 and E2F-1 cooperate to mediate apoptosis. Proc Natl Acad Sci USA 1994; 91: 3602–3606.

71. Lowe SW, Bodis S, McClatchey A, et al. p53 status and the efficacy of cancer therapy in vivo. Science 1994; 266: 807–810.

72. Blandino G, Levine AJ, Oren M. Mutant p53 gain of function: differential effects of different p53 mutants on resistance of cultured cells to chemotherapy. Oncogene 1999; 18: 477–485.

73. Waldman T, Lengauer C, Kinzler KW, Vogelstein B. Uncoupling of S phase and mitosis induced by anticancer agents in cells lacking p21. Nature 1996; 381: 713–716.

74. Lanni JS, Lowe SW, Licitra EJ, Liu JO, Jacks T. p53-independent apoptosis induced by paclitaxel through an indirect mechanism. Proc Natl Acad Sci USA 1997; 94: 9679–9683.

75. Ishikawa J, Xu HJ, Hu SX, et al. Inactivation of the retinoblastoma gene in human bladder and renal cell carcinomas. Cancer Res 1991; 51: 5736–5743.

76. Cordon-Cardo C, Wartinger D, Petrylak D, et al. Altered expression of the retinoblastoma gene product: prognostic indicator in bladder cancer. J Natl Cancer Inst 1992; 84: 1251–1256.

77. Cote RJ, Dunn MD, Chatterjee SJ, et al. Elevated and absent pRb expression is associated with bladder cancer progression and has cooperative effects with p53. Cancer Res 1998; 58: 1090–1094.

78. Grossman HB, Liebert M, Antelo M, et al. p53 and RB expression predict progression in T1 bladder cancer. Clin Cancer Res 1998; 4: 829–834.

79. Benedict WF, Lerner SP, Zhou J, Shen X, Tokunaga H, Czerniak B. Level of retinoblastoma protein expression correlates with p16 (MTS- 1/INK4A/CDKN2) status in bladder cancer. Oncogene 1999; 18: 1197–1203.

12 Clinical Situations for the Role of Radiation Therapy in the Treatment of Bladder Cancer

Mary K. Gospodarowicz, MD,
Michael F. Milosevic, MD,
Padraiq Warde, MD,
and Arthur T. Porter, MD

CONTENTS

INTRODUCTION
SUMMARY
REFERENCES

INTRODUCTION

The majority of bladder cancer patients present with superficial disease and are managed with conservative measures using transurethral resection with or without intravesical chemotherapy. Approximately 20–25% present with muscle invasive bladder cancer, that is potentially life threatening and requires radical treatment. Definitive radiation therapy (RT) has been used for muscle invasive bladder cancer since the early 1900s and there is evidence that patients can achieve durable local control and maintain a functional bladder without a compromise in survival. However, the standard North American approach to the management of bladder cancer not suitable for conservative measures is radical cystectomy *(1)*. In the past few decades, radical radiation therapy has been used in patients who either refused or were not suitable for radical cystectomy. Therefore, there is a limited amount of information on the precise role that radiation therapy plays in the management of bladder cancer.

From: *Current Clinical Urology: Bladder Cancer: Current Diagnosis and Treatment*
Edited by: M. J. Droller © Humana Press Inc., Totowa, NJ

Radiation therapy has been used in the management of bladder cancer in several distinct situations. The most common situation is the use of elective radical RT in muscle invasive bladder cancer in order to eradicate the tumor while preserving normal bladder function. Radical pelvic RT is also used to improve local control following a good response to chemotherapy given as definitive treatment for locally advanced bladder cancer. In both of these situations, salvage cystectomy may be used in the event of an incomplete response to radiation, local recurrence, or the development of a new invasive bladder tumor. Preoperative radiation therapy may be considered in cases of locally advanced bladder cancer, where radical cystectomy alone is associated with a high probability of local failure. Postoperative radiation therapy has also been suggested in this setting, extrapolating from the experience with other tumors. Palliative radiotherapy may be used to alleviate symptoms due to tumor progression in the pelvis in patients with locally advanced bladder cancer not amenable to radical therapy, distant metastasis or coexistent medical conditions that limit survival and the ability to tolerate radical treatment.

To address the role of radiation therapy in bladder cancer, we have asked the following five questions:

1. Is treatment with definitive radiation therapy alone able to eradicate muscle invasive bladder cancer without compromising overall survival? Which patients are the best candidates for bladder conservation with radiation therapy?
2. What is the best prescription for bladder conservation using radiation therapy?
3. When should preoperative RT be considered in locally advanced bladder cancer?
4. What is the role of postoperative RT after radical cystectomy?
5. When should palliative RT be considered in the management of bladder cancer?

These questions will form the basis of this review.

Is Treatment with Definitive Radiation Therapy Alone Able to Eradicate Muscle Invasive Bladder Cancer Without Compromising Overall Survival? Which Patients are the Best Candidates for Bladder Conservation with Radiation Therapy?

Multiple retrospective and several prospective studies have demonstrated high response rates for bladder cancer to treatment with external beam RT (2). For patients with T2–T3 bladder cancer, the reported com-

Table 1
Results of Radical Radiation Therapy
in Patients with Muscle Invasive Bladder Cancer

Author	Centre	# Patients	T2	T3 T3A/T3B	T4 T4A/T4B	Overall
Duncan	Edinburgh	699	40.2%	25.9%	11.6%	30.0%
Gospodarowicz[a]	PMH	121	59.0%	52%/29.7%	50%/16%	44.8%
Pollack	MD Anderson	135	42.0%	20.0%	0.0%	26.0%
Vale	St Barts	60	38.0%	12.0%		
Blandy	London Hospital	614	27.0%	38.0%	9.0%	
Smaaland	Bergen	146	25.7%	9.9%		
Davison[a]	Glasgow	675	49.1%	27.7%	2.3%	
Moonen	Netherlands	379	25.3%	16.9%		22.2%

[a] Cause specific survival.
[b] Results for T3/T4 combined.

plete response rates to RT alone at doses of 50–66 Gy in 1.8–2.5 Gy fractions over 4–6.5 wk have ranged from 30–60%, and the 5-yr actuarial survivals from 9.9–40% (Table 1). Approximately 30% of complete responders subsequently fail, resulting in an actuarial long-term local recurrence free rate of approximately 25%–40%.

Local failure following radical RT may manifest in three forms: 1) failure to control the index primary tumor; 2) residual or recurrent carcinoma *in situ*; or 3) a new superficial or invasive bladder cancer. Failure to control the index tumor or a new invasive cancer requires prompt salvage cystectomy. A new superficial transitional cell cancer may be managed by transurethral resection with or without intravesical chemotherapy. Local failure that presents as carcinoma *in situ* alone can be managed with intravesical BCG *(3,4)*. However, in cases where the original muscle invasive tumor developed on a background of BCG-resistant superficial disease, failure with carcinoma *in situ* is an indication for salvage cystectomy. The above scenarios suggest that not all patients who develop local failure following definitive RT for muscle invasive bladder cancer require immediate salvage cystectomy. However, careful followup after radiation is essential to detect local failure and implement further treatment at an early stage, in order to maximize overall survival.

Shipley et al. demonstrated long-term bladder preservation rates of 40-50% following radical radiotherapy *(5,6)*. The results from the Princess Margaret Hospital showed a 25% long-term cystectomy-free cause-specific survival in 355 unselected patients with T1–T4 bladder cancer who received radical RT in the 1970s *(7)*. However, the precise rate of salvage cystectomy following definitive RT is difficult to estimate. In the past, a large proportion of patients treated with RT were not candidates for cystectomy, and died without attempted salvage *(8)*. In addition, patients may have locally recurrent tumor that is technically amenable to salvage cystectomy but are not offered the procedure because of the early development of distant metastases.

There has been no study directly comparing radical RT to radical cystectomy. However, radical RT with salvage cystectomy has been compared to preoperative RT followed by cystectomy, and preoperative RT followed by cystectomy has been compared to cystectomy alone *(8–12)*. In the UK Institute of Urology trial, patients were randomised to receive preoperative RT of 40 Gy followed by cystectomy or 60 Gy alone with salvage cystectomy for tumor that did not regress or that recurred *(8)*. There was no significant difference in outcome between the arms (5-yr survival 29% for RT and 38% for preoperative RT and cystectomy). A similar trial conducted by the Danish Bladder Cancer Group (DAVECA) confirmed these results, with median survivals of 18 mo following definitive RT and 20 mo following preoperative RT and cystectomy *(9)*. These phase III randomised trials suggest that the strategy of definitive RT followed by selective cystectomy does not adversely affect survival relative to immediate cystectomy.

The criteria used to select patients for definitive RT include a high expectation of durable local control, an ability to deliver treatment in a reproducible fashion, and a low risk of serious complications. Although many prognostic factors have been identified, the response to RT cannot be predicted accurately for an individual patient. The benefit of bladder conservation is limited when bladder function has been irretrievably compromised, when technical problems preclude completion of therapy, or in patients at high risk of intolerable acute or late complications. Radiation therapy will not improve incontinence, nor will it increase the capacity of a bladder damaged by previous interventions. Patients with severe irritable bladder symptoms frequently have intolerable distress during RT and are better served by a cystectomy. Definitive radiation therapy should also be questioned in patients with large bladder diverticula or atonic bladders, in whom reproducible dose delivery may not be possible from day to day during a fractionated course of treatment. These patients may be more likely to suffer local failure or treatment-related complications.

The adverse prognostic factors for complete response to external beam RT include a large tumor volume, as in patients with T3b or multifocal disease, or the presence of ureteric obstruction *(13–16)*. The presence of associated extensive carcinoma *in situ* predicts for the future development of superficial or, if untreated, muscle invasive bladder can-

cer, and possibly a future requirement for salvage cystectomy *(14)*. Therefore, the best candidates for bladder conservation with RT-based protocols are patients with small single T2a–T2b tumors and good bladder
function, who are highly motivated in this regard and accepting of a
prolonged treatment course.

What is the Best Prescription
for Bladder Conservation Using Radiation Therapy?

The traditional approach to bladder conservation revolved around the
use of radical RT alone at a dose that was within the tolerance of the
bladder and surrounding small bowel and rectum. The reported complete response rates following the traditional prescriptions of 50–66 Gy
in 1.8–2.5 Gy daily fractions over 4–6.5 wk ranged between 35% and
60% *(13–15,17–23)*. Altered fractionation schemes and concurrent or
neoadjuvant chemotherapy have been used with the aim of improving
the complete response rate *(24–32)*.

Historically, doses of 52–55 Gy in 2.5–2.75 Gy fractions over 4–
4.5 wk resulted in unacceptable late complication rates *(13,14)*. The use
of lower dose per fraction (1.8–2.0 Gy) and protocols limiting the total
dose to 60–66 Gy in 6–7 wk have more recently resulted in less severe
late intestinal complications, such as bowel obstruction or perforation.
The practice of two-phase treatment with volume reduction at 40–45 Gy
to include the primary tumor alone was pioneered by Shipley *(33)*, and
has resulted in reduced bladder toxicity. The complication of hemorrhagic cystitis with bladder contracture is rarely encountered with modern radiation treatment approaches. The local control rates following
two-phase treatment appear to be equivalent, but different treatment
techniques have not been tested in a prospective randomised trial. Currently, conformal treatment techniques are being tested in bladder cancer to further improve treatment reproducibility and reduce morbidity.

Concurrent cisplatin chemotherapy has been used with RT in an attempt
to improve the therapeutic ratio. A large number of phase II studies of
concurrent cisplatin and RT have shown high complete response rates
with bladder preservation in over 60% of patients. The National Cancer
Institute of Canada phase III randomised trial of concurrent cisplatin and
RT showed improved pelvic recurrence-free survival for the cisplatin
arm (67% vs 47%, $p = 0.038$), but no improvement in overall survival
(34). The optimal dose schedule and method of administration of concurrent cisplatin has not been determined. Eapen investigated the use of
intraarterial cisplatin with concurrent radiation therapy in bladder cancer,
and reported excellent results with an 89% complete response rate and an
80% cause-specific survival *(35,36)*. The strategy of using concurrent

cisplatin or other sensitizing drugs with radiation therapy is promising and requires further study.

A significant proportion of treatment failures in patients with bladder cancer arise from the growth of systemic metastases, which seeded prior to local therapy. This suggests that neoadjuvant chemotherapy given before local treatment may improve outcome. A phase II RTOG study of neoadjuvant CMV chemotherapy followed by RT and concurrent cisplatin showed a 62% 4-yr actuarial survival *(37)*. However, the optimism that neoadjuvant chemotherapy would improve survival in patients with bladder cancer has recently been dashed by the results of the MRC/EORTC trial, where three courses of neoadjuvant CMV had no effect on outcome *(38)*. The 2-yr survival was 62% in the chemotherapy arm, and 60% in the no chemotherapy arm.

Both experimental and clinical data suggest that the use of smaller radiation dose per fraction, in the range of 1.0–1.5 Gy, allows an increased total dose of radiation to be delivered without increasing the risk of late complications. This use of an increased number of small radiation fractions delivered in the same overall time is called "hyperfractionated radiotherapy." Naslund et al. randomised 168 patients with T2–T4 bladder tumors to receive 84 Gy in 84 fractions given 3 times a day, or 64 Gy in 32 fractions given once daily. Both groups were treated over a period of 8 wk with a 2-wk rest interval. There were significant improvements in local control and survival in the hyperfractionated treatment group, that were maintained with 10 yr of follow-up *(39)*. This trial has been criticised for using split-course treatment, which has been abandoned in modern radiotherapy practice because of the potential for tumor regrowth during the rest interval. There is presently no convincing data to support the routine use of hyperfractionated RT, although further study is warranted.

There is abundant evidence that tumor proliferation during a course of RT may lead to lower local control rates. To counteract this, twice daily treatments have been used to deliver the same total dose of radiation over a shorter time. Compression of the overall treatment time in this way without a change in the total radiation dose or the fractional dose is called "accelerated radiotherapy." Several studies have suggested improved local control with accelerated RT *(40–42)*. Horwich et al. recently reported the results of a phase III trial in which 229 patients with locally advanced bladder cancer were randomised to an accelerated RT protocol of 60.8 Gy in 32 fractions over 26 d (1 wk rest interval after 12 fractions), or standard RT with 64 Gy in 32 fractions over 6.5 wk *(41)*. The local control, time to metastasis and overall survival were similar in both arms, but the bowel toxicity was significantly higher in the accelerated fractionation arm.

Tumor hypoxia has been associated with reduced local control following RT, and with an increased risk of distant metastases in a number of human malignancies. There is, as of yet, no direct evidence that clinically significant hypoxia is present in bladder cancer. However, indirect evidence for an important biological effect of hypoxia comes from a meta-analysis of randomised trials of hypoxic radiation sensitizers, which showed significant improvements in both local control and overall survival in patients with bladder cancer *(43)*. Hoskins et al. recently reported a phase II study of carbogen with or without nicotinamide in 61 patients with locally advanced bladder cancer treated with 50–55 Gy in 20 fractions over 4 wk *(44)*. When the results were compared to an earlier cohort of patients treated with RT and either misonidazole or hyperbaric oxygen, major improvements in local control ($p = 0.00001$), progression free survival ($p = 0.001$) and overall survival were observed. However, these results might be explained by changes in RT techniques over the period of the studies, and by patient selection. Further evaluation of this approach in a phase III trial is necessary before any recommendations can be made for routine clinical practice.

The optimal prescription for radical RT in bladder cancer has not been defined. The current standard is to treat the whole bladder to a dose of 40–45 Gy followed by a boost to the primary tumor, giving a further dose of 20–25 Gy. Concurrent cisplatin used in most centres, but other combinations are being investigated.

When Should Preoperative RT be Used in Locally Advanced Bladder Cancer?

The goal of preoperative radiation therapy is to eradicate microscopic extravesical disease and to prevent pelvic recurrence following radical cystectomy. Therefore, only patients who are at high risk of local recurrence in the pelvis can potentially benefit from preoperative RT. Patients with bladder cancer without extravesical extension are at very low risk of pelvic recurrence following cystectomy (<10%), and are not good candidates for preoperative RT. Patients with extensive extravesical disease are at high risk of pelvic recurrence (>30%), but are also at risk of distant failure. In these patients, distant failure will reduce the impact of preoperative RT on overall survival, but the improvement in local control may nevertheless be substantial. Since pelvic recurrence has a considerable adverse effect on quality of life, improvement in local control is a worthwhile goal of treatment.

The Southwest Oncology Group (SWOG) conducted a phase III randomised trial of preoperative RT followed by cystectomy versus cystectomy alone and found no difference in survival *(12)*. Unfortunately, only low dose preoperative RT (20 Gy in 5 fractions over 1 wk) was used, and a large proportion of the patients in the study had T2 disease and were at low risk of pelvic recurrence even without RT. A positive study of preoperative RT was reported by El-Wahidi et al. in which patients with schistosomal bladder cancer were randomised to receive preoperative RT with 44 Gy followed by cystectomy or cystectomy alone *(45)*. Treatment failure was significantly higher in patients treated with surgery alone (29%) compared to those who also received preoperative RT. This study has been published in abstract form only and no details are available on local control or survival. Huncharek et al. reported a meta-analysis of five randomised trials of preoperative RT and cystectomy versus cystectomy alone *(10)*. There was no effect of preoperative RT on survival (odds ratio of 0.71, 95% confidence interval 0.48–1.06), and the impact on local control was not addressed.

There is little modern data dealing with the toxicity of preoperative RT and cystectomy, but the previously conducted randomised trials suggest that this treatment can be delivered safely. Data from several authors, but in particular from Bochner and Mannel, indicate that the use of preoperative RT does not preclude continent urinary diversion *(46,47)*.

There is no rationale for recommending preoperative RT to patients with small T2 tumors. The current approach to the management of patients with more advanced T3 disease that is recognised before surgery most often consists of radical cystectomy and pelvic lymph node dissection followed by adjuvant chemotherapy. Phase II studies have suggested improved survival with this approach. The patterns of failure have not been described in detail, but there may be a reduction in both local and distant recurrence. The role of preoperative RT in this setting of alternate effective treatment remains ill-defined. However, it would be reasonable to recommend preoperative RT to patients with clinical T3 tumors, who are not candidates for adjuvant chemotherapy with the primary aim of reducing pelvic recurrence, if not also improving survival.

What is the Role
of Postoperative RT after Radical Cystectomy?

Postoperative pelvic radiotherapy is used in the management of many pelvic tumors, including prostate, cervix and endometrial cancer. It is most often administered to patients at high risk of pelvic recurrence with the aim of reducing this risk. It has the advantage over preoperative pelvic radiotherapy of allowing treatment to be optimised in individual patients on the basis of surgico-pathologic prognostic factors, and administered only to those who are most likely to benefit. The major disadvantage is the potential for increased toxicity from irradiation of postsurgical tissues.

The rational use of pelvic radiotherapy following radical cystectomy is predicated on knowledge of surgico-pathologic prognostic factors that allow reliable identification of patients who are at high risk of pelvic recurrence. Detailed surgico-pathologic staging studies have not been performed in bladder cancer as for other tumors. However, there are several reports of high pelvic recurrence rates between 30% and 50% in patients with pT3 or pT4 tumors, positive resection margins or involved pelvic lymph nodes. Postoperative pelvic radiotherapy at doses in the range of 40–50 Gy appears to reduce pelvic recurrence in these high risk patients to between 10% and 20% *(11,48,49)*, although the results are difficult to interpret because patients also frequently received preoperative pelvic radiation usually consisting of a single 5 Gy fraction shortly before cystectomy *(11,48)*. The only randomised study of radical cystectomy alone versus cystectomy and postoperative radiation in high risk bladder cancer was reported by Zaghloul et al. *(49)*, and accrued patients with schistosomiasis. The 5-yr pelvic recurrence rate was 50% in the cystectomy arm, but only 7% with the addition of conventionally fractionated radiotherapy. Radiotherapy also appeared to confer a reduction in the risk of metastases in this series, and an improvement in disease-free survival. Notwithstanding these results, which may not necessarily be translatable to patients without schistosomiasis, the factors that predict pelvic recurrence also predict strongly for lymph node and distant recurrence as previously discussed. Therefore, the benefit of pelvic radiation on overall survival is likely to be small.

Postoperative pelvic radiotherapy might be valuable as a means of reducing potentially morbid pelvic recurrences in patients with high risk bladder cancer despite only a small effect on survival, if it were not for the unacceptably high rate of serious late gastrointestinal complications. Several investigators have reported this to be in the range of 20–40%, which is substantially higher than following radical surgery and radiotherapy for other pelvic tumors *(11,48–51)*. Many factors probably contribute to this, but the most important may be the larger volume of small bowel occupying the pelvis following cystectomy. An intact bladder normally displaces small bowel from the pelvis and allows pelvic irradiation at doses necessary for the control of microscopic disease to be administered safely. Surgical techniques that prevent small bowel from

Table 2
Palliative Radiation Therapy in Bladder Cancer

Palliation of local disease
- Hematuria   • Pelvic pain
- Dysuria   • Frequency
- Urgency

Palliation of metastatic disease
- Bone pain   • Spinal cord compression
- Nodal metastasis   • Brain metastases
- Nerve entrapment   • Hemoptysis

filling the void left by the bladder postoperatively may reduce the risk of late complications, as may the use of hyperfractionated radiation *(49)*. However, further study of these approaches, especially the use of altered fractionation schemes, is necessary to define their role in routine clinical practice. Conformal radiation may allow treatment to be administered postoperatively to focal regions within the pelvis, but is unlikely to be helpful in the adjuvant setting where large volumes need to be irradiated. Overall, patients who are at high risk of recurrence following cystectomy are probably better treated with cisplatin-based chemotherapy, which impacts on both local and distant relapse and is usually well tolerated in otherwise healthy patients.

When Should Palliative RT be Considered in the Management of Locally Advanced Bladder Cancer?

It is important to place palliative radiation therapy in the context of total palliative patient care. The Canadian Palliative Care Standards Task Force defined palliative care as "… the combination of active and compassionate therapies intended to comfort and support the patient and family who are living with a life-threatening illness…" *(52)*. Unlike radical treatment, where the objective is tumor control, the goal of palliative therapy is symptom relief and preservation of quality of life. In order to assess the success of palliative intervention, one should evaluate quality of life and symptom relief rather than response of tumor or duration of survival. In bladder cancer, palliative radiation may be used to relieve symptoms caused by local disease, or metastases (Table 2).

The commonly used fractionation schemes for palliative RT include 30 Gy in 10 daily fractions, 35 Gy in 10 fractions, and 20 Gy in 5 fractions. Retrospective studies of palliative radiotherapy administered for local bladder symptoms have documented significant improvement in hematuria, but no improvement in urinary frequency, urgency or nocturia *(53)*. The MRC UK has recently completed a prospective rando-mised trial of two dose prescriptions for palliative RT in bladder cancer, comparing 35 Gy in 10 fractions over 2 wk to 21 Gy in 3 fractions given every second day over 5 d. The endpoints of this trial included duration of symptom relief and toxicity. There was no difference between the two arms, and symptom improvement was observed in 50% of patients *(54)*.

Salminen et al. reported the Australian experience with palliative bladder RT in 94 patients treated with 30 Gy in 6 fractions given twice per wk over 3 wk *(55)*. This treatment provided pain relief and reduced hematuria in over 60% of patients, and reduced urgency in 50%. The authors did not provide data as to the volume treated, but this protocol was associated with considerable toxicity. Sixty-two percent of patients experienced diarrhoea, and 29% reported late toxicity with proctitis, cys-titis, or small bowel injury. Holmang et al. reported the results of pallia-tive RT in 96 patients with locally advanced bladder cancer treated to a dose of 21 Gy in 3 fractions on alternate days *(56)*. Improvement in hema-turia was observed in the majority of patients, but no improvement was noted in urgency, dysuria, or frequency. There were five treatment related deaths, and severe GI toxicity occurred in 26% of patients. Wijkstrom et al. reported the results of palliative RT in 162 patients with locally ad-vanced, incurable bladder cancer unfit for radical therapy who received 21 Gy in 3 fractions over 5 d. Improvement in symptoms was observed in 46% of patients. However, 40% of patients developed significant acute complications, and two patients required colostomy because of late gastrointestinal complications *(57)*.

These results point out several issues that need to be considered in prescribing palliative RT for patients with bladder cancer. The goals of treatment should be clear. In the above series, short palliative fraction-ation schemes were used to relieve symptoms in lieu of conventional frac-tionation. Although, treatment duration was shorter, toxicity was high and counter to the goal of palliation. Therefore, if local tumor control is the desired objective (not just palliation of symptoms), a higher more conven-tional dose with smaller daily fractions should be prescribed. If pallia-tion is the goal, RT appears beneficial to temporarily alleviate hematuria and pain. However, these symptoms will probably recur given sufficient time, as local tumor control is not likely to be achieved. Short-course treatment is therefore most appropriate for patients with pelvic pain or hematuria from bladder cancer, who also have rapidly worsening perfor-mance status, metastases or a limited survival for other reasons. Severe urinary symptoms are rarely adequately controlled with RT, and urinary diversion may be more appropriate in such cases.

SUMMARY

Treatment of muscle invasive bladder cancer with definitive radiotherapy can lead to durable local control and maintain a functional bladder without compromising survival. Patient selection is key. The best candidates for bladder preservation with RT are patients with small vol-ume disease and good bladder function, who are highly motivated. Various strategies to improve local control in patients treated with RT are being investigated and the results of concurrent cisplatin and RT are encouraging. Preoperative RT prior to cystectomy may be useful in patients with locally advanced disease who are at high risk of pelvic failure. Postoperative RT is not currently used because of the high rate of serious late gastrointestinal complications. Palliative radiotherapy to relieve symptoms of local disease or metastasis can be effective, but the toxicity of treatment can be substantial and careful attention to the details of dose-fractionation, treatment volume and technique is essential.

REFERENCES

1. Scher H, Shipley W, Herr W. Cancer of the Bladder. In: *Cancer, Principle and Practice* (De Vita JV, Hellman S, Rosenberg S, eds.). 5th ed. Lippincott-Raven, Philadelphia, PA, 1997, pp. 1300–1322.
2. Gospodarowicz MK, Quilty PM, Scalliet P, Tsujii H, Fossa SD, Horenblas S, et al. The place of radiation therapy as definitive treatment of bladder cancer. Int J Urol 1995; 2(41): 41–48.
3. Palou J, Sanchez-Martin FM, Rosales A, Salvador J, Algaba F, Vicente J. Intravesical bacille Calmette-Guerin in the treatment of carcinoma in situ or high-grade superficial bladder carcinoma after radiotherapy for bladder carcinoma. Br J Urol Int 1999; 83(4): 429–431.
4. Pisters LL, Tykochinsky G, Wajsman Z. Intravesical bacillus Calmette-Guerin or mitomycin C in the treatment of carcinoma in situ of the bladder following prior pelvic radiation therapy. J Urol 1991; 146(6): 1514–1517.
5. Zietman AL, Shipley WU, Heney NM, Althausen AF. The case for radiotherapy with or without chemotherapy in high-risk superficial and muscle-invading bladder cancer. Semin Urol Oncol 1997; 15(3): 161–168.
6. Shipley WU, Zietman AL, Kaufman DS, Althausen AF, Heney NM. Invasive bladder cancer: treatment strategies using transurethral surgery, chemotherapy and radiation therapy with selection for bladder conservation. Int J Radiat Oncol Biol Phys 1997; 39(4): 937–943.
7. Gospodarowicz MK, Rider WD, Keen CW, Connolly JG, Jewett MAS, Cummings BJ, et al. Bladder cancer: long term follow-up results of patients treated with radical radiation. Clin Oncol 1991; 3: 155–161.
8. Bloom HJ, Hendry WF, Wallace DM, Skeet RG. Treatment of T3 bladder cancer: controlled trial of pre-operative radiotherapy and radical cystectomy versus radical radiotherapy. Br J Urol 1982; 54(2): 136–151.
9. Anderstrom C, Johansson S, Nilsson S, et al. A prospective randomised study of preoperative irradiation with cystectomy or cystectomy alone for invasive bladder carcinoma. Eur Urol 1931983; 9: 142–147.

10. Huncharek M, Muscat J, Geschwind JF. Planned preoperative radiation therapy in muscle invasive bladder cancer; results of a meta-analysis. Anticancer Res 1998; 18(3B): 1931–1934.

11. Spera JA, Whittington R, Littman P, Solin LJ, Wein AJ. A comparison of preoperative radiotherapy regimens for bladder carcinoma: The University of Pennsylvania experience. Cancer 1988; 61: 255–262.

12. Smith J, Crawford E, Paradelo J, Blumenstein B, Herschman B, Grossman B, et al. Treatment of advanced bladder cancer with combined preoperative irradiation and radical cystectomy versus radical cystectomy alone: a Phase III Intergroup study. J Urol 1997; 157: 805–808.

13. Duncan W, Quilty PM. The results of a series of 963 patients with transitional cell carcinoma of the urinary bladder primarily treated by radical megavoltage x-ray therapy. Radiother Oncol 1986; 7: 299–310.

14. Gospodarowicz MK, Hawkins NV, Rawlings GA, Connolly JG, Jewett MAS, Thomas GM, et al. Radical radiotherapy for the muscle invasive transitional cell carcinoma of the bladder: Failure analysis. J Urol 1989; 142: 1448–1454.

15. Greven KM, Solin LJ, Hanks GE. Prognostic factors in patients with bladder carcinoma treated with definitive irradiation. Cancer 1990; 65: 908–912.

16. Fung CY, Shipley WU, Young RH, Griffin PP, Convery KM, Kaufman DS, et al. Prognostic factors in invasive bladder carcinoma in a prospective trial of preoperative adjuvant chemotherapy and radiotherapy [see comments]. J Clin Oncol 1991; 9(9): 1533–1542.

17. Davidson SE, Symonds RP, Snee MP, Upadhyay S, Habeshaw T, Robertson AG. Assessment of factors influencing the outcome of radiotherapy for bladder cancer. Br J Urol 1990; 66(3): 288–293.

18. Blandy JP, Jenkins BJ, Fowler CG, Caulfield M, Badenoch DF, England HR, et al. Radical radiotherapy and salvage cystectomy for T2/3 cancer of the bladder. Prog Clin Biol Res 1988; 260: 447–451.

19. Jenkins BJ, Caulfield MJ, Fowler CG, Badenoch DF, Tiptaft RC, Paris AMI, et al. Reappraisal of the role of radical radiotherapy and salvage cystectomy in the treatment of invasive (T2/T3) bladder cancer. Br J Urol 1988; 62: 342–346.

20. Jacobsen AB, Lunde S, Ous S, et al. T2/T3 bladder carcinomas treated with definitive radiotherapy with emphasis on flow cytometric DNA ploidy values. Int J Radiat Oncol Biol Phys 1989; 17: 923–929.

21. Fossa SD, Ous S, Knudsen OS. Radical irradiation of T2 and T3 bladder carcinoma. Acta Radiol Oncol 1985; 24(6): 497–501.

22. Smaaland R, Akslen L, Tonder B, Mehus A, Lote K, Albrektsen G. Radical radiation treatment of invasive and locally advanced bladder cancer in elderly patients. Br J Urol 1991; 67: 61–69.

23. Vale JA, A'Hern RP, Liu K, Hendry WF, Whitfield HN, Plowman PN, et al. Predicting the outcome of radical radiotherapy for invasive bladder cancer. Eur Urol 1993; 24(1): 48–51.

24. Farah R, Chodak GW, Vogelzang NJ, Awan AM, Quiet CA, Moormeier J, et al. Curative radiotherapy following chemotherapy for invasive bladder carcinoma (a preliminary report). Int J Radiat Oncol Biol Phys 1991; 20(3): 413–417.

25. Hall R. Neo-adjuvant CMV chemotherapy and cystectomy or radiotherapy in muscle invasive bladder cancer. First analysis of MRC/EORTC intercontinental trial. Proc Am Soc Clin Oncol 1996; 15: 244; #612.

26. Housset M, Maulard C, Chretien Y, Dufour B, Delanian S, Huart J, et al. Combined radiation and chemotherapy for invasive transitional-cell carcinoma of the bladder: a prospective study. J Clin Urol 1993; 11(11): 2150–2157.

27. Jakse G, Frommhold H. Radiotherapy and chemotherapy in locally advanced bladder cancer. Eur Urol 1985; 14(Suppl 1): 45.

28. Raghavan D, Wallace M. Preemptive (neoadjuvant) chemotherapy: can analysis of eligibility criteria, prognostic factors, and tumor staging from different trials provide valid or useful comparisons? Semin Oncol 1990; 17(5): 613–618.

29. Russell KJ, Boileau MA, Higano C, Collins C, Russell AH, Koh W, et al. Combined 5-fluorouracil and irradiation for transitional cell carcinoma of the urinary bladder [see comments]. Int J Radiat Oncol Biol Phys 1990; 19(3): 693–699.

30. Sauer R, Birkenhake S, Kuhn R, Wittekind C, Schrott KM, Martus P. Efficacy of radiochemotherapy with platin derivatives compared to radiotherapy alone in organ-sparing treatment of bladder cancer. Int J Radiat Oncol Biol Phys 1998; 40(1): 121–127.

31. Shipley WU, Kaufman DS, Heney NM, Althausen AF, Zietman AL. An update of combined modality therapy for patients with muscle invading bladder cancer using selective bladder preservation or cystectomy. J Urol 1999; 162(2): 445–450; discussion 450–451.

32. Vogelzang NJ, Moormeier JA, Awan AM, Weichselbaum RR, Farah R, Straus FD, et al. Methotrexate, vinblastine, doxorubicin and cisplatin followed by radiotherapy or surgery for muscle invasive bladder cancer: the University of Chicago experience. J Urol 1993; 149(4): 753–757.

33. Shipley WU, Van der Schueren E, Kitigawa T, Gospodarowicz MK, Fromhold H, Magno L, et al. (eds). Guidelines for radiation therapy in clinical research on bladder cancer. Alan R. Liss, 1986.

34. Coppin C, Gospodarowicz M, James K, Tannock I, Zee B, Carson J, et al. The NCI-Canada trial of concurrent cisplatin and radiotherapy for muscle invasive bladder cancer. J Clin Oncol 1996; 14: 2901–2907.

35. Eapen L, Stewart D, Crook J, Aitken S, Danjoux C, Rasuli P, et al. Intraarterial cisplatin and concurrent pelvic radiation in the management of muscle invasive bladder cancer. Int J Radiat Oncol Biol Phys 1992; 24(Suppl 1): 211.

36. Eapen LDS, Danjoux C, Genest P, Futter N, Moors D, et al. Intraarterial cisplatin and concurrent radiation for locally advanced bladder cancer. J Clin Oncol 1989; 7(2): 230–235.

37. Tester W, Caplan R, Heaney J, Venner P, Whittington R, Byhardt R, et al. Neoadjuvant combined modality program with selective organ preservation for invasive bladder cancer: results of Radiation Therapy Oncology Group phase II trial 8802. J Clin Oncol 1996; 14(1): 119–126.

38. Ghersi D, Stewart LA, Palmar MKB, et al. Neoadjuvant cisplatin, methotrexate, and vinblastine chemotherapy for muscle-invasive bladder cancer: a randomised controlled trial. International collaboration of trialists. Lancet 1999; 354(9178): 533–540.

39. Naslund I, Nilsson B, Littbrand B. Hyperfractionated radiotherapy of bladder cancer. A ten-year follow-up of a randomised clinical trial. Acta Oncol 1994; 33(4): 397–402.

40. Cole DJ, Durrant KR, Roberts JT, Dawes PJ, Yosef H, Hopewell JW. A pilot study of accelerated fractionation in the radiotherapy of invasive carcinoma of the bladder. Br J Radiol 1992; 65(777): 792–798.

41. Horwich A, Dearnaley D, Huddart R, Graham J, Bessel E, Mason M, et al. A trial of accelerated fractionation in T2/3 bladder cancer. Eur J Cancer 1999; 35(Suppl 4): 5342.

42. Moonen L, van der Voet H, Horenblas S, Bartelink H. A feasibility study of accelerated fractionation in radiotherapy of carcinoma of the urinary bladder. Int J Radiat Oncol Biol Phys 1997; 37(3): 537–542.

43. Overgaard J. Clinical evaluation of nitroimidazoles as modifiers of hypoxia in solid tumors. Oncol Res 1994; 6(10/11): 509–518.

44. Hoskin PJ, Saunders MI, Phillips H, Cladd H, Powell ME, Goodchild K, et al. Carbogen and nicotinamide in the treatment of bladder cancer with radical radiotherapy. Br J Cancer 1997; 76(2): 260–263.

45. El-Wahidi G, Ghoneim MA, Saker H, Fouda MA. Preoperative radiotherapy of schistosomal bladder cancer. Proceedings from ECCO-10 Conference, Vienna, 1999.

46. Bochner BH, Figueroa AJ, Skinner EC, Lieskovsky G, Petrovich Z, Boyd SD, et al. Salvage radical cystoprostatectomy and orthotopic urinary diversion following radiation failure. J Urol 1998; 160(1): 29–33.

47. Mannel RS, Manetta A, Buller RE, Braly PS, Walker JL, Archer JS. Use of ileocecal continent urinary reservoir in patients with previous pelvic irradiation. Gynecol Oncol 1995; 59(3): 376–378.

48. Reisinger SA, Mohiuddin M, Mulholland SG. Combined pre- and postoperative adjuvant radiation therapy for bladder cancer—a ten year experience [see comments]. Int J Radiat Oncol Biol Phys 1992; 24(3): 463–468.

49. Zaghloul MS, Awwad HK, Akoush HH, Omar S, Soliman O, et al. Postoperative radiotherapy of carcinoma in bilharzial bladder: improved disease free survival through improving local control. Int J Radiat Oncol Biol Phys 1992; 23(3): 511–517.

50. Skinner DG, Tift JP, Kaufman JJ. High dose, short course preoperative radiation therapy and immediate single stage radical cystectomy with pelvic node dissection in the management of bladder cancer. J Urol 1982; 127(4): 671–674.

51. Kopelson G, Heaney JA. Postoperative radiation therapy for muscle-invading bladder carcinoma. J Surg Oncol 1983; 23(4): 263–268.

52. Mackillop WJ. The principles of palliative radiotherapy: a radiation oncologist's perspective. Can J Oncol 1996; 6(Suppl 1): 5–11.

53. Fossa SD, Hosbach G. Short-term moderate-dose pelvic radiotherapy of advanced bladder carcinoma. A questionnaire-based evaluation of its symptomatic effect. Acta Oncol 1991; 30(6): 735–738.

54. Duchesne G, Bolger J, Griffiths G, Uscinska B. Preliminary Results of an MRC (UK) Trial of Palliative Radiotherapy in Advanced Bladder Cancer (BA09). In: Royal Australasian Annual Scientific Meeting, 1998; Brisbane, 1998.

55. Salminen E. Unconventional fractionation for palliative radiotherapy of urinary bladder cancer. A retrospective review of 94 patients. Acta Oncol 1992; 31(4): 449–454.

56. Holmang S, Borghede G. Early complications and survival following short-term palliative radiotherapy in invasive bladder carcinoma. J Urol 1996; 155(1): 100–102.

57. Wijkstrom H, Naslund I, Ekman P, Kohler C, Nilsson B, Norming U. Short-term radiotherapy as palliative treatment in patients with transitional cell bladder cancer. Br J Urol 1991; 67(1): 74–78.

58. Moonen L, Voet HVD, de Nijs R, Hart AAM, Horenblas S, Bartelink H. Muscle-invasive bladder cancer treated with external beam radiotherapy: pretreatment prognostic factors and the predictive value of cystoscopic re-evaluation during treatment. Radiot Oncol 1998: 49(2) 145–155.

13 Current Concepts of Urinary Diversion in Men

Courtney M. P. Hollowell, MD,
Gary D. Steinberg, MD,
and Randall G. Rowland, MD, PHD

INTRODUCTION

Prior to the introduction of the ileal conduit more than four decades ago, the options for urinary diversion after cystectomy were extremely limited. Cutaneous pyelostomies and ureterostomies were common forms of urinary diversion. Direct cutaneous anastomoses of the collecting system offered patients a short-term diversion, but the benefits were soon outweighed by significant complications. The relatively poor intrinsic ureteral blood supply frequently lead to distal ureteral slough, recession of the stoma, or stricture formation. Even with the introduction of v-flap techniques designed to widen the stoma, the incidence of stoma stenosis was considerable *(1)*. When diversion of longer duration was required,

From: *Current Clinical Urology: Bladder Cancer: Current Diagnosis and Treatment*
Edited by: M. J. Droller © Humana Press Inc., Totowa, NJ

ureterosigmoidostomy was the popular choice. This allowed for the anal sphincteric mechanism to achieve urinary and maintain fecal continence and was technically simple to perform. Interestingly, the first ureterosigmoidostomy was reported by John Simon in 1852 (2) for the treatment of bladder exstrophy, making ureterosigmoidostomy the first continent urinary diversion. Using a transfixion suture between the ureter and rectum, he noted urine coming from the rectum on the tenth postoperative day. The patient subsequently died within a year.

Since this first attempt, several different modifications were performed with varying degrees of success. For example, Mathesin recognized that, in birds, the ureter opened into the cloaca as a small nipple that was occluded by intraluminal intestinal pressure (3). Even with the addition of antireflux techniques, ureterosigmoidostomy has since fallen in popularity due to the complications associated with urothelium in direct contact with the fecal stream (4). Complications, including pyelonephritis, hyperchloremic metabolic acidosis and an increased risk of adenocarcinoma at the uretero-colic anastomotic junction, have since negated the benefits gained with this procedure. As a result of uniformly poor long-term results, other methods of urinary diversion, such as rectal pouches were developed. Many subsequent contributors have developed literally hundreds of procedures with minor variations since that time.

In 1911, Schoemaker (5) was the first to describe a noncontinent uretero-ileo-cutaneous diversion. The ileal conduit was then popularized in the 1950s by Bricker and associates (6). This technique, which represented a novel approach to urinary diversion, provided a simple but reliable option for supravesical urinary diversion. Interestingly, Gilchrist and Merricks described a continent cutaneous ileocecal reservoir in the same year Bricker published the technique for the ileal conduit (7). The continent cutaneous urinary reservoir was not widely adopted principally because clean intermittent catheterization had not yet been popularized for the management of hypotonic bladders let alone continent urinary reservoirs. The Koch pouch, described in 1975 by Niels Koch and then popularized by Skinner, was the beginning of the continent cutaneous reservoir movement. Significant complication and reoperation rates prompted many modifications in the surgical technique and in the development of several alternatives based on ileocolic and colonic bowel segments.

Despite many early descriptions of continent orthotopic neobladders, this procedure was not widely employed until the late 1980s and the early 1990s. The importance of detubularization of gastrointestinal segments used in urinary reconstruction was not fully appreciated until the

1970s despite early experiences by such authors as Tasker *(8)*, Giertz and Frankson *(9)*, and Goodwin *(10)*. With a better understanding of the effects of detubularization of the bowel, creating a large capacity, high compliance pouch with significantly lower pressures, several orthotopic neobladders have emerged based on ileal, ileocecal or colonic bowel segments.

Presently, patients can be offered a non-continent cutaneous diversion, a continent cutaneous diversion, or an orthotopic neobladder urinary reconstruction. The choice of diversion for each patient is dependent on multiple factors such as tumor stage and location, patient age and comorbidity, renal, hepatic and bowel function, the patients' desires and motivation along with the experience and attitudes of the surgeon. This chapter reviews the results and complications of selected, but representative, techniques for noncontinent cutaneous diversion, continent cutaneous diversion, and orthotopic neobladder reconstruction. In addition, the experience and preferences of the authors are summarized.

INDICATIONS FOR URINARY DIVERSION

Neoplasm

Presently, carcinoma of the bladder is the most common indication for urinary diversion. Less frequently other pelvic malignancies, including carcinoma of the cervix, rectum or prostate may necessitate cystectomy and urinary diversion.

Neurogenic Bladder

Urinary diversion is indicated in those patients who fail conservative management with intermittent catheterization and anticholinergic medications, fail bladder augmentation, and demonstrate deterioration of the upper tracts.

Pretransplantation

Previously, many patients with lower urinary tract anomalies were considered poor candidates for renal transplantation. Small and large bowel segments are now commonly used for urinary diversion of renal allografts when the bladder has been removed or is unsuitable for urinary storage.

Pediatric

The concepts for treating urinary tract abnormalities in children and adolescents have profoundly changed with time. This is true both regarding the type of surgical technique employed for urinary diversion, and our understanding of pediatric pathology and urinary tract dysfunction which has altered the indications leading to urinary diversion. Attempts are now made to preserve bladder function with or without bladder augmentation. The indications for bladder substitution in children include bladder exstrophy, especially if primary bladder closure has failed or continence could not be achieved, neurogenic bladder which has failed conservative management, and malignant tumors such as rhabdomyosarcoma.

Other

Indications including dysfunctional bladders that result in significant persistent bleeding after failed conservative management for a variety of conditions, severe interstitial cystitis that has failed all other treatment modalities, and obstructive uropathy as a consequence of previous radiation or surgery that may necessitate cystectomy and urinary diversion.

NONCONTINENT CUTANEOUS DIVERSIONS

Ileal/Colon Conduit

The Ileal conduit, as described by Bricker (6) has been the mainstay of urinary diversion over the past 45 years. To date, diversions requiring external urinary collecting appliances are the most common. Indeed, it has become a part of every urologic surgeon's armamentarium and, in the authors' opinion, remains the "gold standard" against which all other urinary diversions should be compared. Urinary diversion by ileal conduit consists of diverting urine to a short intestinal segment (15–20 cm in length) brought out through the anterior abdominal wall (Fig. 1).

Fundamentally, there are two types of conduits, one which includes ileum or jejunum and the other in which colon is used. Because of severe electrolyte abnormalities associated with jejunal urinary reconstruction, it is usually not employed, although in cases of regional enteritis, the jejunum may be selected if uninvolved (Table 1). In general, however, jejunum is rarely the only segment available.

The ileum and colon are the two segments most often employed. Ileal resection can result in malabsorption of bile salts and vitamin B_{12}. Resection of greater than 50 cm of terminal ileum, the primary intestinal site for bile salt and vitamin B_{12} absorption, may promote such malabsorption. In addition, unabsorbed bile salts pass into the colon and produce osmotic diarrhea with or without accompanying steatorrhea.

In patients who have undergone extensive pelvic irradiation a portion of transverse colon can be used with confidence. Both ileal and colon conduits result in a similar electrolyte abnormality (Table 1). A nonrefluxing ureterointestinal anastomosis can be performed by reimplanting the ureters into the tenia of colon, a feature which some have suggested

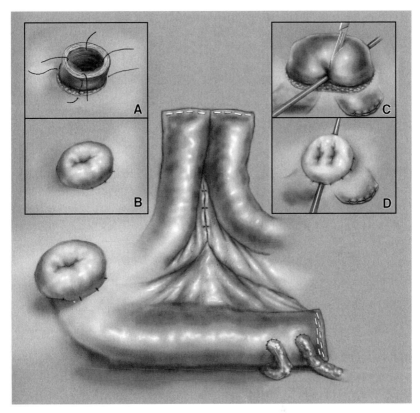

Fig. 1. Operative technique of ileal/colon conduit. A short intestinal segment (15–20 cm in length) is brought out through the anterior abdominal wall. (**A**) and (**B**) Creation of an end "rosebud" stoma. (**C**) and (**D**) Creation of a Turnbull loop stoma.

Table 1
Electrolyte Abnormalities of Urinary Intestinal Diversion

Intestinal segment	Electrolyte abnormality
Stomach	Hypochloremic metabolic alkalosis
Jejunum	Hyponatremic, hyperkalemic metabolic acidosis
Ileum/colon	Hyperchloremic metabolic acidosis

as advantageous in the maintenance of upper urinary tract integrity *(11, 12)*. Currently, there is considerable controversy as to whether a nonrefluxing or refluxing anastomosis is more desirable in any type of urinary tract reconstruction; nevertheless, the colon is more amenable to antireflux ureteral implantation techniques. In general, we have found both ileum and colon to be comparable and to provide a simple and safe means of supravesical urinary diversion.

Complications and Comments

The literature is replete with series reporting experience with non-continent cutaneous urinary diversion. Analysis of the complications in various series of ileal and colonic conduits in adults is summarized in Table 2. Stomal complications are the most frequent problem after cutaneous urinary diversion because of improper construction or placement, poorly fitting urinary appliances and childhood growth rates *(26–28)*. Specific technical points, therefore, must be rigidly adhered to in order to reduce stomal complications. In all elective cases, the stoma site should be selected preoperatively. Extreme care should be used in selecting a location free from abdominal creases in both the standing and sitting position. The location chosen should be away from the belt line, scars, and umbilicus. In general, the stoma should be brought through the belly of the rectus muscle in the right or left lower quadrant. Failure to adhere to these principles may increase the incidence of parastomal hernias *(29)*.

Fundamentally, there are two types of stomas: the end "rosebud" stoma and the loop end ileostomy (Fig. 1) based on a modified Turnbull stoma *(30)*. In the markedly obese patient, the end stoma is difficult to create due to a thick abdominal wall and a short crescent-shape ileal mesentery. Tethering of the distal conduit segment prevents an appropriately protruding stoma. In this circumstance, the loop end ileostomy is easier to perform, achieving a healthy nipple effect without tension. Analysis of the literature reveals that parastomal hernias occur less frequently with conventional end stomas (4–7%) *(21,31)* and are more likely to occur with loop stomas (11%–14%) *(24,32)* due to a larger fascial defect. In contrast, loop stomas have a lower incidence of stomal stenosis than do end stomas, with a reported incidence ranging from 0–5% for the former versus 5–18% for the latter *(15,21,33)*. Children are also particularly susceptible to stomal stenosis because of the disparity of the initial stoma with the ultimate size of intestine. In one large pediatric series, the reported incidence of stomal stenosis was 12.6%, requiring surgical revision in 7.3% of patients *(34)*. In general, enteric urinary conduits can develop segmental or complete stenosis at any time. When obstruction becomes clinically significant due to stomas stenosis, total conduit fibrosis, or the so-called pipe-stem conduit, revision of the conduit or replacement is usually warranted. Uncorrected stomal stenosis may lead to elongation of the conduit, stasis with a predisposition to stone formation, worsening metabolic complications, and upper tract deterioration.

The incidence of intestinal obstruction following supravesical urinary diversion differs depending on which segment of bowel has been used.

Table 2
Complications of Ileal and Colon Conduits (Expressed as Percent)

Author	No. of pts	Yrs of study	Operative mortality	Complication rate		Intestinal obstruction	Wound infection/ dehiscence	Acute pyelonephritis	Ureteral obstructions	Stomal stenosis	Renal calculi	Re-operation rate	
				Early	Late							Early	Late
Ileal Conduits													
Sullivan et al. (1980) (13)	336	1956–1971	14	43	52	0	20	19	15	5	4	–	–
Daughtry et al. (1977) (14)	55	1960–1970	9	22	4	2	18	–	2	–	–	–	–
Johnson and Lamy et al. (1977) (15)	214	1969–1975	3	28	41	10	25	15	18	5	3	–	–
Jaffe et al. (1968) (16)	543	1953–1966	7	–	–	11	11	2.8	–	–	–	–	26
Johnson et al. (1970) (17)	181	1956–1968	14	39	44	10	14	6	16	5	3	–	–
Pernet and Jonas (1985) (18)	132	1958–1981	8	32	32	13	8	20	5	5	8	15	17
Svare et al. (1985) (19)	110	1973–1980	5	28	57	15	19	–	10	5	4	23	22
Butcher and Bricker (1962) (20)	307	1950–1962	12	10	25	–	–	14	2	7	4	–	–
Schmidt (1973) (21)	178	1961–1969	6	50	51	5	9	22	8	18	11	–	–
Colon Conduits													
Schmidt et al. (1976) (22)	22	1970–1975	5	–	–	–	14	–	5	0	–		
Loening et al. (1982) (23)	62	1970–1979	5	25	13	2	6	–	11	0	0		
Morales and Golimbu (1975) (24)	46	1963–1973	15	13	38	7	–	17	20	13	4		
Althausen et al. (1978) (25)	70	1969–1976	0	–	–	6	3	7	6	3	4		

349

Most are temporary episodes of adynamic ileus, which may respond to bowel rest alone. In contrast, others fail conservative management requiring re-exploration. In patients who have had ileum used for diversion, there is a 2–15% incidence of postoperative bowel obstruction requiring treatment. When the colon is used, the incidence of postoperative obstruction is decreased to 2–7% (Table 2). In general, the incidence of postoperative bowel obstruction may be reduced by:

1. Careful handling of tissues.
2. Using transverse colon rather than ileum in patients who have undergone extensive pelvic irradiation.
3. Closure of all mesenteric defects.
4. Complete retroperitonealization of the conduit segment.
5. Placing omentum over the bowel anastomosis.
6. Adequate nasogastric tube decompression (may not be necessary for all patients).

Because proper stomal care is essential for patients undergoing non-continent cutaneous diversion, each patient must be assessed for his or her ability to care for the stomal site and urinary appliance. Patients with severe multiple sclerosis or mentally impaired patients may require that a family member or a visiting nurse assist in caring for the urinary appliance. Dermatitis may be reduced by careful attention to parastomal skin care and by using a properly fitting appliance around a protruding stoma. We have found that both preoperative and postoperative interaction of an enterstomal therapist with the patient is invaluable in minimizing many stomal complications.

The incidence of upper urinary tract deterioration is not insignificant in the patient undergoing conduit urinary diversion. In fact, long term reviews of patients with ileal conduits suggest that one third of renal units undergo some degree of deterioration with time *(35,36)*. Over the long term, about 6% of patients with ileal conduit diversions ultimately die of renal failure *(37)*. Factors that may contribute to upper tract deterioration include ureterointestinal stenosis, chronic bacteruria in association with freely refluxing ureters, stomal stenosis, serious electrolyte abnormalities or upper tract damage present at the time of surgery (Table 3).

Both ileal and colonic segments actively absorb chloride ions in exchange for bicarbonate and a minor degree of hyperchloremic absorption should be anticipated. Hyperchloremic acidosis has been reported with a frequency of 68% in patients with ileal conduits *(38)*. The long-term clinical significance of this minor degree of acidosis is not known. However, bone mineralization may certainly be affected. Severe electrolyte disturbances occur to a lesser degree with the incidence of clini-

Table 3
Factors Which Contribute to Upper Tract Deterioration

1. Ureterointestinal stenosis
2. Recurrent urine infection
3. Ureterointestinal reflux
4. Stomal stenosis
5. Severe electrolyte abnormalities
6. Upper tract damage present at the time of surgery

Table 4
Factors Which Influence Solute Absorption[a]

1. Segment of bowel
2. Renal function
3. Surface area of bowel segment
4. Exposure time of urine to bowel segment
5. Concentration of solutes in urine

[a]Data from McDougal (41).

cal manifestations after conduit diversion ranging from 1.7–16% (39). These electrolyte abnormalities, if significant and allowed to persist, may result in major complications. In fact, severe electrolyte abnormalities secondary to conduit construction have contributed to patient mortality (40).

Fortunately, patients with normal renal function should be able to appropriately buffer the increased acid load and may demonstrate only mild metabolic changes. The factors which influence solute absorption are listed (Table 4). Patients with baseline renal dysfunction, however, may have difficulty excreting the excess solute reabsorbed through the intestine, especially with a continent urinary diversion. In general, we have found that patients with a serum creatinine less than 2.0 mg/dL and minimal proteinuria can tolerate intestine interposed in the urinary tract without significant problems. In patients whose serum creatinine exceeds 2.0 mg/dL, a more detailed assessment of renal function is necessary. Such patients may be a candidate if they can produce a urinary pH of less than 5.8 following an ammonium chloride load, can concentrate their urine to more than 600 mOsm/kg in response to water deprivation, have minimal proteinuria, and have a creatinine clearance that is greater than 35 mL/min (Table 5). In addition, maintaining adequate hydration as well as minimizing bowel redundancy and urinary stasis is crucial to avoid significant metabolic abnormalities.

Table 5
Guidelines for Renal Function
in Patients Undergoing Intestinal Diversion[a]

Serum creatinine < 2.0 mg/dL
If serum creatinine exceeds 2.0 mg/dL
Acidification of urine pH < 5.8
Concentrating ability > 600 mOsm/kg
Minimal proteinuria
Creatinine clearance > 35 mL/min

[a]Data from McDougal *(41)*.

CONTINENT CUTANEOUS DIVERSIONS

The Indiana Pouch

The Indiana pouch was first performed in 1984 by Drs. Rowland and Mitchell. It was first reported in 1985 *(42)*. Several modifications have been made since the original description. Complete detubularization was performed by an ileal patch on the cecal-ascending colonic segment or the colonic segment was incised longitudinally along the antimesenteric surface, folded over, and closed transversely *(43)*. The next major change was the use of staples to taper the efferent limb as described by Bejany and Politano *(44)*. The continence mechanism was still based on the plication of the ileocecal valve with non-absorbable Lembert stitches *(45)*. The most recent modification in 1993 was the use of absorbable staples to detubularize and close the reservoir *(46)*. This change saves approximately one hour of surgical time. The savings in the operating room charges due to the shorter surgical time pays for the cost of the staples.

The clinical results of 81 patients from Indiana University with a minimum of 5-yr followup are presented in Table 6. Table 7 show the reoperation rates of a combined series of Indiana pouches performed at Indian University and University of California, Irvine. Continence is defined as the ability to stay dry for at least 4 h day or night without leaking or having to catheterize. The reoperation rates compare favorably with non-continent cutaneous diversions, other continent cutaneous reservoirs, and orthotopic neobladders *(47)*.

Kock Pouch

The origin of the Kock pouch dates back to the mid 1960s when Kock and Associates began to examine the functional behavior of different types of bladder substitutes *(48)*. The Kock pouch, made from 80 cm of detubularized ileum with an afferent and efferent intussecepted ileal

Table 6
Functional Results of 81 Patients with an Indiana Pouch

Postop time	3 mo	60 mo	>1yr
Daytime catheterization Interval > 4 h	81%	95%	98%
Nighttime catheterization Internal > 4 h	83%	95%	98%
Continent without Catheterization during Normal sleep interval	60%	74%	84%

Table 7
**Open and Percutaneous Procedures
for Complications in 169 Indiana Pouches**[a]

	Early complications	Late complications
	(≤30 d postop)	(≥30 d postop)
Related to pouch	1.2%	12.4%
Not related to pouch	2.4%	3.0%
Total	3.6%	15.4%
Grand total		19.0%

[a] Patients from Indiana University: 69; UC Irvine: 100.
See ref. *(12).*

nipple valve mechanism, is a technically demanding procedure that may require a significant learning curve. The Kock pouch maintains low intraluminal pressures and obtains a large pouch capacity routinely. Average pouch capacities exceed 700 mL and urodynamic evaluations demonstrate pouch pressures ranging between 4–8 cm H_2O in the long-term *(49).* Over the past decade, Skinner and associates have introduced a series of technical modifications in the continence and antireflux mechanism aimed at reducing the incidence of late complications and the need for reoperation. In a six year series of 531 patients undergoing Kock pouch urinary diversion, Skinner and Associates reported an early complication rate of 16.2% and an operative mortality rate of 1.9%. Since the last modification to their surgical technique in July 1985, the late complication rate had decreased to 22%. This report remains the world's largest single institutional experience using the Kock principle. Enthusiasm for this technique, however, remains tempered by a 15% reoperation rate often due to a pinhole fistula at the base of the efferent nipple valve mechanism.

Table 8
Types of Orthotopic Neobladders

Procedure	Segment of bowel
Camey	Ileum
Hautmann	Ileum
Hautmann with chimney	Ileum
Studer	Ileum
Hemi-kock	Ileum
T-Pouch	Ileum
Mainz	Ileocolic
LeBag	Right colon
Reddy	Sigmoid colon

ORTHOTOPIC
NEOBLADDER RECONSTRUCTION

There has long been a need for a method of diversion that does not require an external appliance. It certainly is not disputed that the ileal conduit provides a simple, safe means of diverting urine after cystectomy. Conduits, however, have obvious disadvantages that make orthotopic neobladder reconstruction attractive to some patients. Disadvantages, including a continuously draining, wet abdominal stoma requiring an external urinary appliance may diminish patients' quality of life. However, despite continence of the intra-abdominal urinary reservoirs, the psychological stigma associated with a stoma remains as does the requirement for frequent clean intermittent catheterization.

It is against this backdrop that over the past 10–15 years a plethora of orthotopic urinary reconstructive procedures have been described (Table 8). Efforts have been made to avoid an external stoma and preserve normal volitional voiding. Consequently, patients may have an improved body image, sexuality, sociability, and global sense of well being (51).

Because there have been scores of orthotopic neobladder reconstructions described in the literature, an exhaustive review of all operative techniques is beyond the scope of this section. Our objective is not to champion one technique over the other but rather to illustrate the relative advantages and disadvantages of several commonly performed orthotopic neobladders. After careful review of the literature, it becomes clear that there is no consensus as to which orthotopic urinary reconstruction is superior to any other. The fact that so many procedures have been described suggests that the best has yet to be devised. Other points of controversy include which bowel type is ideal for constructing a urinary reservoir and whether a nonrefluxing or refluxing ureterointestinal anastomosis is desirable in urinary tract reconstruction.

Selection of Patients

All patients must be assessed preoperatively for the ability to perform self-catheterization. Physically or mentally impaired patients may lack adequate motor or cognitive skills to catheterize their urethra, making them poor candidates for any form of continent diversion. Patient gender may also play a part in selecting potential candidates. In the past there was considerable reluctance to create orthotopic neobladders in women due to an increased theoretical risk of urinary incontinence and local tumor recurrence. The concern that women might be incontinent after orthotopic reconstruction has proven to be unfounded. To the contrary, the major concern is hypercontinence, with some series reporting as high as 20% of women requiring long-term intermittent catheterization *(52)*.

An extensive histological review by Stein and associates examined the incidence of concurrent urethral cancer in 56 female patients who underwent cystectomy for transitional cell carcinoma *(53)*. None of the patients were found to have urethral involvement in the absence of tumor at the bladder neck. Equally concerning in women candidates for orthotopic neobladder diversion was the possibility of anterior vaginal wall involvement. Stein and associates identified anterior vaginal wall involvement in four of their female cystectomy specimens. Each of the four specimens also had bladder neck involvement and two had urethral involvement as well. Therefore, we use bladder neck involvement in women as an absolute contraindication to orthotopic diversion.

In the male bladder cancer patient, the risk of urethral recurrence after cystectomy is 5–10% *(54,55)*. Schellhammer and Whitmore demonstrated a 35% risk of urethral recurrence in those patients who had transitional cell carcinoma of the prostatic urethra *(56)*. In contrast, several recent series have found a less than 5% incidence of urethral recurrence in patients with orthotopic neobladder reconstruction, despite the postoperative identification of prostatic stromal involvement *(57,58)*. Skinner and associates theorized that the urine flow through the urethra might decrease the risk of urethral recurrence *(59)*. Recently, they reviewed their clinical and pathological results of 694 men who had undergone cystectomy and either cutaneous diversion (51%) or orthotopic urinary diversion (49%). They found that patients undergoing orthotopic diversion demonstrated a significantly lower incidence of urethral recurrence (2%) compared to those undergoing cutaneous diversion (9%) ($p = 0.001$). Based on these large series, we (GDS and CMPH) recommend orthotopic diversion as an acceptable option if there is no stromal invasion of the prostatic urethra and frozen section analysis of the urethral margin is negative.

Renal and hepatic function must be thoroughly assessed in all potential candidates for continent diversion. We have already outlined our guidelines for renal function in patients undergoing intestinal diversion (Table 5).

Hautmann Neobladder

This operation, popularized at the University of Ulm in Germany, is a product of the enterocystoplasty principles described by Camey and Le Duc (60), who used a loop of detubularized small bowel as a bladder substitute. The Hautmann neobladder consists of 60–80 cm of detubularized ileum oriented into the shape of "W". The ureters are implanted using the Le Duc technique in the posterior margin of the ileal plate. In an 11-yr series of 363 men undergoing cystectomy for invasive bladder cancer, Hautmann and associates (61) reported a perioperative mortality of 3%. The incidence of early and late complications occurred in 39.1% and 32% of patients, respectively. Of the 290 available patients, 95.9% reported good day and nighttime continence and 3.9% performed clean intermittent catheterization in some form. Certainly a major drawback with all series of patients with invasive bladder cancer is a considerable mortality rate, with Hautmann and associates reporting a third of patients dying due to disease progression. Late complications can, therefore, only be examined in those patients that survive. Nevertheless, series with long-term followup are essential to examine possible changes in complication rates over time and to convey accurate expectations to patients regarding long-term results.

Hautmann Neobladder with Chimney Modification

This diversion was initially described by Lippert and Theodorescu (62) in an effort to enhance the flexibility and reduce the pitfalls of Hautmann neobladder reconstruction. Hollowell and associates (63) reported their four-year experience with the chimney modification, in which an 8-12 cm tubularized isoperistaltic ileal chimney was used for the ureterointestinal anastomosis in 50 patients (Fig. 2). Early and late complications occurred in 22% and 20% of patients, respectively, with a perioperative mortality rate of 2%. The early and late (neobladder related and unrelated) complication rates are presented in Table 9. Continence was defined as good if the patient required no protection or wore only a light safety pad, but was otherwise completely dry. Continence was defined as satisfactory if the patient required only one pad during the day or evening and poor if more than one pad was required. After

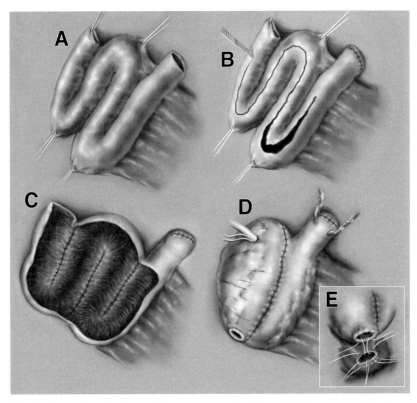

Fig. 2. Operative technique of Hautmann neobladder with chimney modification. The neobladder is constructed by removing an ileal segment 68 cm in length and orienting it into the shape of a "W" with four equal limbs each 15 cm in length. (**B**) The most proximal 8–12 cm of the ileal segment is not detubularized and the remaining 60 cm of bowel is opened along the antimesenteric border. (**C**) The posterior plate of the "W" is sewn together (**D**) and the pouch is closed. (**E**) Ileal urethral anastomosis.

one year 93% of patients reported good daytime continence and 86% reported good nighttime continence. Two patients (4%) performed clean intermittent catheterization in some form.

This modification to the popular Hautmann ileal neobladder has several advantages. First, the isoperistaltic limb allows for less mobilization and more proximal resection of ureters. Second, the ureters do not compete with the bowel mesentery for access to the posterior wall of the neobladder, and are at less risk of angulation and subsequent obstruction in cases of neobladder over distention. Third, we found the chimney modification allows for easier identification and revision of the uretero-intestinal anastomosis should the patient require re-exploration due to

Table 9
Radical Cystectomy and Hautmann
Neobladder with Chimney Modification Study [a]

Early	Less than or equal to 3 mo postop	
	Neobladder related	10%
	Neobladder unrelated	12%
	Total	22%
Late	More than 3 mo postop	
	Neobladder related	16%
	Neobladder unrelated	4%
	Total	20%

[a] Early and late complications of radical cystectomy and Haut-mann neobladder with chimney modification in 50 patients from the University of Chicago.

ureterointestinal stricture or recurrent disease. In the authors' (GDS and CMPH) experience, the chimney modification is simple to perform and compares well with other forms of orthotopic urinary diversion.

Studer Neobladder

This diversion, popularized at the University of Bern, is a variation of the othotopic hemi-Kock procedure. Without the need for an intussuscepted proximal limb, however, this is much simpler in its construction. The Studer neobladder consists of 40 cm of detubularized ileum oriented into the shape of a "U" with a 25 cm isoperistaltic limb to which the ureters are implanted in a refluxing fashion (Fig. 3). In a 10-yr series of 100 consecutive men undergoing cystectomy for invasive bladder cancer, Studer and associates (64) reported major complications in 15% of patients. Daytime continence was 92% at 1 yr and 80% of patients reported good nighttime continence by 2 yr. The major advantage of this diversion is that it allows for significant proximal resection of ureters while still maintaining a tension-free ureterointestinal anastomosis. In addition, the isoperistaltic limb serves to dampen the degree of reflux into the upper urinary tracts.

Hemi-Kock Pouch

In 1987 Ghoneim and associates (65) reported their interim results in 6 patients provided with a urethral Kock pouch. Like the cutaneous Kock pouch reservoir, this diversion employed the use of an intussuscepted nipple valve mechanism to prevent ureteral reflux. The closure of the inferior portion of the pouch left a small aperture patent for the urethral anastomosis. At 3 mo, they reported a mean pouch capacity of 300 mL

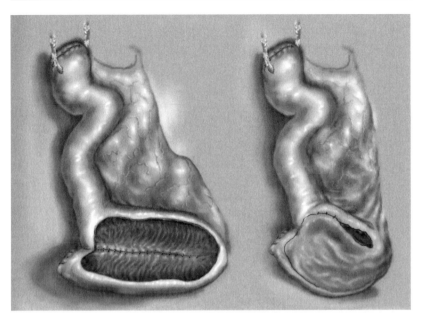

Fig. 3. Operative technique of Studer ileal neobladder. A 60–65 cm ileal segment is excluded from bowel continuity. (**A**) The distal 40 cm are detubularized and oriented into the shape of a "U". Both ureters are anastomosed end-to-side to the remaining 25 cm isoperistaltic limb. (**B**) Closure of the anterior wall of the pouch.

which expanded to 750 mL by 11 mo. Urodynamic assessment showed pouch pressures below 20 cm H_2O at 100% capacity.

The largest single institutional experience with the orthotopic Hemi-Kock pouch was reported by the group at the University of Southern California. Elmajian and associates *(66)* reported their 7-yr experience on 295 consecutive men undergoing orthotopic Hemi-Kock bladder substitution. The early and late complication rates were 15.7 and 13.7%, respectively. Three patients died in the perioperative period, for a mortality rate of 1.0%. Analysis of the pouch-related late complications revealed stone formation (4.1%) along the intussuscepted bowel staple line, afferent nipple stenosis (2.4%) and ureteral reflux (2.0%) as the most frequent. Of the evaluable patients (154), 87% and 86% reported good or satisfactory and day and nighttime continence, respectively. Eight patients (5.3%) performed regular clean intermittent catheterization.

A disadvantage of this diversion was that the afferent nipple valve construction was technically challenging. Interestingly, Kock and associates *(67)* reported a high incidence (53%) of sliding or eversion of the antireflux valve in their experience, suggesting that in the hands of other surgeons results might not be as good as those reported by Elmajian and associates. Perhaps the best reason to suggest that complications associated with the afferent nipple valve remain problematic is evidenced by recent reports that the group at the University of Southern California has developed a new orthotopic ileal neobladder, the T-pouch, with a novel antireflux mechanism *(68)*.

Ileocolic Orthotopic Diversion (Mainz Pouch)

The surgical technique for creation of the Mainz Pouch uses 10–15 cm of cecum as well as 20–30 cm of distal ileum for construction of an ileocolic bladder. Initial applications were for bladder augmentation after subtotal cystectomy and for continent cutaneous urinary diversion. Modifications were then described with the use of a cecourethral anastomosis to allow for normal volitional voiding *(69,70)*. In a series of 27 patients, Fisch and associates *(71)* reported complete daytime continence in 100% of patients and 89% reported complete nocturnal continence, provided they woke two to three times to void each night. In a 4-yr experience with the ileocolic neobladder, Marshall and associates *(72)* reported excellent urodynamic characteristics with a mean pouch capacity of 495 mL and pouch pressures ranging from 10 cm H_2O (50% capacity) to 40 cm H_2O (100% capacity) and no nocturnal enuresis. However, most patients voided once per night. Of this young cystectomy population (mean age 52 yr) 21 were potent preoperatively and 15 remained potent (71%). The author sited two factors for achieving such a high potency rate: 1) preservation of the neurovascular bundles; and 2) patient age.

The major advantage of this diversion is its simplicity in performing a nonrefluxing ureterointestinal anastomosis. Some patients, however, may not be favorable ileocolic bladder candidates, including those with a history of previous colonic surgery, ruptured appendix, extensive diverticulosis, or colonic malignancy. In addition, in some patients it may be difficult to mobilize the cecum into the pelvis for urethral anastomosis. In these situations a small bowel neobladder may be an alternative.

Sigmoid Pouch (Reddy)

A diversion initially popularized by the group at the University of Minnesota, the Sigmoid pouch originally employed a nondetubularized U-shaped sigmoid segment for bladder replacement (similar to the Camey I procedure). After reporting unacceptably high pouch pressures, Reddy *(73)* showed improved urodynamic characteristics using a partially detubularized sigmoid pouch. The pouch eventually evolved into a fully detubularized U-shaped segment approximately 30 cm in length (Fig. 4). In 1994, DaPozzo and associates *(74)* reported on their

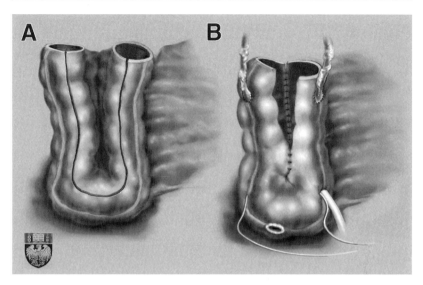

Fig. 4. Operative technique of Sigmoid pouch. (**A**) A 30 cm segment of sigmoid colon is excluded from bowel continuity, detubularized and oriented into the shape of a "U". (**B**) After closing the lower half of the anterior pouch wall, anastomosis of the most dependent portion of the pouch to the membranous urethra is performed.

6-yr experience with the Sigmoid pouch. In 24 consecutive patients, they reported day and nighttime continence rates of 94.1% and 70.6% at 18 mo, respectively. The mean pouch capacity at 18 mo was 492 mL with a pouch pressure of 29 cm H_2O at maximum capacity. The surgical complication rate was reported to be minimal.

The use of sigmoid colon as an orthotopic urinary diversion is advantageous due to the ease with which this segment can be anastomosed to the membranous urethra. It also allows for nonrefluxing submucosal reimplantation. Contraindications include diverticulosis, colon polyps or the presence of inflammatory large bowel disease. The intestinal tract must, therefore, be thoroughly investigated by barium enema or colonoscopy before surgical intervention.

DISTRIBUTION OF TYPES
OF DIVERSION/RECONSTRUCTION

Significant progress and evolution in orthotopic and continent cutaneous urinary reconstruction have occurred over the past several decades due to patient demand for a socially and psychologically more acceptable solution than a continuously draining stomal diversion. Although application of noncontinent cutaneous urinary conduits have diminished, it certainly has its well deserved place in the armamentarium of every urologist. At the University of Chicago, we (GDS and CMPH) estimate that 40% of all cystectomy patients choose an ileal conduit and are well served by a simpler form of diversion. Another 10% of our cystectomy population choose a continent cutaneous reservoir and the remaining 50% choose a neobladder. The reasons for this distribution are unclear, but the surgeons' preferences towards one type of diversion/reconstruction over another may certainly play a major role.

In the third author's (RGR) experience approximately 40% of all cystectomy patients choose an ileal conduit. Another 40% choose a continent cutaneous reservoir, and the remaining 20% choose a neobladder. The choice of type of diversion/reconstruction is closely related to age in this author's experience. In general, patients in their upper 60s or 70s will choose an ileal conduit despite being offered a continent cutaneous reservoir or a neobladder. Most of the patients in this age range do not want to risk incontinence or have to do self-intermittent catheterization regardless of whether it would be through a stoma or the urethra.

Patients in their early to mid 60s are fairly evenly distributed between continent cutaneous reservoirs and neobladders. Patients in their 50s or younger choose a neobladder in a high percentage of cases. Although there are exceptions to this generalization, age is a great predictor of choice.

A patient's tumor stage and location also play a major role in the choices available to the patient. Renal function and bowel function and/or previous bowel surgery or pathologic conditions can limit a patient's options. In any diversion/reconstruction in which the bowel segment serves as a reservoir, absorption of urinary constituents occurs. Renal reserve must be adequate to compensate for this factor. Free water loss occurs from reservoirs and neobladders and can cause problems with dehydration in patients with compromised urine concentrating abilities.

Patients with previous bowel resections of any significant length could potentially suffer from malabsorption if a segment of bowel large enough to create a continent cutaneous reservoir or neobladder is isolated from the intestinal tract. Patients with progressive neurologic disorders such as multiple sclerosis are not good candidates for continent cutaneous reservoirs or neobladders based on the patient's required or possible need to do self-intermittent catheterization in the respective types of diversion/reconstruction.

The proportion of patients who choose the various types of diversion/reconstruction varies in different portions of the country. This may be, in part, due to variations of physician attitudes and experience in different regions and, in part, due to the differences in patients' attitudes in the various regions of the country. In regions where outdoor activities are readily available year round, there seems to be a natural selection process that attracts more active patients who focus on physical fitness, body image, and lifestyle issues. These people are more likely to choose a neobladder with the hope of avoiding a stoma and/or the need to do self-intermittent catheterization.

CONCLUSION

For many years an ileal conduit and ureterosigmoidostomy were the 2 primary options for urinary diversion following cystectomy. Although ureterosigmoidostomy has since fallen out of favor, conduit diversion remains a permanent part of every urologic surgeons' armamentarium. The ultimate goals of urinary tract reconstruction after bladder removal, however, have evolved from simply diverting urine and protecting the upper tracts to creating a socially and psychologically more acceptable solution. Patient survey studies show that patients are more satisfied with continent urinary diversion or neobladder reconstructions *(75)*. Perhaps best evidenced by improved quality of life in those patients whose noncontinent diversions were converted to continent reservoirs *(76)*. Due to the ingenuity and creativity of many urologic surgeons worldwide, there exists a vast array of continent urinary reservoirs, utilizing colon, ileum, ileum and colon, and stomach. Clearly, no single technique is ideal for all patients or clinical situations. This chapter has addressed the clinical results and complications of selected, but representative techniques for noncontinent cutaneous diversion, continent cutaneous diversion and orthotopic neobladder reconstructions. A familiarity with these concepts and a flexible approach to each individual patient is required to obtain the best result.

REFERENCES

1. Chute R, Sallade RL. Bilateral side-to-side cutaneous urethrostomy in the midline for urinary diversion. J Urol 1961; 85: 280.
2. Simon J. Ectopia uesicae (absence of the anterior walls of the bladder and pubic abdominal parietes): operation for directing the orifices of the ureters into the rectum; temporary success; subsequent death; autopsy. Lancet 1852; 2: 568.
3. Mathesin W. New method for ureterointestinal anastomosis. Preliminary report. Surg Gynecol Obstet 1953; 96: 255.
4. Goodwin WE, Scardino PT. Ureterosignoidostomy. J Urol 1977; 118: 169–172.
5. Schoemaker van Stockum WJ, Strater M. Intra-abdominal plastieken. Ned T dschr Geeneekd 1911; 55: 823.
6. Bricker E. Bladder substitution after pelvic evisceration. Surg Clin North Am 1950; 30: 1511.
7. Gilchrist RH, Merricks JW, et al. Construction of a substitute bladder and urethra. Surg Gynecol Obstet 1950; 90: 752.

8. Tasker JH. Ileo-cystoplasty: a new technique. An experimental study with report of a case. Br J Urol 1953; 25: 349.

9. Giertz G, Frankson C. Construction of a substitute bladder, with preservation of voiding, after subtotal and total cystectomy. Acta Chir Scand 1957; 111: 218.

10. Goodwin WE, et al. "Cup-patch" technique of ileocystoplasty for bladder enlargement or partial substitution. Surg Gynecol Obstet 1959; 108: 240.

11. Husmann DA, McLorie GA, Churchill BN. Nonrefluxing colonic conduits: a long-term life-table analysis. J Urol 1989; 142: 1201–1203.

12. Richie JP, Skinner DG. Urinary diversion: the physiological rationale for nonrefluxing colonic conduits. Br J Urol 1975; 47: 269–275.

13. Sullivan JW, Grabstald H, Whitmore WF Jr. Complications of ureteroileal conduit with radical cystectomy: review of 336 cases. J Urol 1980; 124: 797–801.

14. Daughtry JD, Susan LP, Stewart BH, Straffon RA. Ileal conduit and cystectomy: a 10-year retrospective study of ileal conduits performed in conjunction with cystectomy and with a minimum 5-year follow-up. J Urol 1977; 118: 556–557.

15. Johnson DE, Lamy SM. Complications of a single stage radical cystectomy and ileal conduit diversion: review of 241 cases. J Urol 1975; 117: 171–173.

16. Jaffe BM, Bricker EM, Butcher HR Jr. Surgical complications of ileal segment urinary diversion. Ann Surg 1968; 167: 367–376.

17. Johnson DE, Jackson L, Guinn GA. Ileal conduit diversion for carcinoma of the bladder. South Med J 1970; 63: 1115–1118.

18. Pernet F, Jonas U. Ileal conduit urinary diversion: early and late results of 132 cases in a 25-year period. World J Urol 1985; 3: 140.

19. Suare J, Walter S, Kristensen JK, Flemming L. Ileal conduit urinary diversion–early and late complications. Eur Urol 1985; 11: 83.

20. Butcher HR, Sugg WL, McAfee CA, Bricker EM. Ileal conduit method of ureteral urinary diversion. Ann Surg 1962; 156: 68.

21. Schmidt JD, Hawtrey CE, Flocks RH, Culp DA. Complications, results and problems of ileal conduit diversions. J Urol 1973; 109: 210–216.

22. Schmidt JD, Buchsbaum HJ, Jacobo EC. Transverse colon conduit for supravesical urinary tract diversion. Urology 1976; 8: 542–546.

23. Loening SA, Navarre RJ, Narayana AS, Culp DA. Transverse colon conduit urinary diversion. J Urol 1982; 127: 37–39.

24. Morales P, Golimbu M. Colonic urinary diversion: 10 years of experience. J Urol 1975; 113: 302–309.

25. Althansen AF, Hagen-Cook K, Hendren WH. Nonrefluxing colon conduit: experience with 70 cases. J Urol 1978; 120: 35–39.

26. Markland C, Flocks RH. The ileac conduit stoma. J Urol 1966; 95: 355.

27. Kafetsioulis A, Swinney J. Urinary diversion by ileal conduit. A long-term follow-up. Br J Urol 1968. 40: 1.

28. Retik AB, Perlmutter AD, Gross RE. N Engl J Med 1967; 277: 217.

29. Orr JD, Shand J, Watters DA, et al. Ileal conduit urinary diversion in children. An assessment of the long-term results. Br J Urol 1981; 53: 424–427.

30. Turnbull RB, Hewitt CR. Loop-end myotomy ileostomy in the obese patient. Urol Clin North Am 1978; 5: 423–429.

31. Marshall FF, Leadbetter WF, Dretler SP. Ileal conduit parastomal hernias. J Urol 1975; 114: 40–42.

32. Bloom DA, Lieskovsky G, Rainwater G, Skinner DG. The Turnbull loop stoma. J Urol 1983; 129: 715–718.

33. Noble MJ, Mebust WK. Creation of the urinary stoma. AUA Update Series, Lesson 13, Vol 5, 1986.

34. Remigailo RV, Lewis EL, Woodard JR, Walton KN. Ileal conduit urinary diversion. Urology 1976; 7: 343.
35. Middleton AW Jr, Hendren WH. Ileal conduit in children at the Massachusetts General Hospital from 1955 to 1970. J Urol 1976; 115: 591–595.
36. Shapiro SR, Lebowitz R, Colodny AH. Fate of 90 children with ileal conduit urinary diversions a decade later: analysis of complications, pyelography, renal function and bacteriology. J Urol 1975; 114: 289–295.
37. Richie JP. Intestinal loop urinary diversion in children. J Urol 1974; 111: 687–689.
38. Castro JE, Ram MD. Electrolyte imbalance following ileal urinary diversion. Br J Urol 1970; 42: 29–32.
39. Kosko JW, Kursh ED, Resnick MI. Metabolic complications of urologic intestinal substitution. Urol Clin North Am 1986; 13: 193–200.
40. Heidler H, Marberger M, Hohenfellner R. The metabolic situation in ureterosigmoidostomy. Eur Urol 1979; 5: 39–44.
41. McDougal WS. Use of intestinal segments and urinary diversion. In: *Campbell's Urology* (Walsh PC, Retik AB, Vaughan ED, et al., eds.) Vol 3, 7th ed. Philadelphia, PA, WB Saunders, 1997, pp. 3121–3161.
42. Rowland RG, Mitchell ME, Bihrle R. The cecoileal continent urinary reservoir. World J Urol 1985; 3: 185.
43. Rowland RG, Mitchell ME, Bihrle R, et al. The Indiana continent urinary reservoir. J Urol 1987; 137: 1136–1139.
44. Bejany DE, Politano VA. Stapled and nonstapled tapered distal ileum for construction of a continent colonic urinary reservoir. J Urol 1988; 140: 491–494.
45. Rowland RG, Bihrle R, Scheidler D, et al. Update on the Indiana continent urinary reservoir. Prob Urol 1991; 5: 269.
46. Rowland RG, Kropp BP. Evolution of the Indiana continent urinary reservoir. J Urol 1994; 152: 2247–2251.
47. Rowland RG. Complications of continent cutaneous reservoirs and neobladders-series using contemporary techniques. AUA Update Series 14: lesson 25. 1995.
48. Kock NG. Intra-abdominal "reservoir" in patients with permanent ileostomy: preliminary observations on a procedure resulting in fecal "continence" in five ileostomy patients. Arch Surg 1969. 99: 223.
49. Chen KK, Chang LS, Chen MT. Urodynamic and clinical outcome of Kock pouch continent urinary diversion. J Urol 1989; 141: 94–97.
50. Skinner DG, Lieskovsky G, Boyd S. Continent urinary diversion. J Urol 1989; 141: 1323–1327.
51. Weijerman PC, Schurmans JR, Hop WC, Schroder FH, Bosh JL. Morbidity and quality of life in patients with orthotopic and heterotopic continent urinary diversion. Urology 1998; 51(1): 51–56.
52. Stein JP, Stenzl A, Grossfeld GD, et al. The use of orthotopic neobladders in women undergoing cystectomy for pelvic malignancy. World J Urol 1996; 14: 9–14.
53. Stein JP, Stenzl A, Esrig D, et al. Lower urinary tract reconstruction in women following cystectomy using the Kock ileal reservoir with bilateral ureteroilealurethrostomy: initial clinical experience. J Urol 1994; 152: 1404–1408.
54. Cordonnier JJ, Ssjut HJ. Urethral occurrence of bladder carcinoma following cystectomy. Trans Am Assoc Genitourin Surg 1961; 52: 13.
55. Freeman JA, Esrig D, Stein JP, et al. Management of the patient with bladder cancer: urethral recurrence. Urol Clin North Am 1994; 21(4): 645–651.
56. Schellhammer PF, Whitmore WF Jr. Transitional cell carcinoma of the urethra in men having cystectomy for bladder cancer. J Urol 1976; 115: 56–60.

57. Freeman JA, Tarter TA, Esrig D, et al. Urethral recurrence in patients with ortho-topic ileal neobladders. J Urol 1996; 156: 1615–1619.
58. Iselin CE, Robertson CN, Webster GD, et al. Does prostate transitional cell carci-noma preclude orthotopic bladder reconstruction after radical cystoprostatectomy for bladder cancer? J Urol 1997; 158: 2123–2126.
59. Stein JP, Ginsberg D, Groshen S, Fang AC, Bochner B, Skinner E, et al. Urethral tumor recurrence following cystectomy and urinary diversion: clinical and patho-logical characteristics in 694 patients. J Urol, part 2, 161:264A, abstract 1020, 1999.
60. Camcy M, LeDuc A. L'entro-cystoplastic apres cystoprostatectomie totale pour cancer de la uessie. Indications, technique operatoire, surveilance et resultants sur quatre-uingt-sept cas. Ann Urol 1979; 13: 114.
61. Hautmann RE, Depetriconi R, Gottfried H, Kleinschmidt K, Mattes R, Paiss T. The ileal neobladder: complications and functional results in 363 patients after 11 years of follow-up. J Urol 1999; 161: 422–428.
62. Lippert CM, Theodorescu D. The Hautmann neobladder with chimney: a versatile modifications. J Urol 1997; 158: 1510–1512.
63. Hollowell CMP, Christiano AP, Steinberg, GD. Technique of Hautmann ileal neobladder with chimney modification: interim results in 50 patients. J Urol 2000; 163: 47–51.
64. Studer UR, Danuser H, Merz VW, Springer JP, Zingg EJ. Experience in 100 patients with an ileal low pressure bladder substitute combined with an efferent tubular isoperistaltic segment. J Urol 1995; 154: 49–56.
65. Ghoneim MA, Kock NG, Kycke G, Shehab El-Din AB. An applicance-free, sphinc-ter-controlled bladder substitute: the urethral Kock pouch. J Urol 1987; 138: 1150–1154.
66. Elmajian DA, Stein JP, Esrig D, Freeman JA, Skinner EC, Boyd SD, et al. The Kock ileal neobladder: updated experience in 295 male patients. J Urol 1996; 156: 920–925.
67. Kock NG, Ghoneim MA, Lycke KG, Mahran MR. Replacement of the bladder by the urethral Kock pouch: Functional results, urodynamics and radiological features. J Urol 1989; 141: 1111–1116.
68. Stein JP, Lieskovsky G, Ginsberg DA, Bochner BH, Skinner DS. The T-pouch: an orthotopic ileal neobladder incorporating a serosal lined ileal antireflux tech-nique. J Urol 1998. 159: 1836–1842.
69. Thuroff JW, Alken P, Riedmiller H, Jacobi GH, Hohenfellner R. 100 cases of Mainz Pouch: continuing experience and evolution. J Urol 1988; 140: 283–288.
70. Marshall FF. Creation of an ileocolic bladder after cystectomy. J Urol 1988; 139: 1264–1268.
71. Fisch M, Wammack R, Hohenfellner R. Seven years experience with the Mainz pouch procedure. Archivos Españoles de Urologia 1992; 45: 175.
72. Marshall FF, Mostwin JL, Radebaugh LC, Walsh PC, Brendler CB. Ileocolic neobladder post-cystectomy: continence and potency. J Urol 1991; 145: 502–504.
73. Reddy PK. Detubularized sigmoid reservoir for bladder replacement after cysto-prostatectomy. Urology 1987; 29(6): 625–628.
74. DaPozzo LF, Colombo R, Pompa P, Montorsi F, et al. Detubularized sigmoid colon for bladder replacement after radical cystectomy. J Urol 1994; 152: 1409–1412.
75. Gerharz EW, Weingartner K, Dopatka T, Kohl UN, Basler HD, Riedmiller HN. Quality of life after cystectomy and urinary diversion: results of a retrospective interdisciplinary study. J Urol 1997; 158: 778–785.
76. Boyd SD, Feinberg SM, Skinner DG, Lieskovsky G, Baron D, Richardson J. Qual-ity of life survey of urinary diversion patients: comparison of ileal conduits versus continent Kock ileal reservoirs. J Urol 1987; 138: 1386–1389.

14 Current Concepts for Urinary Diversion in Women

Arnulf Stenzl, MD and Georg Bartsch, MD

CONTENTS

INTRODUCTION

Although intestinal continent reservoirs to the urethra have been used now successfully in the male for several years *(1,2)* its use in females undergoing cystectomy for bladder cancer has not routinely been considered till recently. An undefined risk of the extent of transitional cell cancer (the most common type of bladder cancer) into the female urethra was probably the reason for almost unequivocally performing total urethrectomy in combination with anterior pelvic exenteration. The lack of a remnant portion of the urethra, no data about secondary urethral tumors, and insufficient knowledge about the functional anatomy of the isolated female urethra and its sphincter were the biggest obstacles in the development and common use of an orthotopic reconstruction of the lower urinary tract after cystectomy for bladder cancer. The use of intestinal pouches with ileal segments as a urethral substitute with or without an artificial urinary sphincter had not gained wide acceptance either *(3)*.

From: *Current Clinical Urology: Bladder Cancer: Current Diagnosis and Treatment*
Edited by: M. J. Droller © Humana Press Inc., Totowa, NJ

EVOLUTION OF URINARY DIVERSION IN WOMEN

The first cystectomy in a female is attributed to Pawlick *(4)* more than a century ago. The ureters in this patient were diverted into the vagina and he reported continence and patient survival of 16 yr. Others, however, were not able to achieve similar results and this technique of urinary diversion was subsequently abandoned. Ureteral implantation techniques into the large bowel as published by Lotheisen *(5)* and Coffey *(6)* at the turn of the century remained the only stoma-free form of urinary diversion throughout most of this century. Despite an increasing popularity in recent years of orthotopic lower urinary tract reconstruction to the urethra *(7)* for male patients with bladder neoplasms, a similar approach for female patients with bladder cancer was thought not to be feasable because of the need to perform a concomitant total urethrectomy. A larger combined series of 2 institutions and several anecdotal reports *(8,9)* had indicated, however, that selected women with TCC undergoing radical cystectomy could be spared a portion of their urethra safely and this could be enough to render them continent when anastomosed to a low pressure intestinal reservoir *(10)*.

The risk of synchronous and metachronous urethral tumors in female bladder cancer patients has been the subject of several studies *(11–13)*. In addition we performed extensive anatomical and histological studies of the female urethra and its relationship to surrounding structures to assess the optimal level of urethral dissection in order to obtain a minimal risk for both residual tumor in the remnant urethra and postoperative incontinence in case of a planned orthotopic neobladder *(14,15)*. This resulted in a clinical protocol applying urethral-sparing surgery for cystectomy in women with orthotopic reconstruction of the lower urinary tract as described in previous reports *(16,17)*. Documented additional experience with regards to anatomy of the remnant urethra, patient selection, refinements of the surgical technique, patient outcome with regard to their underlying disease, risk of tumor recurrence, and postoperative continence in more than hundred patients operated on in recent years *(8,18–21)* has shown that roughly the same results as reported with male patients with an orthotopic neobladder can be achieved.

INCIDENCE OF URETHRAL
TUMORS IN FEMALE BLADDER TCC

One of the most important questions when considering an orthotopic neobladder in females is whether the oncological outcome can be compromised in any way. About 80% of the urethra can be preserved in this type of surgery. However, only a very short segment (in some patients

Table 1
Review of the Literature with Documented Cases of Overt Tumor
or Carcinoma *in situ* of the Urethra in Female Patients with Bladder Cancer

Author	Study period	No. of pts.	No. BN tumors	Urethral tumors	Urethral cis
Riches et al. *(21)*	ng	19[a]	3	3	–
Ashworth *(1)*	ng	293	ng	4	–
Richie et al *(22)*	1969–1971	21[a]	ng	–	1
Coutts et al. *(6)*	1974–1983	18[a]	ng	2	1
De Paepe et al. *(7)*	1974–1988	22[a]	ng	5	3
Coloby et al. *(5)*	1970–1990	47[a]	9	3	–
Stein et al. *(26)*	1982–1992	65[a]	16	7	–
Stenzl et al. *(34)*	1973–1992	356	49	6	–
Total		841		30 (3.6%)	5

[a]Heterogeneously selected bladder cancer study populations.
[b]ng = no data were given, BN = bladder neck. Adapted from *(22)*.

even none) of the remnant urethra is covered by transitional cell epithelium. The major part of the urethral mucosa consists of either regular or metaplastic squamous epithelium. The level of transition between squamous and transitional epithelium varies considerably. With increasing age, this transition zone moves cranially, covering at times the whole urethra, bladder neck, and part of the trigone *(23,24)*. This is probably due to estrogen influence and would also explain why often only squamous metaplasia is found at the level of urethral dissection in these patients, most of them being in the sixth and seventh decade at the time of surgery. To our knowledge no data exist as to whether a TCC recurrence ever occurred or is possible on squamous epithelium if removal of the primary cancer together with the entire urothelium of the bladder was achieved.

The problem of defining the risk of urethral tumors in the remnant female urethra after cystectomy has been approached in several ways (Table 1). Stein et al. *(12)* and Coloby et al. *(11)* in a recent retrospective analysis step-sectioned urethrocystectomy specimens of female bladder cancer patients and found urethral tumor involvement in 7 of 65 (10.7%) and 3 of 47 (6.4%) patients, resp. In both studies these urethral tumor occurrence strongly correlated with a location of the primary bladder cancer at the bladder neck and/or the trigone. Therefore a subtotal urethrectomy in patients without primary tumor involvement of the bladder neck was favourably discussed. On the other hand De Paepe et al. *(25)* in a similar study found carcinoma *in situ* or overt papillary tumor in the urethra in 36% (8/22 patients) and concluded that the urethra should be removed in all women undergoing radical cystectomy for TCC of the bladder. Unfortunately in this study comprising only 22 cases treated over a period of 15 yr no details regarding localization of either primary tumors in the bladder or secondary tumors in the urethra were provided. Ashworth *(26)* and Stenzl et al. *(22)* looked at the incidence of secondary urethral tumors in *all* patients treated for bladder cancer at a single institution over a longer period of time. Ashworth reported urethral tumors in 1.4% of 293 female patients, but no further details with regards to stage or localization of the primary tumor were given. In 356 female patients with different stages of bladder cancer followed for up to 33 yr, Stenzl et al. found an incidence of urethral tumor involvement in 2% of the entire study group, and in 1% of patients with localized (T2 to T3b, N0, M0) invasive cancer amenable to radical cystectomy. The only consistent risk factor for urethral tumors in this study was simultaneous primary tumor involvement of the bladder neck. It was therefore concluded that a large caudal segment of the urethra could safely be spared in selected cystectomy female patients undergoing orthotopic urinary reconstruction to the remnant urethra, provided neither preoperative biopsies of the bladder neck nor intraoperative frozen sections of the urethra at the level of dissection showed any tumor or atypia. In the same institution the overall incidence of secondary urethral tumors in 910 male patients was 6.1% *(27)*.

From these studies it can be concluded that the incidence of urethral cancer in female bladder cancer patients is lower than in male patients. Orthotopic reconstruction of the lower urinary tract in the male is almost a standard operation now with a high acceptance rate both by patients and doctors and an acceptably low local recurrence rate *(1,28,29)*. A strong correlation seems to exist in both sexes between urethral tumors and bladder neck involvement of the primary bladder tumor. Bladder neck atypia or overt tumors should therefore be a contraindication in females to subtotal urethrectomy and orthotopic neobladders. A similar approach is currently practiced in males with prostatic urethral tumor involvement without resulting in increased local recurrence rates so far *(30)*.

It is still advisable to remove as much urethra covered by transitional epithelium as possible. When performing a nerve-sparing technique more proximal urethra (and hence amount of transitional epithelium) can be removed while still maintaining perfect continence.

ANATOMY OF THE FEMALE URETHRA

The female urethral sphincter system consists of layers of smooth musculature controlled by autonomic nerves and striated muscle innervated by somatic nerves. It is generally agreed that the autonomic nerve branches for the urethral smooth muscle sphincter originate from the pelvic plexus *(31)*. The innervation of the voluntary urinary sphincter system is considered controversial. Most authors assume that the nerve supply to this sphincter is provided by branches of the pudendal nerve *(32,33)*. However, an innervation of the striated sphincter system in the male under the control of the autonomic nervous system has also been described *(34)*.

It is well known that women treated with a distal partial urethrectomy for problems such as complicated diverticula and tumors may remain continent unless a major portion of the middle third of the urethra has been removed *(35,36)*. It always seemed to be a given fact that the bladder neck together with an adequate length of cranial urethra were mandatory for urinary continence in women.

Recent fetal and adult cadaver dissection studies have shown that the entire rhabdosphincter, which is innervated by the pudendal nerve from below, is located in the caudal half of the urethra and merges approximately halfway with the mid-layer of the proximal smooth musculature. Smooth muscle of the outer and inner layer innervated by the autonomic nerve system, however, is present throughout the whole length of the urethra.

Nerve fibers from the pelvic plexus located dorso-lateral to the rectum have been traced all the way to the bladder neck and urethra running dorsal to the distal ureter, underneath the lateral vesical pedicle, and alongside the lateral walls of the vagina *(14)*. Performing an anterior exenteration with complete resection of the vagina, and with the caudal border of resection being just below the bladder neck would result in dissection of the majority if not all autonomic nerves to the female urethra. However, leaving the lateral vaginal walls intact and with careful dissection of the bladder neck and cranial urethra the majority of plexus fibers to the urethra can be preserved (Fig. 1).

The suspensory fascial reinforcements of the remnant urethra will not be severed when performing a nerve-sparing cystectomy since care is taken to stay as close as possible to the urethra proximally and to abstain completely from any dissection caudal to the level of urethral severing.

Another consideration is the lymphatic drainage of the remnant urethra after cystectomy. Any bladder tumor close to (but not at) the bladder neck with grossly enlarged lymph nodes may cause a reversed lymphatic tumor cell drainage to the external inguinal lymph nodes *(37)* with a chance of periurethral tumor cell nests in the remnant urethra. Preoperatively one should therefore pay attention to enlarged pelvic and inguinal lymph nodes. If biopsies show tumor involvement this should be a relative contraindication for an orthotpic urinary diversion.

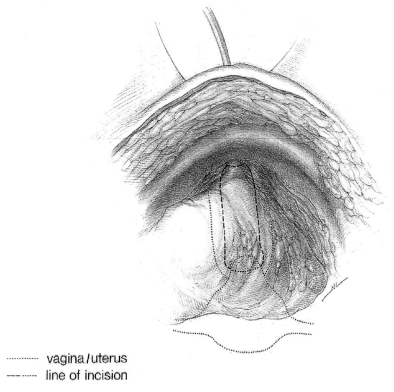

·········· vagina / uterus
— · — ······ line of incision

Fig. 1. Line of incision during nerve-sparing cystectomy in order to preserve autonomous nerve fibers to the remnant urethra. Reproduced with permission from
ref. *(15)*.

PATIENT SELECTION

Female candidates for an orthotopic neobladder to the urethra should be
selected according to tumor extension, urethral competence, general performance status, and motivation (Table 2). We unconditionally exclude
patients with tumor at the bladder neck and/or in the urethra, any positive
surgical margin on intraoperative frozen section, patients with grossly
enlarged positive lymph nodes, and patients with distant metastasis. Apart
from the usual preoperative staging with bimanual and transurethral
tumor evaluation, abdominal and thoracic imaging, and bone scan biopsies of the bladder neck are therefore necessary. Any suspicious lymph
nodes are checked either intraoperatively by frozen section or, e.g.,
inguinally by preoperative biopsy under local anesthesia.

Urethral competence is assessed by the patients' history, endoscopy,
radiography, and intraluminal pressure profile (UPP). Patients with either
a history of stress incontinence of grade II or more due to an incompetent

Table 2

Exclusion Criteria for an Orthotopic Reconstruction of the Lower Urinary
Tract to the Urethra in Female Patients with Bladder or Other Pelvic Tumors

---

Tumor related criteria
Tumor/cis at the bladder neck
Urethral tumor
Any positive surgical margin (frozen section)
$\geq=N_2$
Any tumor involvement of inguinal nodes
M+

Urethral competence
h/o of stress incontinence >= grade 2 due to sphincteric incompetence
Marked urethral hypermobility
$P_{rest} < 30$ cm H_2O in the UPP
Full dose radiation to the urethra

Performance status, motivation
Any reduced performance status (e.g., Karnofsky <=90%)
No motivation to undergo intensive continence training if necessary
No motivation to wear pads if necessary
No motivation or dexterity for clean intermittent catheterization if necessary

---

[a]Cis= carcinoma *in situ*; UPP = intraluminal pressure profile. Adapted from *(16)*.

sphincter, marked urethral hypermobility, or maximal resting pressure
in the UPP of less than 30 cm H_2O are generally excluded.

The preoperative general performance status of patients where an
orthotopic reconstruction to the urethra is anticipated should not be
reduced because they need their strength, among other things, for continence training. Motivation includes the understanding and handling of
specific problems of orthotopic neobladders in females such as possible
urinary retention or post void residuals, and at least initially nocturnal
and diurnal incontinence.

SURGICAL TECHNIQUE

The technique of anterior exenteration together with lymphadenectomy is described elsewhere in this book as well as in the literature. We
therefore describe only variations from this technique for female patients
undergoing an orthotopic reconstruction of the lower urinary tract. All
our patients received an ileal low pressure reservoir—either a so-called
Hemi-Kock *(1)* or a T-pouch *(38)*—with an antireflux protection for the
upper urinary tract and direct anastomosis of the pouch to the remnant
urethra. However, any low pressure reservoir that can be brought to the
remnant urethra is probably suitable *(8,18)*.

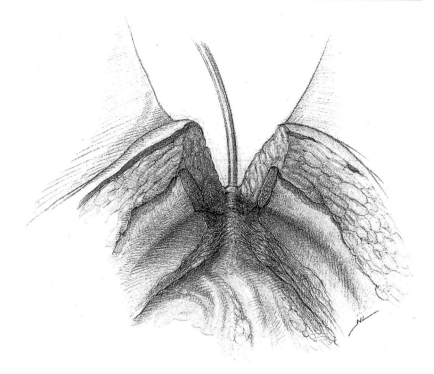

Fig. 2. Schematic drawing of an adult anatomic specimen of the bladder neck and urethra with part of the pubic bone removed. When following the dashed line of incision (---) during dissection and staying close to the urethra and bladder neck, resp., neither the majority of the autonomous nerves to the remnant urethra nor the urethral suspensory system will be destroyed. Reproduced with permission from ref. *(16)*.

To facilitate intraoperative catheterization of the pouch after severing the Foley catheter during cystectomy patients can be placed in a low lithotomy position. In most cases, however, we place the patients in a simple supine position, thus avoiding any possible damage to the lower limbs in connection with positioning.

When performing pelvic lymphadenectomy care is taken to minimize dissection in the region of the upper hypogastric nerve crossing the common iliac artery. Special attention is then directed towards dissection and resection of the inner female genitalia. After the usual mobilization of ovaries, tubes and uterus only the vaginal fundus and the anterior vaginal wall down to the level of the subsequent urethral dissection are resected (Fig. 1). The dorsal half of the vaginal fundus is incised circumferentially around the cervical insertion or scar from a previous hysterectomy. The line of incision is continued ventrally and caudally to include

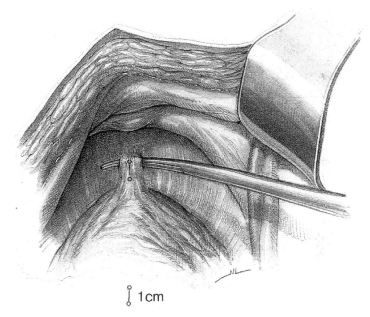

Fig. 3. The urethra is clamped and dissected approximately 0.5–1 cm caudal of the bladder neck. Reproduced with permission from ref. *(15)*.

an approximately 2 cm wide strip of the ventral wall of the vagina. Bladder neck and proximal urethra are then carefully "peeled" out of the surrounding connective tissue and fascia. Care is taken to incise the endopelvic fascia medially where it leaves the bladder surface. Dissection of the proximal urethra is performed by incising the fascia longitudinally in the midline and staying as close to the urethral wall as possible, thereby not destroying the majority of nerve fibers coursing to the remnant urethra (Fig. 2). The proximal urethra with its Foley catheter is clamped with a strong Overholt-clamp and severed approximately 0.5–1 cm distal to the bladder neck (Fig. 3). The operative specimen is then removed and a transverse frozen section of the urethra is sent for an intraoperative pathological diagnosis.

In all our specimens squamous metaplasia was present but no tumor or dysplasia was seen at the level of urethral dissection. In obese patients an ureteral catheter placed antegrade may be an additional help in guiding the final pouch catheter transurethrally prior to closing the urethroileal anastomosis. The vaginal defect is closed transversely with a 0 running polyglycolic acid (PGA) suture (Fig. 4). Into the resulting small vaginal pouch continence training devices may be introduced if necessary. If these women are sexually active the vaginal defect might also be closed with a small detubularized ileal patch.

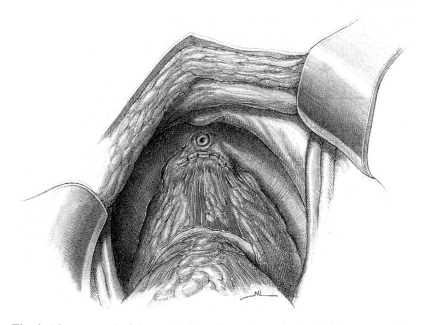

Fig. 4. After removal of the surgical specimen the vagina is closed transversely. Any low-pressure reservoir can now be anastomosed to the remnant urethra. A "J"-omentum flap or additional attachment sutures of the pouch to the pelvic wall are advocated to improve postoperative micturition results. Reproduced with permission from ref. *(15)*.

Any low pressure reservoir can be anastomosed to the remnant urethra, preferably with six 2-0 synthetic absorbable sutures. We have seen that downward migration of the pouch into the wide female pelvis may result in intestinal folds which cause intermittent obstructive valves at the ileo-urethral anastomosis. Instead of anastomosing the spout-like residual opening which is anastomosed to the urethra in the Hemi-Kock or T-pouch, we therefore now use a technique as used in the creation of other pouches in males. Here, a circular ileal opening close to the mesentery at the lowest part of the pouch is anastomosed to the urethra *(39)*.

At the end of the procedure a J-omentum flap is brought down and placed around the bottom part of the pouch *(17)*. Alternatively portions of the ileal pouch adjacent to this anastomosis are sutured to the anterior and lateral pelvic walls as well as the remnant vaginal sac both to avoid the formation of obstructive folds over the urethral anastomosis and to reduce the possibility of creating a "pouchocele" due to descensus of the reservoir postoperatively. Initial attempts to perform a "neobladder neck suspension" in order to improve early continence have failed. These patients went into urinary retention. Suspension of the vaginal vault with remnant portions of the round ligaments or fascial strips in order to prevent kinking of the pouch and accumulation of subsequent residual urine have recently been suggested, but long term data are not available yet.

Both uretero-ileal anastomosis are stented with 7 Fr. single J ureteral catheters which are brought out either transurethrally alongside the urethral catheter or through the lower abdominal wall. Pelvic drains are removed after 5 d, ureteral catheters after approximately 8–10 d and the 20 Fr. urethral catheter after 14 d, provided a previous pouchogram shows no extravasation.

POSTOPERATIVE URODYNAMICS AND CONTINENCE

A routine postoperative urodynamic assessment of the pouch and remaining urethra is not necessary, but was initially performed in 15 patients. The voiding pattern including documented volumes at each micturition was determined by a detailed questionnaire. In order to obtain the maximum pouch volume the average of the 3 maximum volumes were calculated. This served as a value up to which the pouch was filled during urodynamic testing. The calculated bladder capacity in these women ranged from 400–750 cc (mean 560) and post void residuals ranged from 0–150 cc.

The intraluminal pouch pressures at rest were below 30 cm H_2O in all patients but one, who had intermittent peak pressures of up to 38 cm H_2O after 6 mo. Maximum intraluminal urethral pressures in the UPP ranged from 30–35 cm H_2O (mean 32), which was virtually unchanged from preoperative values with an average of 33.4 cm H_2O (range 28–42 cm H_2O).

In evaluating diurnal and nocturnal continence we used definitions from the recent literature (20). In patients followed for more than 6 mo daytime continence was achieved in 87.5%, and nocturnal continence in 79%. It is interesting to note that only 25% of the patients with preoperative radiation (all of them due to gynecological tumors) had regained diurnal continence whereas all the others had grade I–II stress incontinence. Therefore a full course of preoperative radiation may be seen as a relative contraindication for this type of surgery unless the patient is willing to take the risk of placement of an artificial sphincter.

Urinary retention or post void residuals of 50%+ of the voided volume was successfully treated in patients with an ileal valve partially or totally obstructing the neobladder outlet. This entity, which was first described in one of our recent publications (16), is seen endoscopically when putting the cystoscope just below the bladder neck and draining the pouch.

These valves can be carefully incised, thereby correcting the problem completely.

SUMMARY

Recent larger series seem to confirm the initial preliminary results showing that sparing the urethra at cystectomy will not compromise oncological outcome and can be satisfactorily used for orthotopic reconstruction of the lower urinary tract. Diurnal and nocturnal continence rates of 87.5% and 79%, respectively, and clean intermittent catheterization in approximately 10% after 6 mo are results easily comparable to larger male series and justify the use of orthotopic neobladders as the procedure of choice in selected females as well.

We know now that urinary continence of any bladder substitution can be maintained despite removal of the bladder neck and the adjacent proximal urethra. In our anatomical studies as well as those of others no prominent sphincteric structure was present either in the female bladder neck or cranial urethra. The bulk of the striated intrinsic sphincter (Rhabdosphincter) lies in the mid to caudal third of the urethra and is not removed with proximal urethrectomy as described above. Its innervation via the pudendal nerve is not disturbed during this type of surgery.

Controversy still exists whether dissecting the autonomic nerves to the urethra originating in both pelvic plexus when performing a subtotal vaginectomy and resection of the bladder neck including a wide margin of surrounding tissue compromises long term results. We do not know if these autonomic nerves are needed for a satisfactory function of the urethral smooth muscles. Nor can we say to what extent we are able to spare these nerves at each individual surgery. Based on our antomical and functional studies, however, we believe that most of the autonomic innervation of the remnant urethra should stay intact postoperatively in order to preserve both muscular resistance and continence despite removal of a safe segment the proximal urethra for oncological reasons.

Postoperative results can be optimized by:

1. Performing a nerve-sparing anterior exenteration leaving posterior and lateral vaginal walls intact, carefully dissecting out bladder neck and proximal urethra.
2. Removal of 0.5–1 cm of cranial urethra *en bloc* with the cystectomy specimen and obtain a frozen section of the whole urethral circumference.
3. Use of a low pressure reservoir for urinary diversion.
4. Prevention of complications due to a downward migration of the pouch either with a J-omentum flap or with stay sutures between pouch wall and surrounding pelvic structures.

REFERENCES

1. Skinner DG, Boyd SD, Lieskovsky G, Bennett C, Hopwood B. Lower urinary tract reconstruction following cystectomy: experience and results in 126 patients using the Kock ileal reservoir with bilateral ureteroileal urethrostomy. J Urol 1991; 146: 756–760.

2. Studer UE, Danuser H, Merz VW, Springer JP, Zingg EJ. Experience in 100 patients with an ileal low pressure bladder substitute combined with an afferent tubular isoperistaltic segment. J Urol 1995; 154: 49–56.

3. Light K. Long term results using the artificial sphincter around bowel. Br J Urol 1989; 64: 56.

4. Pawlick K. Exstirpace mechyre mocoveho. Lekaru Ceskych, 1890; xxix: 705–706.

5. Lotheissen G. Ueber Uretertransplantationen. Wiener Klin Wochenschrift 1899; 12: 883–889.

6. Coffey R. Physiologic implantation of the severed ureter or common bile duct into the intestine. JAMA 1911; 56: 397–401.

7. Skinner DG, Studer UE, Okada K, Aso Y, Hautmann H, Koontz W, et al. Which patients are suitable for continent diversion or bladder substitution following cystectomy or other definitive local treatment? Int J Urol 1995; 2: 105–112.

8. Cancrini A, de Carli P, Fattahi H, Pompeo V, Cantiani R, von Heland M. Orthotopic ileal neobladder in female patients after radical cystectomy: 2-year experience. J Urol 1994; 153: 956–958.

9. Tobisu K-I, Coloby P, Fujimoto H, Miutani T, Kakizoe T. An ileal neobladder for a female patient after radical cystectomy to ensure voiding from the urethra: a case report. Jpn J Clin Oncol 1992; 22: 359–363.

10. Stein J, Stenzl A, Esrig D, Freeman J, Boyd S, Lieskovsky G, et al. Lower urinary tract reconstruction following cystectomy in women using the Kock ileal reservoir with bilateral ureteroileal urethrostomy: initial clinical experience. J Urol 1994; 152: 1404–1408.

11. Coloby P, Kakizoe T, Tobisu K-I, Sakamoto M. Urethral involvement in female bladder cancer patients: mapping of 47 consecutive cysto-urethrectomy specimens. J Urol 1994; 152: 1438–1442.

12. Stein J, Cote R, Freeman J, Esrig D, Skinner E, Boyd S, et al. Lower urinary tract reconstruction in women following cystectomy for pelvic malignancy: a pathologic review of female cystectomy specimens. J Urol 1994; 151: 304A, abstract 308.

13. Stenzl A, Draxl H, Posch B, Colleselli K, Falk M, Bartsch G. The risk of urethral tumors in female bladder cancer: can the urethra be used for orthotopic reconstruction of the lower urinary tract? J Urol 1995; 153: 950–955.

14. Colleselli K, Stenzl A, Eder R, Strasser H, Poisel S, Bartsch G. The female urethral sphincter: a morphological and topographical study. J Urol 1998; 160: 49–54.

15. Stenzl A, Colleselli K, Poisel S, Feichtinger H, Pontasch H, Bartsch G. Rationale and technique of nerve sparing radical cystectomy before an orthotopic neobladder procedure in women. J Urol 1995; 154: 2044–2049, © Springer-Verlag GmbH & Co. KG, Germany.

16. Stenzl A, Colleselli K, Bartsch G. Update of urethra-sparing approaches in cystectomy in women. World J Urol 1997; 15: 134–138.

17. Stenzl A, Colleselli K, Poisel S, Feichtinger H, Bartsch G. The use of neobladders in women undergoing cystectomy for transitional-cell cancer. World J Urol 1996; 14: 15–21.

18. Hautmann R, Paiss T, Kleinschmidt K, de Petriconi R. The ileal neobladder in the female: why it works or not. J Urol 1995; 153: 243A, abstract 58.

19. Jarolim L, Babjuk M, Hanus T, Jansky M, Skrivanova V. Female urethra-sparing cystectomy and orthotopic bladder replacement. Eur Urol 1997; 31: 173–177.

20. Stein JP, Grossfeld GD, Freeman JA, Esrig D, Ginsberg DA, Cote RJ, et al. Orthotopic lower urinary tract reconstruction in women using the Kock ileal neobladder: updated experience in 34 patients. J Urol 1997; 158: 400–405.

21. Stenzl A, Colleselli K, Poisel S, Feichtinger H, Bartsch G. Anterior exenteration with subsequent ureteroileal urethrostomy in females. Anatomy, risk of urethral recurrence, surgical technique, and results. Eur Urol 1998; 33: 18–20.

22. Stenzl A, Draxl H, Posch B, Colleselli K, Falk M, Bartsch G. The risk of urethral tumors in female bladder cancer: can the urethra be used for orthotopic reconstruction of the lower urinary tract? J Urol 1995; 153: 950-955 issn: 0022-5347.

23. Packham D. The epithelial lining of the female trigone and urethra. Br J Urol 1971; 43: 201.

24. Wiener D, Koss L, Salaby B, Freed S. The prevalence and significance of Brunn´s nests, cystitis cystica, and squamous metaplasia in normal bladders. J Urol 1979; 122: 317.

25. De Paepe M, André R, Mahadevia P. Urethral involvement in female patients with bladder cancer. A study of 22 cystectomy specimens. Cancer 1990; 65: 1237–1242.

26. Ashworth A. Papillomatosis of the urethra. Br J Urol 1956; 28: 3–11.

27. Erckert M, Stenzl A, Falk M, Bartsch G. The incidence of urethral tumor involvement in male bladder cancer patients. World J Urol 1996; 14; 3–8.

28. Hautmann RE. Neobladder and bladder replacement. Eur Urol 1998; 33: 512.

29. Studer UE, Danuser H, Hochreiter W, Springer JP, Turner WH, Zingg EJ. Summary of 10 years' experience with an ileal low-pressure bladder substitute combined with an afferent tubular isoperistaltic segment. World J Urol 1996; 14: 29–39.

30. Iselin CE, Robertson CN, Webster GD, Vieweg J, Paulson DF. Does prostate transitional cell carcinoma preclude orthotopic bladder reconstruction after radical cystoprostatectomy for bladder cancer? J Urol 1997; 158: 2123–2126.

31. Wein A, Levin R, Barrett D. Voiding function: relevant anatomy, physiology, and pharmacology. In: *Adult and Pediatric Urology* (Gillenwater J, Grayhack J, Howards S, Duckett J, eds.) 2nd ed, Chicago, IL, Year Book, 1991, pp. 933–999.

32. Gosling JA, Dixon JS, Critchley HO, Thompson SA. A comparative study of the human external sphincter and periurethral levator ani muscles. Br J Urol 1981; 53: 35–41.

33. Tanagho EA, Meyers FH, Smith DR. Urethral resistance: its components and implications. II. Striated muscle component. Invest Urol 1969; 7: 195–205.

34. Donker P, Droes J, Van Ulden B. Anatomy of the musculature and innervation of the bladder and the urethra. In: *Scientific Foundations of Urology* (Williams D, Chisthol G, eds.). Heinemann, London, 32. vol II, 1976.

35. Neuwirth H, Stenzl A, de Kernion J. Urethral cancer. In: *Cancer Treatment* (Haskell C, ed.). WB Saunders, Philadelphia, PA, 1990, pp. 762–764.

36. Spence H, Duckett J. Diverticulum of the female urethra: clinical aspects and presentation of a simple operative technique for cure. J Urol 1970; 104: 432.

37. Reiffenstuhl G. Das Lymphsystem des weiblichen Genitale. Urban & Schwarzenberg, Munich, 1957.

38. Stein JP, Lieskovsky G, Ginsberg DA, Bochner BH, Skinner DG. The T pouch: an orthotopic ileal neobladder incorporating a serosal lined ileal antireflux technique. J Urol 1998; 159: 1836–1842.

39. Studer U, Ackermann D, Casanova G, Zingg E. Three year´s experience with an ileal low pressure bladder substitute. Br J Urol 1989; 63: 43–52.

15 Current Prospects for the Use of Molecular Markers in Treatment of Bladder Cancer by Cystectomy or Bladder-Conserving Approaches

Guido Dalbagni, MD,
Carlos Cordon-Cardo, MD, PHD,
and Joel Sheinfeld, MD

Contents

INTRODUCTION

Clinically, "superficial" bladder tumors (stages Ta, Tis, and T1) account for 75% to 85% of urothelial neoplasms, while the remaining 15–25% are invasive (T2, T3, T4) or metastatic (N+,M+) lesions at the time of initial presentation *(1)*. Over 70% of patients with superficial tumors will have one or more recurrences after initial treatment, and about one-third of those patients will progress and eventually succumb to their disease *(2)*. It is for these reasons that new methods are being developed to identify and monitor those patients presenting with superficial tumors who are likely to develop recurrent and invasive carcinoma.

In patients who present initially with invasive disease, we are faced with two major problems. First, despite aggressive surgical resection and adjuvant radiotherapy and/or chemotherapy, the overall cure rate

From: *Current Clinical Urology: Bladder Cancer: Current Diagnosis and Treatment*
Edited by: M. J. Droller © Humana Press Inc., Totowa, NJ

remains in the range of 20–50%. In addition, distant micrometastatic disease, unrecognized at the time of initial diagnosis and treatment, occurs in a substantial percentage of patients and is the major cause of treatment failure and subsequent death.

It is becoming increasingly evident that morphological changes and their clinical manifestations are preceded by molecular and biochemical alterations. Since selection criteria to determine treatment for a particular tumor in a particular patient are incompletely defined, new biological determinants are needed for proper selection and monitoring of therapy.

It is well known that morphologically similar tumors may behave in radically different fashions, a fact that seriously hampers the ability to accurately predict clinical outcome and properly designed therapeutic intervention in a given case. The use of modern molecular and immunochemical techniques has led to remarkable progress in our understanding of cell growth and differentiation, these being key issues in tumor development and progression. Biologic markers that correlate with tumor behavior and response to therapy are constantly being identified. The implementation of objective predictive assays to our armamentarium of diagnostic and prognostic tools will enhance our ability to assess tumor biological activities and to design effective treatment regimens.

We will discuss new markers, in the context of the cell cycle, that might help identifying molecular subgroups with similar clinical behavior. These new markers, if prospectively validated, will help tailoring treatment according to the predicted clinical outcome.

THE CELL CYCLE (FIG. 1)

Cyclins and Cyclin-Dependent Kinases (Cdk)

Cellular proliferation follows an orderly progression through the cell cycle, which is controlled by protein complexes composed of cyclins and cyclin-dependent kinases (Cdk) *(3–5)*. The cyclins can be defined as a set of periodic proteins that are synthesized at determined phases of the cell cycle and then suddenly degraded *(6)*. The current model for the enzymatically active complexes consist of a cyclin as regulatory molecule and a Cdk as catalytic subunit. Their regulatory function is achieved by phosphorylation of fundamental elements involved in cell cycle transitions, such as the retinoblastoma protein. An analogy may be drawn between these cyclin-Cdk complexes and those formed by growth factor receptors with kinase activity upon binding to their corresponding physiological ligands, the end result being the phosphorylation of particular substrates.

Multiple cyclins have been isolated and characterized, and a temporal map of their expression during cell cycle progression delineated.

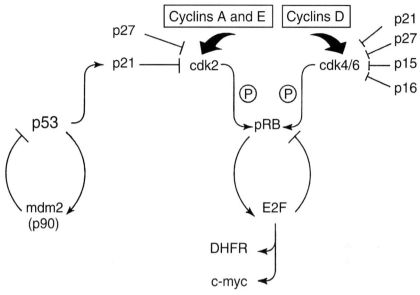

Fig. 1. The cell cycle.

Briefly, five major classes of mammalian cyclins (termed A–E) have been described. Cyclins C, D1–3 and E reach their peak of synthesis and activity during the G1 phase and apparently regulate the transition of a cell from G1 to S phase. On the other hand, cyclins A and B1–2 achieve their maximal levels later in the cycle, during S and G2 phases, and are regarded as regulators of the transition to mitosis.

Similarly, multiple Cdk molecules are being identified and their cyclin partners and patterns of cell cycle specificity distinguished. It is postulated that the complexes formed by cyclin D1 and Cdk4 govern G1 progression, while cyclin E-Cdk2 controls entry into S phase. Cyclin A-Cdk2 units effect their regulation through S phase, and cyclin B-cdc2 (also known as Cdk1) control entry into mitosis (4,7). Several studies have suggested that gene amplification and overexpression of cyclin D1 and Cdk4 are oncogenic events in certain tumors, probably related to tumor progression.

p53 and pRB are Cell Cycle Regulators

Findings from several lines of investigation suggest that p53 controls a cell cycle checkpoint responsible for maintaining the integrity of the genome. It has been shown that wild-type *p53* mediates arrest of the cell cycle in the G1 phase after sublethal DNA damage (8). In addition, p53 appears to be involved in transcriptional control (9,10). Like most of the well-characterized transcription factors, p53 proteins possess a nuclear localization signal and a sequence-specific DNA-binding domain (11).

The retinoblastoma gene encodes an approximately 105 kDa nuclear phosphoprotein *(12–14)*. While the amount of pRB does not change during progression of the cell cycle, the phosphorylation state of pRB is cell cycle dependent, and is a target for the enzymatic activity of cyclin-Cdk complexes *(15–17)*. pRB is in the underphosphorylated form in G1, and as cells progress into late G1 and early S phase, pRB becomes highly phosphorylated and remains phosphorylated in G2. The underphosphorylated form of pRB is believed to be the functionally active form of pRB in G0/middle G1 *(18)*. pRB can complex stably by the interaction of this region with cellular proteins, including members of the E2F family *(19–20)*.

E2F is a 60 kDa transcription factor originally identified through its role in transcriptional activation of the adenovirus E2 promoter *(21)*. Unbound E2F transcription factors could stimulate transcription of cellular genes. E2F sites are present in genes implicated in induction of S phase, such as thymidine kinase, Myc, Myb, dihydrofolate reductase and DNA polymerase *(22)*. This suggests that E2F family members may be responsible for traversing the G1/S restriction point of the cell cycle *(23)*.

A relationship between *p53* and *pRB* in cell cycle regulation is suggested based on the action of two novel genes that are regulated by p53: the *MDM2* and the *p21* (also known as *WAF1*, *Cip1* and *Sdi1*) genes. The *MDM2* gene maps to the long arm of chromosome 12 and is under transcriptional control by wild-type p53 (wt p53) *(24–26)*. The product encoded by *MDM2* is a 90 kDa zinc-finger protein (mdm2), that also contains a p53-binding site *(26)*. It has been shown that mdm2 proteins bind to p53 and act as a negative regulator, inhibiting wt p53 transcriptional regulatory activity and creating an autoregulatory feedback loop. It is postulated that overexpression of mdm2 inactivates both p53 and Rb.

An alternative pathway of p53-pRB interaction is mediated by *p21*. (The *p21* gene belongs to a new family of negative cell cycle regulators, functioning as cyclin-dependent kinase inhibitory molecules.) *p21* inactivates cyclin-Cdk complexes that, as described, target pRB phosphorylation *(27–29)*. In that context, *p21* serves as an effector of cell cycle arrest in response to activation of the p53 G1 phase checkpoint pathway. These findings imply a potential link between p53 and pRB in cell cycle regulation, apoptosis, and tumor progression.

Cyclin-Dependent Kinase Inhibitors: Negative Regulators

A new family of negative cell cycle regulators which functions as Cdk-inhibitory molecules has been identified, and the genes that encode these proteins designated *CKI* genes. The mechanism whereby they achieve their function appears to be through the formation of stable complexes that inactivate the catalytically operative units. The first and probably best characterized member of this family is *p21* (described above), which inactivates cyclin E-cdk2, cyclin A-cdk2, and cyclins D1-, D2- and D3-cdk4 complexes *(28–30)*. As mentioned, these are components of the regulatory kinases that target pRB for phosphorylation.

Another member of the *CKI* group is p16, which encodes a 148 aa protein of Mr 15,845 *(31)*. Unlike *p21*, p16 forms binary complexes specifically with Cdk4 and Cdk6, inhibiting their activity and, by doing so, also inhibiting pRB phosphorylation. However, p16 does not interact with Cdc2 or Cdk2 *(31)*.

Very recently, the *p15/INK4B* gene has been reported, which encodes a protein of 137 aa with Mr 14,700, and shown to be a potential effector of TGFβ induced cell cycle arrest *(32)*. *p15* has substantial homology to p16. *p15* has the ability to form binary complexes, to bind and inactivate Cdk4 and Cdk6, inhibiting pRB phosphorylation. These two genes map to the short arm of chromosome 9 (9p21), a region that accounts for loss of heterozygosity and homozygous deletions in various human tumor cell lines. Since these genes are also mutated in primary tumors, they are likely to be relevant candidate tumor suppressor genes.

Two new members have been added to this rapidly growing group of Cdk-inhibitors: p27/Kip1 *(33–35)* and p18 *(36)*. p27 is a negative regulator implicated in G1 phase arrest by TGFβ, cell–cell contact, agents that elevate cyclic AMP, and the growth inhibitory drug rapamycin. p27/Kip1, which shares sequence homology with p21/WAF and its encoded product (198 aa–Mr 22,257), associates with cyclin E-Cdk2, cyclin A-Cdk2, and cyclin D-Cdk4 complexes, abrogating their activity *(37)*. Recently, the cloning of *p18* has been reported *(36)*. This gene encodes a 168 aa protein (Mr 18,116) that is a homolog of p16/INK4A. *p18* interacts with Cdk4 and Cdk6 and inhibits the kinase activity of cyclin D-Cdk4 and -Cdk6 complexes.

ALTERATIONS
OF THE CELL CYCLE AND BLADDER CANCER
Cyclin Dependent Kinases (CDK)

Loss of genetic material on chromosome 9 is an early abnormality detected in bladder tumors *(38–41)*. More recently, the existence of two altered loci, one in each of both chromosome 9 arms, was postulated *(42, 43)*. A detailed analyses conducted by Orlow et al. on 73 bladder tumors showed that two regions, one on 9p at the IFN cluster (9p21), and the other on 9q associated with the q34.1–2 bands, had the highest frequencies of allelic losses *(44)*.

The 9p21 region has been found to be mutated frequently in a wide variety of human tumor cell lines, and the search for a putative tumor suppressor gene in this region led to the characterization of the so-called multiple tumor suppressor 1 (*MTS1*) gene *(45)*. It was confirmed that the *MTS1* gene was the previously identified *p16/INK4A/CDKN2* (*p16*) gene *(46)*. In addition to the p16, the p15/INK4B/MTS2 (*p15*) gene is found in tandem at 9p21 *(47)*. These genes encode members of a new family of negative cell cycle regulators, which products function as cyclin-dependent kinase inhibitory molecules *(46–48)*. The initial enthusiasm over the high frequency of mutations of these genes in cell lines was restrained by reports from a number of investigators who failed to observe appreciable frequencies in primary human tumor material. Nevertheless, several independent groups of investigators have shown more recently that genetic alterations mainly of *p16*, as well as deletions of *p15*, are common events in certain human primary tumors, including bladder cancer *(49–54)*. Moreover, it has been shown that genetic alterations of *p16* are independent of TP53 mutations, suggesting that *p16* and *p53* function in separate pathways of tumor suppression *(53)*. Orlow et al. have very recently reported an overall frequency of deletions and rearrangements for the *p16* and *p15* genes in bladder cancer of 19% and 18%, respectively *(54)*. Moreover, this study revealed that *p16* and *p15* alterations were associated with low stage, low grade bladder tumors.

It should be emphasized that only Ta and T1, but not Tis, lesions showed deletions of either *p16* or *p15*. Since *p16* alterations occur independently of *p53* mutations *(53)*, and *p53* mutations are frequent events in Tis bladder tumors *(55)*, data from that report further support the hypothesis that bladder carcinogenesis may develop through two distinct molecular pathways *(39,56)*. Taken together, the results suggest that *p16* and *p15* alterations confer selective growth advantage to urothelial tumor cells, but mutations in other genes are required to produce an overt malignant phenotype.

P53, RB

The potential relevance of RB alterations in bladder cancer was disclosed in two independent studies *(57,58)*. Using a mouse monoclonal antibody (mAB) and IHC in frozen tissue sections of 48 primary bladder tumors, Cordon-Cardo and collaborators *(57)* found normal levels of pRB expression in 34 cases. However, a spectrum of altered patters of expression, from undetectable pRB levels to heterogeneous expression of pRB, was observed in 14 patients. Thirteen of the 38 patients diagnosed with muscle invasive tumors were categorized as pRB altered, while only one of the 10 superficial carcinomas had the altered pRB phenotype. The survival was significantly decreased in pRB altered patients compared to those with normal pRB expression ($p < 0.001$) *(57)*.

Similarly, Logothetis et al. found altered pRB expression in locally advanced bladder cancer *(58)*. Forty-three patients were evaluated using the Rb-WL-1 polyclonal antiserum and IHC. These investigators reported altered pRB expression in 37% of the tumor specimens analyzed. There was a significant decrease in disease-free survival for patients with documented abnormal pRB levels. Taken together, these data suggested that altered pRB expression occurred in all grades and stages of bladder cancer, but was more commonly associated with muscle invasive tumors. Moreover, altered patterns of pRB may become an important prognostic variable in patients presenting with invasive bladder cancer.

The clinical implications of detecting TP53 mutations and altered patterns of its encoded product (*p53*) in bladder tumors has been the focus of a series of investigations *(59–68)*. Early studies revealed that *p53* mutations were common events in bladder cancer and associated with tumor stage and grade *(59,60)*. Dalbagni et al. correlated alterations of chromosome 17 with p53 nuclear overexpression in a cohort of 60 bladder tumors *(61)*. Deletion of 17p correlated with grade ($p = 0.039$) and stage ($p = 0.004$), while p53 nuclear overexpression correlated with grade ($p = 0.027$), stage ($p = 0.008$), vascular invasion ($p = 0.021$) and the presence of nodal metastases ($p = 0.007$). There was a strong correlation between the p53 overexpression and *p53* deletions ($p < 0.001$).

Following this study, Cordon-Cardo et al. designed a study to evaluate the sensitivity and specificity of different laboratory assays directed to the identification of *p53* mutations (including IHC with mAB PAb1801, RFLP, PCR-SSCP, and sequencing) *(62)*. Using this approach, they also tested the hypothesis that p53 nuclear overexpression detected by IHC can reliably identify the presence of mutant *p53* products in bladder neoplasms. Nuclear immunoreactivities were observed in 26 of 42 bladder tumors analyzed. Abnormal shifts in mobility were noted in 14 of the 42 cases in distinct exons. There was a strong association between p53 nuclear overexpression and 17p LOH ($p < 0.001$), as well as p53 nuclear overexpression and detection of *p53* mutations by SSCP and sequencing ($p < 0.001$). Using receiver operating curve (ROC) statistical analysis the accuracy of detecting *p53* mutations by IHC was estimated to be 90.3%. In addition, this study defined 20% tumor cells displaying nuclear immunoreactivities as an appropriate cutoff point for IHC (p53-positive phenotype).

The aim of a subsequent group of analyses was to investigate the hypothesis that altered patterns of p53 expression correlated with tumor progression in patients with superficial bladder tumors. Detection of p53 nuclear overexpression was evaluated by IHC using mAB PAb1801 on deparaffinized tissue sections in tumors from 43 patients with T1 bladder cancer *(63)*, 54 patients with Ta neoplasms *(64)*, and 33 patients affected with pure Tis *(65)*. Nuclear *p53* overexpression was correlated with clinicopathological variables, and results submitted to Fisher exact test, as well as univariate and multivariate *(63–65)*. The median followup for these cohorts of patients was 119, 110, and 124 mo, respectively. Patients in each stage were stratified into two groups, utilizing the cutoff point identified through the ROC analysis previously conducted (20% nuclear positive tumor cells) *(62)*. A strong association was found between tumor progression and *p53*-positive phenotype in the three studies ($p < 0.01$). Moreover, nuclear overexpression of p53 was an independent variable associated with disease progression and death due to bladder cancer.

Two studies dealing with p53 nuclear overexpression conducted in unselected bladder cancer patients were recently reported. Lipponen analyzed 212 bladder tumors, using IHC and 20% positive nuclear staining as the cutoff value *(56)*. However, the primary antibody used was a purified rabbit polyserum (NCL-CM1-1:150 dilution). The mean followup time was over 10 yr. Nuclear overexpression of p53 was associated with tumor grade and disease progression. In univariate analysis p53 overexpression predicted poor outcome in the entire cohort. However, overexpression of p53 had no independent prognostic value over clinical stage and mitotic index in a multivariate survival analysis. Esrig et al. determined the relation between nuclear accumulation of p53 and tumor progression in a cohort of 243 patients treated by radical cystectomy utilizing IHC and antibody PAb1801 *(67)*. These investigators noticed that detection of nuclear p53 was significantly associated with an increased risk of recurrence ($p < 0.001$) and decreased overall survival ($p < 0.001$). Moreover, *p53*-positive phenotype was an independent predictor of recurrence and survival.

CONCLUSION

The neoadjuvant use of chemotherapy offers the advantages of bladder preservation and early treatment of micrometastases in patients diagnosed with invasive bladder cancer. However, despite the chemosensitivity of invasive urothelial neoplasms, complete pathologic response in the primary lesion occurs in only 20–30% of patients. In order to determine whether aberrant p53 expression has independent significance for response, relapse, and survival in patients with muscle-invasive bladder cancer treated with neoadjuvant M-VAC chemotherapy, Sarkis et al. evaluated 90 patients who received this regimen with a median followup of 5.8 yr *(68)*. Patients whose tumors had *p53*-positive phenotype ($n = 47$) had a significantly higher proportion of cancer deaths. Multivariate analysis revealed that *p53* overexpression had independent significance for long-term survival ($p < 0.001$) *(68)*.

The proper diagnosis, management, and overall control of cancer is a major challenge in clinical oncology. Because the modality of therapy primarily depends on morphological evaluation and clinical staging, the diagnosis carries significant consequences. However, it is well known that morphologically similar tumors presenting in any assigned stage may behave in radically different fashions, a fact that seriously hampers the ability to accurately predict clinical behavior in a given case. The use of modern molecular and immunohistochemical techniques has led to remarkable progress in our understanding of cell growth, differentiation, and programmed cell death, these being key issues in tumor development and progression.

Biological markers, such as alterations of *p53* and *RB*, that correlate with tumor behavior when detected in specific tumor types await validation studies. Similarly, prospective clinical analyses utilizing well characterized cohorts of patients and properly selected normal and tumor paired samples are needed to better delineate the role of mutations occurring in these genes, as they may impact on the management of patients affected with cancer. The implementation of objective predictive assays to our diagnostic and prognostic tools will enhance our ability to assess tumor biological activities and to design effective treatment regimens. The need now is to translate this newly developed scientific information into diagnostic and prognostic strategies. Other challenges that we are facing relate not only to the clinical applicability of these tools, but also to the ethical issues that are raised when these genetic aberrations are detected.

REFERENCES

1. Prout GR. Bladder carcinoma and a TNM system of classifiction. J Urol 1977; 117: 583–588.
2. Reuter VE, Melamed MR. The lower urinary tract, In: *Diagnostic Surgical Pathology* (Sternberg SS, ed.). Raven, New York, NY, pp. 1355.
3. Murray AW, Hunt T. The cell cycle, an introduction. Freeman, New York, NY, 1993.
4. Nurse P. Universal control mechanism in regulating onset of M-phase. Nature 1990; 344: 503–508.
5. Reed SI. The role of p34 kinases in the G1 to S-phase transition. Ann Rev Cell Biol 1992; 8: 529–561.
6. Evans T, Rosenthal ET, Youngblom J, Distel D, Hunt T. Cyclin: a protein specified by maternal mRNA in sea urchin eggs that is destroyed at each cleavage division. Cell 1983; 33: 389–396.

7. Lewin B. Driving the cell cycle: M phase kinase, its partners, and substrates. Cell 1990; 61: 743–752.

8. Kastan MB, Onkyekwere O, Sidransky D, Vogelstein B, Craig RW. Participation of p53 protein in the cellular response to DNA damage. Cancer Res 1991; 51: 6304–6311.

9. Zambetti G, Bargonetti J, Walker K, Prives C, Levine AJ. Wild-type p53 mediates positive regulation of gene expression through a specific DNA sequence element. Genes Dev 1992; 6: 1143–1152.

10. Kern SE, Pietenpol JA, Thiagalingam S, Seymour A, Kinzler KW, Vogelstein B. Oncogenic forms of p53 inhibit p53-regulated gene expression. Science 1992; 256: 827–830.

11. Fields S, Jang SK. Presence of a potent transcription activating sequence in the p53 protein. Science 1990; 249: 1046–1049.

12. Friend SH, Horowitz JM, Gerber MR, Wang XF, Bogenmann E, Li FP, Weinberg RA. Deletions of a DNA sequence in retinoblastomas and mesenchymal tumors: organization of the sequence and its encoded protein. Proc Natl Acad Sci USA 1987; 84: 9059–9063.

13. Lee W-H, Shew J-Y, Hong FD, Sery TW, Donoso LA, Young LJ, et al. The retinoblastoma susceptibility gene encodes a nuclear phosphoprotein associated with DNA binding activity. Nature 1987; 329: 642–645.

14. Fung Y-K, Murphree AL, T'Ang A, Qian J, Hinrichs SH, Benedict WF. Structural evidence for the authenticity of the human retinoblastoma gene. Science 1987; 236: 1657–1661.

15. DeCaprio JA, Ludlow JW, Lynch D, Furukawa Y, Griffin J, Piwnica-Worms H, et al. The product of the retinoblastoma susceptibility gene has properties of a cell cycle regulatory element. Cell 1989; 58: 1085–1095.

16. Buchkovich K, Duffy LA, Harlow E. The retinoblastoma protein is phosphorylated during specific phases of the cell cycle. Cell 1989; 58: 1097–1105.

17. Chen PL, Scully P, Shew J-Y, Wang JY, Lee WH. Phosphorylation of the retinoblastoma gene product is modulated during the cell cycle and cellular differentiation. Cell 1989; 58: 1193–1198.

18. Mittnacht S, Weinberg RA. G1/S phosphorylation of the retinoblastoma protein is associated with an altered affinity for the nuclear compartment. Cell 1991; 65: 381–393.

19. DeFeo-Jones D, Huang PS, Jones RE, Haskell KM, Vuocolo GA, Hanobik MG, et al. Cloning of cDNAs for cellular proteins that bind to the retinoblastoma gene product. Nature 1991; 352: 251–254.

20. Chellappan SP, Hiebert S, Mudryj M, Horowitz JM, Nevins JR. The E2F transcription factor is a cellular target for the RB protein. Cell 1991; 65: 1053–1061.

21. Kovesdi I, Reichel R, Nevins JR. Identification of a cellular transcription factor involved in E1A trans-activation. Cell 1986; 45: 219–228.

22. Johnson DJ, Schwarz JK, Cress WD, Nevins JR. Expression of transcription factor E2F1 induces quiescent cells to enter S phase. Nature 1993; 365: 349–352.

23. Weintraub SJ, Prater CA, Dean C. Retinoblastoma protein switches the E2F site from positive to negative element. Nature 1992; 358: 259–261.

24. Fakharzadeh SS, Trusko SP, George DL. Tumorigenic potential associated with enhanced expression of a gene that is amplified in a mouse tumor cell line. EMBO J 1991; 10: 1565–1569.

25. Momand J, Zambetti GP, Olson DC, George D, Levine AJ. The mdm-2 oncogene product forms a complex with the p53 protein and inhibits p53-mediated transactivation. Cell 1992; 69: 1237–1245.

26. Oliner JD, Kinzler KW, Metlzer PS, George DL, Vogelstein B. Amplification of a gene encoding a p53 associated protein in human sarcomas. Nature 1992; 358: 80–83.

27. Xiong Y, Zhang H, Beach D. Subunit rearrangement of the cylin-dependent kinases is associated with cellular transformation. Genes Dev 1993; 7: 1572–1583.

28. Harper JW, Adami GR, Wei N, Keyomarsi K, Elledge SJ. The p21 cdk-interacting protein Cip1 is a potent inhibitor of G1 cyclin-dependent kinases. Cell 1993; 75: 805–816.

29. El-Deiry WS, Tokino T, Velculescu VE, Levy DB, Parsons R, Trent JM, et al. WAF1, a potential mediator of p53 tumor suppression. Cell 1993; 75: 817–825.

30. Xiong Y, Hannon GJ, Zhang H, Casso D, Kobayashi R, Beach D. p21 is a universal inhibitor of cyclin kinases. Nature 1993; 366: 701–704.

31. Serrano M, Hannon GJ, Beach D. A new regulatory motif in cell-cycle control causing specific inhibition of cyclin D/CDK4. Nature 1993; 366: 704–707.

32. Hannon GJ, Beach D. p15^{INK4B} is a potential effector of TGF-β-induced cell cycle arrest. Nature 1994; 371: 257–261.

33. Polyak K, Kato J-Y, Solomon MJ, Sherr CJ, Massague J, Roberts JM, Koff A. p27^{Kip1}, a cylin-Cdk inhibitor, links transforming growth factor-β and contact inhibition to cell cycle arrest. Genes Develop 1994; 8: 9–22.

34. Polyak K, Lee M-H, Erdjument-Bromage H, Koff A, Roberts JM, Tempst P, Massague J. Cloning of p27^{Kip1}, a cyclin-dependent kinase inhibitor and a potential mediator of extracellular antimitogenic signals. Cell 1994; 78: 59–66.

35. Toyoshima H, Hunter T. p27, a novel inhibitor of G1 cyclin-cdk protein kinase activity, is related to p21. Cell 1994; 78: 67–74.

36. Guan K-L, Jenkins CW, Li Y, Nichols MA, Wu X, O'Keefe CL, et al. Growth suppression by p18, a p16$^{INK4/MTS1}$- and p14$^{INK4B/MTS2}$-related CDK6 inhibitor, correlates with wild-type pRB function. Genes Develop 1994; 8: 2939–2952.

37. Gibas Z, Prout GR, Connolly JG, Pontes JE, Sandberg AA. Nonrandom chromosomal changes in transitional cell carcinoma of the bladder. Cancer Res 1984; 44: 1257.

38. Tsai YC, Nichols PW, Hiti AL, Williams Z, Skinner DG, Jones PA. Allelic losses of chromosomes 9, 11, and 17 in human bladder cancer. Cancer Res 1990; 50: 44.

39. Dalbagni G, Presti J, Reuter V, Fair WR, Cordon-Cardo C. Genetic alterations in bladder cancer. Lancet 1993; 324: 469.

40. Habuchi T, Ogawa O, Kakehi Y, et al. Accumulated allelic losses in the development of invasive urothelial cancer. Int J Cancer 1993; 53: 579.

41. Miyao N, Tsai YC, Lerner SP, et al. Role of chromosome 9 in human bladder cancer. Cancer Res 1993; 53: 4066.

42. Cairns P, Shaw ME, Knowles MA. Preliminary mapping of the deleted region of chromosome 9 in bladder cancer. Cancer Res 1993; 53: 1230.

43. Ruppert JM, Tokino K, Sidransky D. Evidence for two bladder cancer supressor loci on human chromosome 9. Cancer Res 1994; 53: 5093.

44. Orlow I, Lianes P, Lacombe L, Dalbagni G, Reuter VE, Cordon-Cardo C. Chromosome 9 deletions and microsatellite alterations in human bladder tumors. Cancer Res 1994; 54: 2848.

45. Kamb A, Gruis NA, Weaver-Feldhaus J, et al. A cell cycle regulator potentially involved in genesis of many tumor types. Science 1994; 264: 436.

46. Serrano M, Hannon GJ, Beach D. A new regulatory motif in cell-cycle control causing specific inhibition of cyclin D/CDK4. Nature 1993; 366: 704.

47. Hannon GJ, Beach D. p15^{INK4B} is a potential effector of TGF-β-induced cell cycle arrest. Nature 1994; 371: 257.

48. Cordon-Cardo C. Mutation of cell cycle regulators: biological and clinical implications for human neoplasias. Am J Path 1995; 147: 545.

49. Kamb A, Liu Q, Harshman K, Tavtigian S, Cordon-Cardo C, Skolnick MH. Rates of p16 (MTS1) mutations in primary tumors with 9p loss. Science 1994; 265: 416.
50. Spruck CH, Gonzalez-Zulueta M, Shibata A, et al. p16 gene in uncultured tumours. Nature 1994; 370: 183.
51. Williamson M, Elder PA, Shaw ME, Devlin J, Knowles M. p16(CDKN2) is a major deletion target at 9p21 in bladder cancer. Hum Mol Genet 1995; 4: 1569.
52. Cairns P, Polascik TJ, Eby Y, et al. Frequency of homozygous deletion at p16/CDKN2 in primary human tumours. Nature Genet 1995; 11: 210.
53. Gruis NA, Weaver-Feldhaus J, Liu Q, et al. Genetic evidence in melanoma and bladder cancers that p16 and p53 function in separate pathways of tumor suppression. Am J Pathol 1995; 146: 1199.
54. Orlow I, Lacombe L, Hannon GJ, et al. Deletion of the p16 and p15 genes in human bladder tumors. J Natl Cancer Inst 1995; 87: 1524.
55. Sarkis AS, Dalbagni G, Cordon-Cardo C, et al. Association of p53 nuclear overexpression and tumor progression in carcinoma in situ of the bladder. J Urol 1994; 152: 388.
56. Spruck CH, Ohneseit PE, Gonzalez-Zulueta M, et al. Two molecular pathways to transitional cell carcinoma of the bladder. Cancer Res 1994; 54: 784.
57. Cordon-Cardo C, Wartinger D, Petrylak D, et al. Altered expression of the retinoblastoma gene product is a prognostic indicator in bladder cancer. J Natl Cancer Inst 1992; 84: 1251.
58. Logothetis CJ, Xu H-J, Ro JY, et al. Altered retinoblastoma protein expression and known prognostic variables in locally advanced bladder cancer. J Natl Cancer Inst 1992; 84: 1257.
59. Sidransky D, Von Eschenbach A, Tsai YC, et al. Identification of p53 gene mutations in bladder cancers and urine samples. Science 1991; 252: 706.
60. Fujimoto K, Yamada Y, Okajima E, et al. Frequent association of p53 gene mutation in invasive bladder cancer. Cancer Res 1992; 52: 1393.
61. Dalbagni G, Presti JC, Reuter VE, et al. Molecular genetic alterations of chromosome 17 and p53 nuclear overexpression in human bladder cancer. Diag Mol Pathol 1993; 2: 4.
62. Cordon-Cardo C, Dalbagni D, Saez GT, et al. TP53 mutations in human bladder cancer: genotypic versus phenotypic patterns. Int J Cancer 1994; 56: 347.
63. Sarkis AS, Dalbagni G, Cordon-Cardo C, et al. Nuclear overexpression of p53 protein in transditional cell bladder carcinoma: a marker for disease progression. J Natl Cancer Inst 1993; 85: 53.
64. Sarkis AS, Zhang Z-F, Cordon-Cardo C, et al. p53 nuclear overexpression and disease progression in Ta bladder carcinoma. Int J Oncol 1993; 3: 355.
65. Sarkis AS, Dalbagni G, Cordon-Cardo C, et al. Association of p53 nuclear overexpression and tumor progression in carcinoma in situ of the bladder. J Urol 1994; 152: 388.
66. Lipponen PK. Over-expression of p53 nuclear oncoprotein in transitional-cell bladder cancer and its prognostic value. Int J Cancer 1993; 53: 365.
67. Esrig D, Elmajian D, Groshen S, et al. Accumulation of nuclear p53 and tumor progression in bladder cancer. N Engl J Med 1994; 331: 1259.
68. Sarkis AS, Bajorin DF, Reuter VE, et al. The prognostic value of p53 nuclear overexpression in patientes with invasive bladder cancer treated with neoadjuvant M-VAC. J Clin Oncol 1995; 13: 1384.

16 New Possibilities in Systemic Treatment for Metastatic Bladder Cancer

Randall Millikan, MD, PHD
and Simon J. Hall, MD

INTRODUCTION

Transitional cell carcinoma of the urothelium is a chemosensitive malignancy. It is well established that combination chemotherapy routinely alters the natural history of both locally unresectable and metastatic disease. Unfortunately, substantial clinical advances in the treatment of urothelial cancer with cytotoxics have not been apparent since the advent of combination therapy a generation ago. Despite high response rates, and the appearance of second, third, and even fourth-line regimens that produce objective responses, the median survival of patients with metastatic urothelial cancer has consistently been reported in the range of 12–14 mo. Even though this is more than double the expectation of survival with no therapy, and a reliable, palliative benefit is beyond question,

From: *Current Clinical Urology: Bladder Cancer: Current Diagnosis and Treatment*
Edited by: M. J. Droller © Humana Press Inc., Totowa, NJ

systemic therapy with cytotoxic agents is nonetheless stranded on a very modest plateau *(1)*.

To date, there is no material advance from the benchmark established by M-VAC *(2)*. This venerable combination of methotrexate (30 mg/m^2 d 1, 15, and 22), vinblastine (3 mg/m^2 d 2, 15, and 22), doxorubicin (30 mg/m^2 d 2) and cisplatin (70 mg/m^2 d 2) has been shown to be superior to single agent cisplatin *(3)*, the combination of cyclophosphamide, doxorubicin and cisplatin (CisCA) *(4)*, several variants of the original using escalated doses with or without growth factor support *(5–7)*, and the combination resulting from replacement of cisplatin with carboplatin *(8)*. A Phase 3 trial comparing M-VAC to gemcitabine and cisplatin has appeared *(9)*, and no incremental improvement was noted. A trial of 5-FU, interferon-alpha and cisplatin is expected to be reported within the next year. Unfortunately, no preliminary communication from these trials has foreshadowed the establishment of a new benchmark in overall survival. Despite the failure (so far) to demonstrate improved survival, it is clear that some of the newer combinations are less toxic than M-VAC and comparably active *(9)*. Remarkably, some phase 3 trials have even been designed primarily to test a toxicity hypothesis, which speaks volumes about the widely felt frustration that we may have reached the limits of conventional cytotoxic therapy.

This sentiment notwithstanding, active agents continue to be identified, and remarkably high response rates are reported. Significant single-agent activity is seen with the vinca alkaloids, cisplatin, methotrexate and other antifolates, anthracyclines, taxanes, gemcitabine and ifosfamide—more than a dozen agents *(10)*. Even leaving aside the important issues of dose, schedule and sequence, there are an astonishing number of 2, 3, or 4-component regimens (>10^5) that can be derived from such a pool of building blocks. Exploring this number of regimens far exceeds the capacity of academic oncology, to say nothing of poster space at ASCO.

Further, we do not really know the rules for making profitable multi-agent combinations. For example, there are now several useful combination regimens that violate the purported "Cardinal Principle" that each agent within a combination should have significant single-agent activity: 5-FU/leucovorin in colon cancer (no activity for leucovorin), paclitaxel/estramustine in prostate cancer (no single agent activity for either drug), 5-FU/interferon-alpha/cisplatin in bladder cancer (no activity for interferon, and almost none for 5-FU) to name but a few. Apparently, given the possibilities for synergy and "biomodulatiton," the pool of building blocks is even larger than it seems at first glance. Soon, the combinatorial problems will be even worse, as agents based on new paradigms become available. Preliminary results suggest that most of these newer agents will be more effective when applied in combination with traditional cytotoxics. Once again however, we do not really know how to develop these combinations or how to optimally evaluate them.

A final complication in the setting of urothelial cancer arises from the ethical problem of foregoing standard therapy in untreated patients (which is known to triple life expectancy) in favor of new agents of unknown efficacy. It is apparent that the traditional paradigm of evaluating single agents in phase 2 studies of previously untreated patients no longer serves us. Central to the problem of therapy improvement in urothelial cancer will be refinement of methodology for clinical investigation.

Our main task in this chapter is to provide an overview of emerging therapies beyond the traditional cytotoxic paradigm, with a particular emphasis on the possibilities for gene therapy. Nonetheless, it is useful to take brief account of the state of the art with conventional chemotherapy. In so doing, we will highlight challenges (and opportunities) for optimizing use of existing agents, and set the context for the development of new methodology.

NEW CYTOTOXIC AGENTS FOR BLADDER CANCER

Ifosfamide

Currently, one of the most promising regimens for urothelial cancer is a product of the ongoing efforts at Memorial Sloan-Kettering and consists of ifosfamide, paclitaxel, and cisplatin (ITP) *(11,12)*. This regimen produces a major response in about 70% of patients with locally unresectable or metastatic urothelial cancer. Unfortunately, it requires growth factor support and is quite expensive—just the pharmacy charges for this regimen are about $16,000 per cycle (this compares to about $3100 for a cycle of M-VAC). To date, the observed median survival is roughly 18 mo. Only future comparative trials will establish if this apparent improvement reflects stage migration due to improved followup and imaging; improved supportive care; patient selection; or a real incremental advance from the well established historical benchmark of 13.5 mo associated with M-VAC given in this setting at Memorial Sloan-Kettering.

In part, the ITP regimen reflects a renewed interest in the use of ifosfamide for urothelial cancer (Table 1). Investigators at Indiana University have provided a review of this topic *(22)*, and have contributed an active regimen built from ifosfamide, vinblastine and gallium nitrate (VIG) *(21)*. Unfortunately, gallium nitrate is associated with potentially severe and unpredictable retinal toxicity. Furthermore, the VIG regimen did not appear to represent an advance over M-VAC in further experi-

Table 1
Ifosfamide in Urothelial Cancer

Ifosfamide (g/m2)	Other agents	Untreated	Salvage	Ref.
1 × 5 d	–	0/15		(13)
1.8 × 5 d	–	8/20		(14)
1 × 5 d	–	–	1/20	(15)
1.5 × 5 d	–	–	11/56	(16)
1 × 4 d	Paclitaxel 135 mg/m^2 over 24 h, d 1	2/11	2/9	(17)
1 × 5 d	5-FU 350 mg/m2 × 5d	–	0/15	(18)
1.5 × 5 d	VP-16 120 mg/m^2 × 5 d	12/25	–	(19)
1.8 × 5 d	Epirubicin 80 mg/m^2 d 1	11/17	–	(20)
1.5 × 3 d	Paclitaxel 200 mg/m^2 over 3 h, d 1 Cisplatin 70 mg/m^2 d 1	30/44	–	(12)
1.2 × 5 d	Vinblastine 0.11 mg/kg d 1 and d 2 Gallium Nitrate 300 mg/m^2 × 5 d	18/27	–	(21)

ence in the cooperative group setting, and no further development of this regimen is planned. Nonetheless, there is sufficient interest in ifosfamide that other combinations are in development. An intriguing early report from Egypt *(20)* suggested very promising results from the combination of ifosfamide and epirubicin. Anecdotal experience at MD Anderson has shown significant "salvage" activity for the combination of ifosfamide and doxorubicin, and trials building on this observation are in progress. The remarkable dose/response relationship seen for ifosfamide in the context of soft-tissue sarcomas has recently been re-emphasized *(23)*. The data collected in Table 1 suggest that a similar relationship may obtain in the context of urothelial cancer.

Taxanes

The taxanes are active and generally well-tolerated *(24)*. Indeed, many taxane based regimens have been described (Table 2) and some of these have become front-line at many centers. Investigators at Mayo have reported on the doublet of paclitaxel and cisplatin, which they find to be active and well tolerated in previously untreated patients. Updated information with this regimen in the setting of metastatic disease suggests that the median survival is indeed comparable to that obtained with M-VAC *(29)*. A regimen of paclitaxel, methotrexate and cisplatin (TMP) was developed at MD Anderson *(32)*. This regimen was promising in the salvage setting, producing several responses in patients that progressed during therapy with front-line M-VAC. The regimen has since evolved and

Table 2
Taxanes in Urothelial Cancer

Taxane (mg/m^2)	Other agents	Untreated	Salvage	Median survival	Ref.
Paclitaxel 250 over 24 h, d1, q 21 d	–	11/26	–	8.4 mo	(25)
Paclitaxel 200 over 3 h, d 1, q 21 d	–	–	1/14	NR[b]	(26)
Docetaxel 100 d 1, q 21 d	–	9/29	–	NR[b]	(27)
Docetaxel 100 d 1, q 21 d	–	–	4/30	NR[b]	(28)
Paclitaxel 135 over 3 h, d 1, q 21 d	Cisplatin 70 mg/m^2 d 1	19/29	–	13.6 mo	(29)
Paclitaxel 200 over 3 h, d 1, q 21 d	Carboplatian AUC 5	18/36	–	9.5 mo	(30)
Paclitaxel 200 over 3 h, d 1, q 21 d	Carboplatian AUC 5	4/29	–	9.4 mo	(31)
Paclitaxel 200 over 3 h, d 1, q 21 d	Methotrexate 30 mg/m^2 d 1 Cisplatin 70 mg/m^2 d 1	–	10/25	NR[b]	(32)
Paclitaxel 100 over 1 h, d 1 and d 8, q 21 d	Methotrexate 30 mg/m^2 d 1 and d 8 Cisplatin 40 mg/m^2 d 1and d 8	11/33[a]	–	NR[b]	(33)
Docetaxel 75 d 1, q 21 d	Cisplatin 75 mg/m^2 d 1	15/25	–	13.6 mo	(34)
Docetaxel 75 d 1, q 21 d	Cisplatin 75 mg/m^2 d 1	10/19	–	NR[b]	(35)

[a]Refers to patients with cT3b or T4a disease rendered pT ≤ T1 after 4–5 cycles of neoadjuvant therapy.

[b]NR = Not reported.

is now front-line neoadjuvant therapy for patients with locally advanced disease at MD Anderson (Table 2). The doublet of paclitaxel and carboplatin requires special comment. We find that many physicians use this combination as first-line therapy, despite published data relating survival results well below the historical benchmark of 12–14 mo (30). Recently, a trial performed in the Southwest Oncology Group failed to confirm adequate activity (overall response rate <20%; median survival 9.4 mo) for this combination (31). At present, available data do not support off-protocol use of this regimen as front-line therapy. The experience with paclitaxel and carboplatin is an important reminder that "response" as an endpoint of clinical investigation is of limited value. It is clearly important to keep watch on median survival as well as overall response rate in phase 2 trials.

Table 3
Gemcitabine in Urothelial Cancer

Gemcitabine (mg/m²)	Other agents	Untreated	Salvage	Ref.
1200 over 30 min d 1, 8, 15 q 28 d	–	11/39	–	(37)
1200 over 30 min d 1, 8, 15 q 28 d	–	–	7/35	(38)
1000 over 30 min d 1, 8, 15 q 28 d	Cisplantin, 35 mg/m² d 1, 8, 15	11/37	–	(39)
1000 over 30 min d 1, 8, 15 q 28 d	Cisplantin, 75 mg/m² d 1	12/16	–	(40)
1000 over 30 min d 1, 8, 15 q 28 d	Paclitaxel, 200 mg/m² over 1 h, d 1	–	15/25	(41)
2500–3,000 over 30 min, d 1, q 14 d	Paclitaxel, 150 mg/m² over 3 h, d 1	–	8/15	(42)
2000 over 30 min d 1, q 14 d	Doxorubicin, 50 mg/m² d 1	5/6	–	(43)
1000 over 30 min d 1 and d 8, q 21 d	Cisplatin, 70 mg/m² d 1 Paclitaxel, 80 mg/m² over 1 h, d 1 and d 8	23/29	–	(44)
800 over 30 min d 1 and d 8, q 21 d	Carboplatin, AUC 5 d 1 Paclitaxel, 200 mg/m² over 3 h, d 1	11/19	–	(45)

Gemcitabine

The recent availability of gemcitabine *(36)*, which is strongly synergistic with cisplatin and other DNA damaging agents, and does have single-agent activity in urothelial cancer, has led to multiple phase 2 studies (Table 3). Gemcitabine has relatively modest non-hematologic toxicity, and thus several well tolerated regimens have been put forward. The best studied of these is the combination of gemcitabine and cisplatin *(40)*. In fact, as mentioned above, an international phase 3 trial of this doublet versus M-VAC has already completed accrual. Combinations of gemcitabine with paclitaxel are especially noteworthy, as this doublet not only shows promising activity, but can also be applied to patients with compromised renal function. Despite intense clinical research activity with gemcitabine combinations, it is not yet clear what the optimal doublet or triplet based on gemcitabine may be, and the complex issues surrounding the drug's schedule dependency and drug-drug interactions *(46)* suggest that we have much yet to learn about applying this agent in the clinic.

NEW APPROACHES TO COMBINATION CHEMOTHERAPY

While necessarily highly selective, this brief overview serves to illustrate the point that three whole families of new combinations (i.e., those based on ifosfamide, taxanes and gemcitabine) have been reported in the last few years, unfortunately without generating much evidence that survival is improving. It seems less and less likely that the next cytotoxic drug will provide a means to advance beyond the current therapeutic plateau. This is not to say that work to develop cytotoxic chemotherapy should not continue. With so many active drugs, and having explored such a tiny fraction of the combinatorial space available, one can be certain that we have not yet discovered the optimal use of available agents. For example, we still do not know if bringing more of the available agents to bear will lead to improved outcome, nor do we know the best strategy for including more agents.

In general, complex, multicomponent regimens usually force compromise from the optimal dose and schedule of some of the components, and it is often the case that additional agents add toxicity without improving outcome. A better strategy for bringing more active agents to bear is likely to be the combination of individually optimized doublets or triplets applied sequentially. This is nicely illustrated by the recent experience in small cell lung cancer in which a 4-component regimen ("CODE") was found to be more toxic but no more effective than sequential treatment with two well established regimens "CAV/EP" *(47)*.

The concept of sequential or "modular" therapy is just now starting to be applied to urothelial cancer, led, once again, by the group at Sloan-Kettering. They have developed a doublet of gemcitabine and doxorubicin, with a view toward combining a block of this regimen with a block of ITP *(43)* (Fig. 1). Preliminary results show that this approach is not only feasible, but may in fact be less toxic than prolonged exposure to multiple cycles of ITP. The group at MD Anderson is also conducting a pilot study of a "modular" approach to systemic chemotherapy (Fig. 1). In the latter approach, platinum-based regimens are alternated with non-platinum-containing regimens. As expected, these preliminary studies show high clinical activity and one can expect more reports along these lines.

Even within this concept of combining regimens, we are still left with the daunting task of sorting out which regimens (or combinations of regimens) are the most promising and worthy of further development. Selecting from the myriad of phase II studies being reported is in fact a more formidable problem than the initial development of novel combinations for phase I and phase II testing. Clearly, it is not possible to do pairwise phase III comparisons on even a fraction of the novel combinations being reported. The pressing issue therefore is to develop some basis for comparison short of a phase III trial. In particular, the devel-

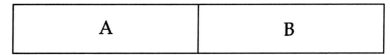

Memorial "Modular" Program:
A = Gemcitabine/Adriamycin (12 wks)
B = Ifosfamide/Taxol/Cisplatin (12 wks)

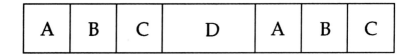

MD Anderson "Modular" Program:
A = Ifosfamide/Adriamycin (3 wks x 2)
B = Taxol/Methotrexate/Cisplatin (3 wks x 2)
C = Taxol/Adriamycin (3 wks x 2)
D = Gemcitabine/Cisplatin (6 wks)

Fig. 1. The concept of sequential or "modular" therapy as applied to urothelial cancer.

opment of methods to overcome the pitfalls of multiple small phase 2 studies, usually done at referral centers with ill-defined patient selection factors at work, is of fundamental importance. A brief review of some emerging solutions to this problem is the subject of the following chapter.

LESSONS FROM TUMOR BIOLOGY

Even while we work to optimize the impact of existing chemotherapy however, it is all too evident that we need to expand our horizons beyond the cytotoxic paradigm. Thus it is timely to ask: What of our improving understanding of tumor biology can we apply in the clinic today?

Marker Directed Therapy

One of the first applications of our burgeoning understanding of tumor biology to clinical practice has been the ability to characterize tumors on the basis of specific molecular phenotypes. This can be done at the DNA, RNA or protein level, using many different experimental techniques. Indeed, the study of "markers" and their correlation with clinical outcome now constitutes the bulk of "translational" cancer research, and is rapidly becoming a new paradigm for the pathologic classification of malignancy.

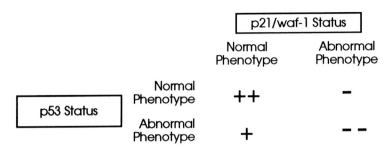

Fig. 2. Stratification of prognosis by p53 and p21/waf-1 status. ++ Especially good prognosis. +/− Intermediate prognosis. − − Especially poor prognosis.

For muscle-invasive urothelial cancer, it is known that the protein phenotype (by immunohistochemical staining of paraffin embedded tumor tissue) corresponding to the products of the p53 and Rb genes is strongly prognostic. While individually informative, the combination of these markers is especially striking. Patients with a normal phenotype for both markers (i.e., <10% of cells showing nuclear staining for p53 and, for Rb, heterogeneous nuclear staining) have a very favorable prognosis with cystectomy alone. Those with one abnormal marker have an intermediate prognosis, and those with both markers abnormal have an especially poor outcome *(48)*. That both of these genes are involved in cell-cycle control makes such an "interaction" quite reasonable. Recently, p21/waf1 status has also been investigated in urothelial tumors. This gene is transcriptionally upregulated by p53, and thus the status of p21 protein may provide additional insight into the "p53 pathway." Indeed, Cote *(49)* found that p21 status does further stratify the group with a normal p53 immunohistochemical phenotype (Fig. 2). It seems likely that these and other ongoing studies will eventually allow individually optimized therapy on the basis of tumor phenotype (and genotype) *(50)*.

In the context of specific therapies, it is of interest to find markers that correlate with response. The p53, Rb and p21 markers are all related to "apoptotic threshold" and are therefore of great interest from the viewpoint of chemosensitivity. However, initiation of apoptosis is an extremely complex event, and thus the influence of these genes on sensitivity to chemotherapy is expected to be both cell type and context dependent. These issues for p53 were recently reviewed *(51)*.

To date, clinical information about marker status in relation to sensitivity to chemotherapy is quite limited. Cote et al. *(52)* have studied a cohort of patients that participated in the USC trial of adjuvant chemotherapy for locally advanced bladder cancer *(53)*. In that study, it was found that among those that received chemotherapy, 10 of 18 patients with normal p53 staining relapsed, while only 6/14 patients with abnormal p53 phenotype relapsed. This finding led to the hypothesis that an abnormal p53 phenotype predisposes to chemosensitivity in patients with urothelial cancer treated with cisplatin based therapy. This hypothesis is now being tested prospectively in a multi-center randomized trial. This important trial should provide substantial information about the clinical implications, including chemosensitivity, of p53 (and several other markers).

By contrast, Wu et al. have shown in a retrospective review that abnormal p53 phenotype is associated with a decreased probability of response to radiotherapy (54) in patients with cT3b bladder cancer. Also, a recent report from the University of California at Davis (55) found no association of p53 immunostaining and the probability of response to paclitaxel based therapy.

Clearly, the issue of sensitivity to chemotherapy is complex. It seems unlikely that any single marker will provide a broadly applicable indicator of benefit from cytotoxic therapy. The emerging technology of characterizing expression of up to several thousand genes on a chip array is expected to be especially fruitful for the task of defining molecular phenotypes that relate to complex endpoints such as sensitivity to chemotherapy or the probability of benefiting from adjuvant therapy.

Growth Factors

Beyond the use of markers to inform prognosis and to guide therapy, is the promise of finding more specific and effective therapies by exploiting our developing knowledge of the molecular effectors of carcinogenesis and the malignant phenotype. The recognition that many oncogenes and tumor suppressor genes code for components necessary for the reception and transduction of growth factor signals led to great expectations for new cancer therapies. It is now known that many growth factor receptors are expressed on urothelial cancers, and that various approaches targeting these pathways show antitumor effects in preclinical models. Moreover, it is well established that over-expression of growth factor receptors is a marker for progression to an invasive phenotype in early stage urothelial disease (56).

The epidermal growth factor (EGF) related pathways (57), and specifically the c-erbB related genes her-1 and her-2, are the best studied. The products of these genes are receptors that typically function as homo- or hetero-dimers. They signal by means of autophosphorylation of tyrosine residues on the cytoplasmic side of the receptor, which in turn can interact with multiple transduction pathways. There are multiple possibilities for therapeutic intervention in this cascade, ranging from blockade of ligand/receptor interaction, such as by antibodies or small molecule antagonists; inhibition of the receptor's tyrosine kinase activity; interfering with physical association of transduction elements, as for example by blocking farnesylation of membrane associated components such as ras; interfering with "downstream" kinases; or interfering with coupled systems such as calcium homeostasis or the regulation of protein serine/threonine phosphorylation.

The therapeutic potential of agents interfering with EGF receptor (EGF-R) mediated signaling has been extensively investigated in pre-clinical models, and in some early clinical studies. Mendelsohn has shown *(58)* that antibodies directed to the extracellular portion of EGF-R have potent growth-inhibitory effects in vitro. Blocking EGF-R signaling has been shown to have multiple therapeutically relevant consequences, including G1 arrest (+/- apoptosis), Rb hypophosphorylation, increased p27, decreased matrix metalloprotease expression and decreased angiogenesis *(59)*. More importantly, in combination with cytotoxics, durable complete remissions have been observed in murine models *(60)*. A humanized antibody (C225) is now in phase 2 human trials, but unfortunately there are as yet no data in urothelial cancer. Blocking the tyrosine kinase activity of the EGF-R is an alternative strategy for therapeutic intervention. Several small molecules with such activity have been described. Dinney et al. *(61)* have reported anti-tumor effects with staurosporine analogs in an orthotopic mouse model of using human urothelial cancer lines. To date however, there is no clinical experience with EGF-R (or her-2/neu) antagonists in urothelial cancer.

In addition to interfering with EGF-R signaling, an alternate strategy is to use the receptor for physically targeting therapeutic interventions to cells that overexpress the receptor. Many examples of this strategy are based on bioconjugates of EGF (or transforming growth factor-alpha, another high affinity ligand for EGF-R) to various biologic effectors—ranging from toxins to genes to radioisotopes. It has been shown that such conjugates can selectively deliver effectors to cells expressing EGF-R, and that relevant biologic effects are seen in model systems *(62)*. Human trials of such approaches are just getting underway.

Molecular Therapies

Beyond the interruption of growth factor receptor function, there are many approaches to the problem of interfering with the intracellular transduction apparatus. For example, farnesyl transferase inhibitors have been shown to have protean metabolic effects, and can be synergistic with cytotoxic agents *(63)*. In addition, protein tyrosine kinase inhibitors could have the advantage of working at a confluence of multiple signaling pathways, and thereby exert a more general therapeutic effect. The pharmacology of "fine-tuning" the specificity of protein tyrosine kinase inhibitors is an active area of investigation *(64)*.

Recently, the central role of regulated proteolytic destruction by means of the proteasome has been recognized as an integral feature of cell cycle control *(65)*. Inhibitors of the proteasome are strikingly cytotoxic, and have shown promise in pre-clinical studies *(66)*. Agents in this class are now in human trials. Although not yet tested in the context of urothelial cancer, these agents represent an exciting and entirely novel paradigm for systemic therapy.

Antiangiogenesis

Perhaps the most compelling insight of tumor biology has been the recognition that angiogenesis is an absolutely essential step for cancers to become macroscopic, and therefore life-threatening *(67)*. Indeed, once the pathways of angiogenesis were appreciated, it was shown that many known therapies demonstrate "antiangiogenic" effects as part of their overall anti-tumor activity. Prevention of tumor induced angiogenesis is an especially appealing therapeutic strategy because for most cancers we already have the means to very effectively "debulk" the tumor by means of surgery and chemotherapy. In fact, most patients with urothelial cancer can now be successfully treated to the point of microscopic residual disease. A therapy that would keep such residual disease from growing beyond the size limitations of nutrient diffusion would effectively cure the vast majority of patients that now relapse and die of metastatic urothelial cancer. Unfortunately, no trials of agents in this class have been reported in patients with urothelial cancer.

Antimetastasis Therapy

The process whereby tumors establish metastases is highly selective and requires the specific expression of multiple genes *(68)*. Especially targeted for anti-metastasis therapy have been the matrix metalloproteases (MMP), a group of enzymes capable of digesting collagen and other connective tissue proteins *(69)*. Although activated in various ways, a common feature of the metastatic phenotype is expression of proteolytic activity of this class, often associated with suppression of the inhibitors of these enzymes. Recently, small molecule inhibitors of MMPs have come into clinical trials *(70)*. So far, it appears that these agents are safe, but only very modest clinical activity has been seen in single agent trials. Once again however, synergy with cytotoxics has been seen in preclinical models, and combination studies in humans are ongoing. No reports of such combination therapy in urothelial cancer have appeared.

Immunotherapy

Finally, the use of agents such as interferons and interleukins continues to be of interest in the systemic therapy of urothelial cancer. Interferon has been studied in combination with cytotoxics by Logothetis et al. *(71)*. Preliminary results in patients having failed traditional chemotherapy were sufficiently promising that a phase III trial of 5-FU, interferon-alpha and cisplatin vs M-VAC has been completed. The results of this study are expected within the next year. Recent results combining interferon with other cytotoxics *(72)* suggest that this concept is worthy of further exploration. In view of the profound anti-tumor benefit sometimes observed with BCG therapy of superficial bladder cancer, the possibility that systemic immunotherapy could be beneficial for metastatic urothelial cancer is of substantial interest. Given the ready availability of tumor tissue, bladder cancer would seem to be an ideal context for investigations of tumor antigen vaccines and immunomodulatory gene therapy *(see below)*.

GENE THERAPY

Many novel approaches to cancer treatment are based on the rapidly evolving technology for gene manipulation and delivery to represent the ultimate form of molecular therapy. As outlined below, growth suppression within directly inoculated tumors has already been documented with most forms of locally applied gene therapy. However, the treatment of metastatic disease is much more challenging, requiring the gene of interest to either be delivered to disseminated lesions or to generate systemic antitumor activity despite anatomically localized expression.

Methods of Gene Delivery

Whatever the strategy, in order to be used therapeutically, genes must first be delivered to relevant target cells. Thus, methods for gene delivery, vectors, are fully as important as the genes themselves (Table 4). A thorough discussion of vector technology is beyond the scope of this chapter, but several general points are worthy of emphasis. Vectors may be broadly classified according to their requirement for integration into chromosomal DNA prior to gene expression. Some, such as retroviruses, must integrate into cellular DNA, while genes delivered by means of liposomes and adenoviruses can be expressed episomally, that is, within the cytoplasm, without a requirement for DNA integration.

Chromosomal integration results in long term expression and heritability *(73)*. However, successful retroviral integration depends on the breakdown of the nuclear membrane during mitosis, and thus applica-

Table 4
Gene Therapy Vectors

Delivery vector	Advantages	Disadvantages
Naked DNA/ liposome plasmids	Very large genes Non-immunogenic Non-toxic Potentially targetable	Extremely inefficient
Retrovirus	Permanent expression Relatively non-immunogenic Ideal for ex vivo selection	Express only post-mitosis Inefficient in vivo Random integration
Adenovirus	Episomal expression Efficient transduction of most cells Produced in high titers Toxic at high doses	Transient expression Immunogenic
AAV	Expression for cell lifetime Expression independent of mitosis Site-specific integration	Low titer production
Herpes virus	Cell-specific affinity	Toxic

tion of retroviral vectors is limited to cells undergoing mitosis directly related to the period of exposure to virus. Nonetheless, retroviral vectors may be ideal for ex vivo gene therapy. In this approach, a patient's cells are removed and made to express a particular gene product by in vitro transduction and selection, producing altered cells to be given back to the patient. The cell cycle limitations of retroviral vectors can be overcome by use of adeno-associated virus (AAV) *(74)*. AAV gains access to the nucleus and stably integrates at a site specific locus on chromosome 19, in both replicating and senescent cells. Unfortunately, production of high titers of AAV necessary for directly cytotoxic or tumor suppressor gene therapy is difficult with existing methods. However, AAV may be a suitable method for generating stable expression of a systemically active substance.

Of the nonintegrating vectors, replication incompetent adenovirus has already been widely used for gene therapy of cancer, since it can be produced in large quantities, and can infect a wide variety of tissues *(73)*. Interestingly, some bladder cancer cell lines do not express adenoviral receptors, and thus may have limited value as a vector for bladder cancer *(75)*. Since adenovirus-mediated gene expression is not dependent on DNA integration, transgenes are expressed in both replicating and non-replicating cells, but are diluted with successive mitoses *(73)*. In general, adenoviruses elicit both humoral and cellular immune responses, which may limit the duration of gene expression and the ability to re-dose. In order to avoid this immune response, a "gutless" adenovirus vector, which expresses essentially no viral proteins, is being developed. Liposome vectors can potentially deliver genes of unlimited size and are non-immunogenic *(73)*. However, classical liposome-mediated transfection is extremely inefficient, thus far limiting in vivo use. Newer variants utilizing liposomes expressing targeting molecules may make this approach more attractive.

In order for gene therapy to specifically target metastatic tumor cells, genes must be delivered systemically. However, for therapeutic and toxicity considerations, restriction of gene expression to tumor cells is a necessity. A tissue specific promoter will limit gene expression only to those cells which can activate that particular promoter. Uroplakin is expressed only by the transitional epithelium and bladder cancers *(76, 77)*, and has a candidate restricted promoter *(78,79)*. So far, tissue specific give low levels of gene expression compared to standard viral promoters. Furthermore, promoter restriction limits gene expression, not vector entry into the cell, such that vector related toxicities to other tissues will not be limited by such a method.

The direct targeting of cancer cells for gene delivery is dependent on the identification of unique surface markers on tumor cells to direct preferential vector binding. Significant progress has been made with adenovirus which infects cells by the coordination of two independent events: the binding of the knob on the virus surface to the coxsackie-adenovirus receptor and the interaction the penton base with specific integrins on the cell surface to direct internalization (Fig. 3). Specific antibodies against the knob can be conjugated to receptor ligands so adenovirus binding is now mediated by ligand to receptor binding; internalization occurs through the normal mechanism *(80)*. A "tropism modified" adenovirus can then target cells which overexpress particular receptors. For bladder cancer, epidermal growth factor receptor is overexpressed by many transitional cell cancers *(57)* and may serve as the target for an adenoviral conjugate expressing EGF *(81)*. Phage display libraries, bacterophages conjugated to random sets of peptides, when sequentially passaged through vascular beds of normal or cancerous have identified distinct vascular endothelial fingerprints between different tissues and normal tissues and cancers *(82)*. These peptides may be used to target gene delivery to tumor vasculature. Indeed, adenoviral knobs have been engineered to express such a peptide to direct endothelial specific vector binding *(83)*. This concept may also be applied to cationic liposomes, by incorporating targeting molecules on the surface of the liposome.

A final example of cell-specific expression exploits the natural lytic life cycle of viruses. The ONYX-015 is a replication competent mutant adenovirus which will only replicate in cells lacking functional p53 *(84)*

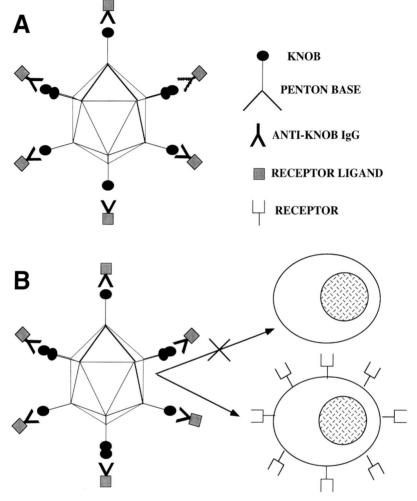

Fig. 3. "Tropism Modified" Adenovirus. Specific antibodies to the knob block binding to the cell surface. With the conjugation of the antibody to receptor ligand the adenovirus binds to a cell only with the receptor for that ligand. Internalization occurs through the normal mechanism.

(Fig. 4), a common finding in advanced and metastatic bladder cancers. ONYX-015 suppresses tumor growth following both local and systemic delivery by repetitive dosing without significant toxicity *(84–86)*. However, these experiments were performed in immunocompromised mice which have a blunted response to the viral vector. Nevertheless, second generation p53 restricted vectors are being developed to express therapeutic genes *(87,88)*.

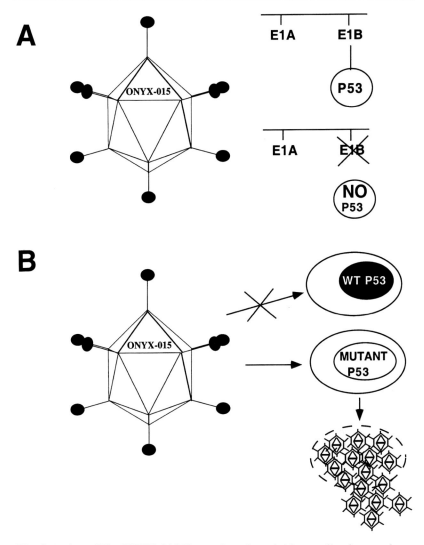

Fig. 4. Action of The ONYX-015 Vector. In order to initiate replication an adenovirus must inactivate p53 thorough binding of the E1B gene product. The ONYX-015 has a mutated E1B, such that it cannot inactivate wild type p53. Consequently, it may not replicate in p53 wildtype cells but is able to replicate in p53 mutant cells. The vector kills by cell lysis.

METHODS OF ANTICANCER GENE THERAPY

Tumor Suppressor Gene Therapy

The discovery that many cancers develop in concert with the loss of function of specific genes, dubbed "tumor suppression genes," suggested that replacement of such genes should be therapeutically useful. Studies of bladder cancer have yielded several candidate genes for therapeutic replacement. Among them are the cell-cycle related genes Rb, p53, p21/waf1 and p16 *(48,49,89)*. Loss of function of these genes, by means of allelic loss, mutation or methylation is thought to disrupt cell cycle control, allowing uncontrolled growth and/or promotion of further mutation. In many tumor models, p53 replacement results in growth suppression of injected tumors *(90–95)*. Likewise, experience in humans has been shown p53 therapy to be safe with some responses *(96,97)*. In bladder cancer, p53 gene therapy has focused on intravesical treatment. The ability to infect both normal mucosa and tumors has been demonstrated *(98)*. While attractive for ease and practicality, the potential for intravesical gene delivery is diminished by protective mechanisms within the mucosa, resulting in inconsistent transfection, usually confined to superficial cell layers. The use of ethanol has dramaticaly improved gene expression within mucosa and established tumors, but it remains to be seen if transduction is sufficient to impact the growth of an established tumor *(99)*. A human phase I trial of an adenoviral-p53 construct as an intravesical therapy is underway at MD Anderson.

Although not yet in human trials, both Rb and p16 gene therapies have been explored as potential approaches for the treatment of bladder cancer. Transduction of the Rb gene results in growth arrest but not death of both Rb– and Rb+ cells, though effects in Rb– cells are more pronounced *(100,101)*. Interestingly, a truncated Rb gene has been shown to be a more potent inhibitor of growth arrest than the full length gene, pointing to molecular mechanisms to enhance activity *(100)*. Introduction of the p16 gene also results in growth arrest of bladder cancer cells, though only in those which are p16 mutant *(102)*. Combining p53 and p16 gene transduction may result in supra-additive growth suppression via the induction of apoptosis *(103)*. These results suggest that combinations of genes, directed by the genetic damage harbored by the particular tumor being treated, may be more successful than using a single therapeutic gene. As noted previously, the relationship between p53 mutation and sensitivity to radiation and chemotherapy is complex *(51, 54,104–106)*. Nonetheless, combination of p53 gene replacement and chemotherapy or radiation therapy has shown enhanced cell kill in p53 mutant cells *(107–110)*. However, the complexity is underscored by the observation that some combinations with other tumor suppressor genes may demonstrate antagonism *(102)*.

In principle, effective tumor eradication by means of tumor suppressor gene replacement requires that virtually 100% of the tumor be transduced. However, even by direct injection into established tumor masses, only 20-30% transduction is observed. Despite this, it is clear that more cells are killed than are actually transduced, the so-called "bystander effect" which is invoked to explain better than expected results for p53 gene therapy *(91,94,111)*. While perhaps related to a loco-regional anti-angiogenic effect *(112)*, this phenomemeon is largely ill-defined with regard to tumor suppressor gene therapy and the subject of intense investigation.

Pro-Drug Activation Gene Therapy

Pro-drug activation gene therapy refers to the expression of a gene product that converts an inactive pro-drug into a cytotoxic substance. Of the several systems under investigation, only Herpes Simplex Virus-thymidine kinase gene (HSV-tk) transduction in combination with systemic ganciclovir (GCV) has been studied in bladder cancer. The HSV-tk product phosphorylates GCV, converting it into a nucleoside analogue (pGCV) which inhibits DNA synthesis *(114)* and generates a defined bystander effect. The latter is mediated by several mechanisms including gap junction transport of the nondiffusible pGCV to nontransduced cells; the endocytosis of cellular vesicles containing pGCV by nontransduced cells, and the induction of an immune response *(114–118)*. Preclinical studies of this system in bladder cancer have documented local tumor growth suppression in both subcutaneous and orthotopic models sufficient to yield a survival advantage but not cures *(119,120)*. Significant, but incomplete, growth suppression of synchronous and asynchronous tumor deposits has been observed following treatment of the primary tumor *(115,121–127)*. This "action at a distance" appears to be mediated by an immune mechanism. This suggests that further modulation of this immune effect may provide a means of enhancing response to such therapy.

Immunomodulatory Gene Therapy

While the growth suppressive activities of both tumor suppressor and pro-drug activation gene therapy are primarily local, immunomodulatory gene therapy can generate a systemic response from local gene expression, and is thus an attractive concept for treating disseminated cancers. A variety of methods have been explored to generate cellular antitumor activity through either ex vivo or *in situ* manipulations. Gene therapy mediated expression of immunomodulatory cytokines may have some advantages over systemic cytokine administration, including less morbidity and the physical localization of cytokine in the presence of putative tumor antigens.

Tumor vaccines have been created by subcutaneous injection of lethally irradiated tumor cells which have been transduced with a cytokine gene with the intent of generating an immune response against the injected cells which will also recognize tumor distant from the site of vaccination. Preclinical studies in a bladder cancer model have shown that vaccine therapy results in the rejection of cytokine producing cells, generation of a cellular immune response against tumor cell challenge, and growth suppression of established orthotopic bladder tumors *(128,129)*. Clinical trials of this approach in non-urothelial cancers have documented safety and cellular immune responses, but have shown low response rates *(130,131)*. Novel approaches to enhance efficacy are under study, including combination of vaccinations with systemic cytokine administration, cytokines and MHC class I genes, and cytokines with co-stimulatory molecules *(132– 135)*. In instances where specific tumor antigens have been identified, such as PSA for prostate cancer, vector mediated expression of the tumor antigen has the ability to generate immune responses *(136)*. To enhance the probability of immune recognition of tumor specific antigens, second generation vaccines use dendritic cells, professional antigen presenting cells, pulsed with candidate tumor antigens *(131,137)*. In instances where tumor antigens remain unidentified, as with transitional cell carcinoma, pulsing with tumor mRNAs extracted and amplified from small tumor samples have been performed in animal models with encouraging results *(138)*.

To avoid the costly and time consuming process of tumor harvest and ex vivo culture to produce tumor vaccine, *in situ* strategies to promote immune response have been proposed. For example, direct injection of adenoviral vectors containing genes for cytokines such as IL-2 or IL-12 into a tumor can lead to complete regression, generation of cellular immunity and systemic activity against challenge tumors *(139–141)*. Often however, mono-cytokine gene therapy engenders only incomplete growth suppression. This observation has led to the development of combination strategies which mirror those being explored with vaccine therapy. Also under development is combination of cytokines with HSV-tk gene therapy, since incomplete immune responses are generated by HSV-tk+GCV alone. Addition of cytokines improves tumor growth sup-pression and generates sustained, profound immunity in murine models *(142–144)*.

Antiangiogenesis Gene Therapy

Angiogenesis is critical to the growth and metastasis of tumor cells, leading to the identification of an ever enlarging list of both promoters and inhibitors of this fundamental process *(67)*. Gene therapy strategies include both inhibition of pro-angiogenic factors or overexpression of inhibitors of angiogenesis. Vascular endothelial growth factor (VEGF) is an important promoter of angiogenesis. Gene therapy-mediated expression of soluble VEGF receptor (sFLT-1) sequesters soluble VEGF and in a dominant negative fashion inactivates VEGF through formation of heterodimers; suppression of primary and metastatic tumor growth has been achieved by such treatment *(145,146)*. However, the activities of sFLT-1 are not systemic following local expression and would therefore only be active for metastatic lesions following regional vascular delivery.

Treatment with the potent angiogenesis inhibitors angiostatin or endostatin results in reduction of local and metastatic tumors to microscopic remnants without toxicity *(147, 148)*. A gene therapy approach has been entertained, mainly due to problems producing the large quantities of protein required for clinical application. Expression of endostatin or angiostatin by tumor cells, or by transfected muscle cells remote from the site of tumor, can significantly suppress the growth of local and disseminated lesions *(149–151)*. So far, the results of gene therapy are not as impressive as those reported with protein treatment *(147,148)*; however, systemic growth inhibition has been demonstrated following transduction of only a small percentage of cells.

CONCLUSIONS

There has been rapid progress in the discovery of novel therapeutic targets for disseminated bladder cancer. Preclinical and early clinical trials have provided proof-of-principle for many approaches. However, it will undoubtedly require several more years to develop these leads into genuine therapies that produce clinically relevant alteration of the natural history of metastatic urothelial cancer. The work ahead will provide ample challenge for the intellect and resolve of urologic oncologists—and we think, considerable hope for our patients.

REFERENCES

1. Levine EG, Raghavan D. MVAC for bladder cancer: time to move forward again. J Clin Oncol 1993; 11: 387–389.
2. Sternberg CN, Yagoda A, Scher HI, et al. M-VAC (methotrexate, vinblastine, doxorubicin and cisplatin) for advanced transitional cell carcinoma of the urothelium. J Urol 1988; 139: 461–469.
3. Loehrer PJ, Einhorn LH, Elson PH, et al. A randomized comparison of cisplatin alone or in combination with methotrexate, vinblastine, and doxorubicin in patients with metastatic urothelial carcinoma: a cooperate group study. J Clin Oncol 1992; 10: 1066–1073.
4. Logothetis CJ, Dexeus FH, Finn L, et al. A prospective randomized trial comparing MVAC and CISCA chemotherapy for patients with metastatic urothelial tumors. J Clin Oncol 1990; 8: 1050–1055.

5. Loehrer PJ, Elson R, Dreicer R, et al. Escalated dosages of methotrexate vinblastine doxorubicin and cisplatin plus recombinant human granulocyte colony-stimulating factor in advanced urothelial carcinoma: an Eastern Cooperative Oncology Group trial. J Clin Oncol 1994; 12: 483–488.

6. Logothetis CJ, Finn LD, Smith T, et al. Escalated MVAC with or without recombinant human granulocyte-macrophage colony-stimulating factor for the initial treatment of advanced malignant urothelial tumors: results of a randomized trial. J Clin Oncol 1995; 13: 2272–2277.

7. Dodd PM, McCaffrey JA, Mazumdar M, et al. Phase II trial of intermediate dose methotrexate in combination with vinblastine, doxorubicin, and cisplatin in patients with unresectable or metastatic transits with transitional-cell carcinoma of the urothelial tract with ifosfamide, paclitaxel, and cisplatin: a phase II trial. J Clin Oncol 1998; 16: 2722–2727.

8. Bellmunt J, Ribas A, Eres N, et al. Carboplatin-based vs cisplatin-based chemotherapy in the treatment of surgically incurable advanced bladder carcinoma. Cancer 1997; 80: 1966–1972.

9. von der Maase H, Hansen SW, Roberts JT, et al. Gemcitabine and cisplatin versus methotrexate, vinblastine, doxorubicin and cisplatin in advanced or metastatic bladder: results of a large, randomized multinational, multicenter, phase III study. J Clin Oncol 2000; 18: 3068–3077.

10. Kirsh EJ, Baunoch DA, Stadler WM. New chemotherapy regimens for advanced bladder cancer. Sem Urol Oncol 1998; 16: 23–29.

11. Bajorin DF, McCaffrey JA, Hilton S, et al. Treatment of patients with transitional-cell carcinoma of the urothelial tract with ifosfamide, paclitaxel, and cisplatin: a phase II trial. 1998; 16: 2722–2727.

12. McCaffrey JA, Dodd PM, Hilton S, et al. Ifosfamide + paclitaxel + cisplatin (ITP) chemotherapy for patients (pts) with unresectable or metastatic transitional cell carcinoma (TCC). Proc Am Soc Clin Oncol 1999; 18: 1267.

13. Gad-el-Mawla N, Ziegler J, Hamza R, et al. Phase II chemotherapy trials of 5-FU, cyclophosphamide, ifosfamide, and vincristine in carcinoma of the bilharzial bladder. Cancer Treat Rep 1984; 68: 419–420.

14. Gad-el-Mawla N, Hamza MR, Zikri ZK, et al. Chemotherapy in invasive carcinoma of the bladder. Acta Oncol 1989; 28: 73–76.

15. Pronzato P, Vigani A, Pensa F, Vanoli M, Tani F, Vaira F. Second line chemotherapy with ifosfamide as outpatient treatment for advanced bladder cancer. Am J Clin Oncol 1997; 20: 519–521.

16. Witte RS. ECOG phase II trial of ifosfamide in the treatment of previously treated advanced urothelial carcinoma. J Clin Oncol 1997; 15: 589–593.

17. Roth BJ, Finch DE, Birhle R, et al. A phase II trial of ifosfamide + paclitaxel (IT) in advanced transitional cell carcinoma of the urothelium. Proc Am Soc Clin Oncol 1997; 16: 1156 abstract.

18. Kattan J, Culine S, Theodore C, Droz JP. Phase II trial of ifosfamide, fluorouracil, and folinic acid (fifo regimen) in relapsed and refractory urothelial cancer. Cancer Invest 1995; 13: 276–279.

19. Ruther U, Schmidt A, Rothe B, Seessler R, Eisenberger F, Jipp P. Preliminary results of chemotherapy with ifosfamide and VP-16 in advanced urothelial carcinoma. Fourth International Congress on Anti-Cancer Chemotherapy, February 2–5, 1993, Paris, France. p. 105.

20. Gad-el-Mawla N, Khaled H, Abdel-Wareth A. Epirubicin, Ifosfamide combination chemotherapy in invasive bladder cancer. Proc Am Soc Clin Oncol 1990; 9: 137.

21. Einhorn LH, Roth BJ, Ansari R, Dreicer R, Gonin R, Loehrer PJ. Phase II trial of vinblastine, ifosfamide, and gallium combination chemotherapy in metastatic urothelial carcinoma. J Clin Oncol 1994; 12: 2271–2276.

22. Roth BJ. Ifosfamide in the treatment of bladder cancer. Sem Oncol 1996; 23: 50–55.

23. Patel SR, Vadhan-Raj S, Burgess MA, et al. Results of two consecutive trials of dose-intensive chemotherapy with doxorubicin and ifosfamide in patients with sarcomas. Am J Clin Oncol 1998; 21: 317–321.

24. Vaughn DJ. Review and outlook for the role of paclitaxel in urothelial carcinoma. Sem Oncol 1999; 26: 117–122.

25. Roth BJ, Dreicer R, Einhorn LH, et al. Significant activity of paclitaxel in advanced transitional-cell carcinoma of the urothelium: a phase II trial of the Eastern Cooperative Oncolgy Group. J Clin Oncol 1994; 12: 2264–2270.

26. Papamichael D, Gallagher CJ, Oliver RT, Johnson PW, Waxman J. Phase II study of paclitaxel in pretreated patients with locally advanced/metastatic cancer of the bladder and ureter. Br J Cancer 1997; 75: 606–607.

27. de Wit R, Kruit WH, Stoter G, de Boer M, Kerger J, Verweij J. Docetaxel (Taxotere): an active agent in metastatic urothelial cancer; results of a phase II study in non-chemotherapy-pretreated patients. Br J Cancer 1998; 78: 1342–1345.

28. McCaffrey JA, Hilton S, Mazumdar M, Sadan S, Kelly WK, Scher HI, Bajorin DF. Phase II trial of docetaxel in patients with advanced metastatic transitional-cell carcinoma. J Clin Oncol 1997; 15: 1853–1857.

29. Burch PA, Richardson RL, Cha SS, et al. Phase II trial of combination paclitaxel and cisplatin in advanced urothelial carcinoma (UC). Proc Am Soc Clin Oncol 1999; 18: 1266.

30. Redman BG, Smith DC, Flaherty L, Du W, Hussain M. Phase II trial of paclitaxel and carboplatin in the treatment of advanced urothelial carcinoma. J Clin Oncol 1998; 16: 1844–1848.

31. Small EJ, Lew D, Redman BG, et al. Southwest oncology group study of paclitaxel and carboplatin for advanced transitional-cell carcinoma: the importance of survival as a clinical trial end point. J Clin Oncol 2000; 18: 2537–2544.

32. Tu SM, Hossan E, Amato R, Kilbourn R, Logothetis CJ. Paclitaxel, cisplatin and methotrexate combination chemotherapy is active in the treatment of refractory urothelial malignancies. J Urol 1995; 154: 1719–1722.

33. Unpublished results from University of Texas, MD Anderson Cancer Center protocol ID 95–198. Study Chairman: Randall Millkan.

34. Sengelov L, Kamby C, LUnd B, Engelholm SA. Docetaxel and cisplatin in metastatic urothelial cancer: a phase II study. J Clin Oncol 1998; 16: 3392–3397.

35. Garcia del Muro X, Marcuello E, Climent MA, et al. Phase II Study of Docetaxel and Cisplatin in Advanced Urothelial Cancer: Preliminary Results. Proc Am Soc Clin Oncol 1999; 18: 1306.

36. Vogelzang NJ, Stadler WM. Gemcitabine and other new chemotherapeutic agents for the treatment of metastatic bladder cancer. Urology 1999; 53: 243–250.

37. Stadler WM, Kuzel T, Roth B, Raghavan D, Dorr FA. Phase II study of single-agent gemcitabine in previously untreated patients with metastatic urothelial cancer. J Clin Oncol 1997; 15: 3394–3398.

38. Lorusso V, Pollera CF, Antimi M, et al. A phase II study of gemcitabine in patients with transitional cell carcinoma of the urinary tract previously treated with platium. Italian Co-operative Group on Bladder Cancer. Eur J Cancer 1998; 34: 1208–1212.

39. von der Maase H, Andersen L, Crino L, Weissbach L, Dogliotti L. A phase II study of gemcitabine and cisplatin in patients with transitional cell carcinoma. Proc Am Soc Clin Oncol 1997; 16: 1155.

40. Stadler WM, Murphy B, Kaufman D, Raghavan D. Phase II trial of gemcitabijne (GEM) plus cisplatin (CDDP) in metastatic urothelial cancer (UC). Proc Am Soc Clin Oncol 1997; 16: 1152.

41. Meluch AA, Greco FA, Burris HA III, O'Rourke TO, Ortega G, Morrissey LH, et al. Gemcitabine and paclitaxel in combination for advanced transitional cell carcinoma (TCC) of the urothelial tract: a trial of the Minnie Pearl Research Network. Proc Am Soc Clin Oncol 1999; 18: 1338.

42. Marini L, Sternberg CN, Sella A, Calabro F, van Rijn A. A new regimen of gemcitabine and paclitaxel in previously treated patients with advanced transitional cell carcinoma. Proc Am Soc Clin Oncol 1999; 18: 1335.

43. Dodd PM, McCaffrey JA, Hilton S, Mazumdar M, Icasiano E, Higgins G, et al. Phase I evaluation of sequential doxorubicin + Gemcitabine (AG) then ifosfamide + paclitaxel + cisplatin (ITP) for patients (pts) with unresectable or metastatic transitional cell carcinoma (TCC). Proc Am Soc Clin Oncol 1999; 18: 1268.

44. Bellmunt J, Guillem V, Paz-Ares L, et al. A phase II trial of paclitaxel, cisplatin and gemcitabine (TCG) in patients (pts) with advanced transitional cell carcinoma (TCC) of the urothelium. Proc Am Soc Clin Oncol 1999; 18: 1279.

45. Vaishampayan U, Smith D, Redman B, Kucuk O, Ensley J, Hussain M. Phase II evaluation of carboplatin, paclitaxel and gemcitabine in advanced urothelial carcinoma. Proc Am Soc Clin Oncol 1999; 18: 1282.

46. Noble S, Goa KL. Gemcitabine. A review of its pharmacology and clinical potential in non-small cell lung cancer and pancreatic cancer. Drugs 1997; 54: 447–472.

47. Murray N, Livingston RB, Shepherd FA, et al. Randomized study of CODE versus alternating CAV/EP for extensive-stage small-cell lung cancer: an Intergroup study of the National Cancer Institute of Canada Clinical Trials Group and Southwest Oncology Group. J Clin Oncol 1999; 17: 2300–2308.

48. Cote RJ, Dunn MD, Chatterjee SJ, et al. Elevated and absent pRb expression is associated with bladder cancer progression and has cooperative effects with p53. Cancer Res 1998; 58: 1090–1094. See also: Cordon-Cardo C, Zhang ZF, Dalbagni G, Drobnjak M, Charytonowicz E, Hu SX, Xu HJ, Reuter VE, Benedict WF. Cooperative effects of p53 and pRB alterations in primary superficial bladder. Cancer Res 1997; 57: 1217–1221.

49. Stein JP, Ginsberg DA, Grossfeld GD, et al. Effect of p21WAF1/CIP1 expression on tumor progression in bladder. J Natl Cancer Inst 1998; 90: 1072–1079.

50. Stein JP, Grossfeld GD, Esrig D, Freeman JA, Figueroa AJ, Skinner DG, Cote RJ. Prognostic markers in bladder cancer: a contemporary review of the literature. J Urol 1998; 160: 645–659.

51. Keegan PE, Lunec J, Neal DE. p53 and p53-regulated genes in bladder. Br J Urol 1998: 82: 710–720.

52. Cote RJ, Esrig D, Goshen S, Jones PA, Skinner DG. p53 and treatment of bladder cancer. Nature 1997; 385: 123–125.

53. Skinner DG, Daniels JR, Russell CA, Lieskovsky G, Boyd SD, Nichols P, et al. The role of adjuvant chemotherapy following cystectomy for invasive bladder cancer: a prospective comparative trial. J Urol 1991; 145: 459–467.

54. Wu CS, Pollack A, Czerniak B, Chyle V, Zagars GK, Hu SX, Benedict WF. Prognostic value of p53 in muscle-invasive bladder cancer treated with preoperative radiotherapy. Urology 1996; 47: 305–310.

55. Meyers FJ, Miller TR, Williams SG, Gandour-Edwards R, Edelman MJ, DeVere White RW. Response to a Taxol based chemotherapy regimen in advanced transitional cell carcinoma is independent of p53 expression. Proc Am Soc Clin Oncol 1999; 18: 1283.

56. Neal DE, Sharples L, Smith K, Fennelly J, Hall RJ, Harris AL. The epidermal growth factor receptor and the prognosis of bladder cancer. Cancer 1990; 65: 1619–1625.

57. Ravery V, Grignon D, Angulo J, Pontes E, Montie J, Crissman J, Dhopin D. Evaluation of epidermal growth factor receptor, transforming growth factor alpha, epidermal growth factor and fc-erbB2 in the progression of invasive bladder cancer. Urol Res 1997; 25: 9–17.

58. Fan Z, Mendelsohn J. Therapeutic application of anti-growth factor receptor antibodies. Curr Opinion Oncol 1998; 10: 67–73.

59. Perrotte P. Matsumoto T, Inoue K, Kuniyasu H, Eve BY, Hicklin DJ, et al. Anti-epidermal growth factor receptor antibody C225 inhibits angiogenesis in human transitional cell carcinoma growing orthotopically in nude mice. Clin Cancer Res 1999; 5: 257–265.

60. Fan Z, Baselga J, Masui H, Mendelsohn J. Antitumor effect of anti-epidermal growth factor receptor monoclonal antibodies plus cis-diaminedichloroplatinum on well established A431 cell xenografts. Cancer Res 1993; 53: 4637–4642.

61. Dinney CPN, Parker C, Dong Z, Fan D, Eve BY, Bucana C, Radinsky R. Therapy of human transitional cell carcinoma of the bladder by oral administration of the epidermal growth factor receptor protein tyrosine kinase inhibitor 4,5-dianilino-phthalimide. Clin Cancer Res 1997; 3: 161–168.

62. Siegall CB, FitzGerald DJ, Pastan I. Selective killing of tumor cells using EGF or TGF alpha-Pseudomonas exotoxin chimeric molecules. Semin Cancer Biol 1990; 1: 345–350.

63. Moasser MM, Sepp-Lorenzino L, Kohl NE, Oliff A, Balog A, Su DS, et al. Farnesyl transferase inhibitors cause enhanced mitotic sensitivity to taxol and epothilones. Proc Natl Acad Sci USA 1998; 95: 1369–1374.

64. Klohs WD, Fry DW, Kraker AJ. Inhibitors of tyrosine kinase. Current Opin Oncol 1997; 9: 562–568.

65. Spataro V, Norbury C, Harris AL. The ubiquitin-proteasome pathway in cancer. Br J Cancer 1998; 77: 448–455.

66. Adams J, Palombella VJ, Sausville EA, et al. Proteasome inhibitors: a novel class of potent and effective antitumor agents. Cancer Res 1999; 59: 2615–2622.

67. Fidler IJ, Kumar R, Bielenberg DR, Ellis LM. Molecular determinants of angiogenesis in cancer metastasis. Cancer J Sci 1998; 4: 58–66.

68. Fidler IJ. Critical determinants of cancer metastasis: rationale for therapy. Cancer Chemo Pharmacol 199; 43(Suppl): S3–S10.

69. Wojtowicz-Praga SM, Dickson RB, Hawkins MJ. Matrix metalloproteinase inhibitors. Invest New Drugs 1997; 15: 61–75.

70. Steward WP. Marimastat (BB2516): current status of development. Cancer Chemo Pharm 1999; 43(Suppl): S56–S60.

71. Ellerhorst JA, Sella A, Amato RJ, Tu S-M, Millikan RE, Finn LD, et al. Phase II trial of 5-fluorouracil, interferon-a and continuous infusion interleukin-2 for patients with metastatic renal cell carcinoma. Cancer 1997; 80: 2128–2132.

72. Rohde D. Thiemann D. Wildberger J. Wolff J. Jakse G. Treatment of renal cancer patients with gemcitabine (2',2'-difluorodeoxycytidine) and interferons: antitumor activity and toxicity. Oncol Rep 1998; 5: 1555–1560.

73. Verma IM, Somia N. Gene therapy: promises, problems and prospects. Nature 1997; 389: 239–242.

74. Linden RM, Berns KI. Adeno-associated virus: a basis for a potential gene therapy vector. Gene Ther 1997; 4: 4–5.

75. Li Y, Pong RC, Bergelson JM, Hall MC, Sagalowsky AI, Tseng CP, et al. Loss of adenoviral receptor expression in human bladder cancer cells: a potential impact on the efficacy of gene therapy. Cancer Res 1999: 59: 325–330.

76. Moll R, Wu XR, Lin JH, Sun TT. Uroplakins, specific membrane proteins of uro-thelial umbrella cells, as histological markers of metastatic transitional cell carci-nomas. Am J Pathol 1995; 147: 1383–1397.

77. Wu RL, Osman I, Wu XR, et al. Uroplakin II gene is expressed in transitional cell carcinoma but not in bilharzial bladder squamous cell carcinoma: alternative path-ways of bladder epithelial differentiation and tumor formation. Cancer Res 1998; 58: 1291–1297.

78. Lin JH, Zhao H, Sun TT. A tissue specific promoter that can drive a foreign gene to express in the suprabasal urothelial cells of transgenic mice. Proc Natl Acad Sci USA 1995; 92: 679–683.

79. Kerr DE, Bondioli KR, Zhao H, Kreibich G, Wall RJ, Sun TT. The bladder as a bioreactor: urothelial production and secretion of growth hormone into urine. Natl Biotechnol 1998; 16: 75–79.

80. Douglas JT, Rogers BE, Rosenfeld ME, Michael SI, Feng M, Curiel DT. Targeted gene delivery by tropism-modified adenoviral vectors. Nat Biotechnol 1996; 14: 1574–1579.

81. Cristiano RJ. Targeted, non-viral gene delivery for cancer gene therapy. Front Biosci 1998; 3: D1161–D1170.

82. Arap W, Pasqualini R, Ruoslahti E. Cancer treatment by targeted drug delivery to tumor vasculature in a mouse model. Science 1998; 279: 377–380.

83. Krasnykh V, Mitriev I, Mikheeva G, Miller CR, Belousova N, Curiel DT. Char-acterization of an adenovirus vector containing a heterologous peptide epitope in the H1 loop of the fiber knob. J Virol 1998; 72: 1844–1852.

84. Bischoff JR, Kirn DH, Williams A, et al. An adenovirus mutant that replicates selectively in p53-deficient human tumor cells. Science 1996; 274: 373–376.

85. Heise C, Sampson-Johannes A, Williams A, McCormick F, Von Hoff DD, Kirn DH. ONYX-015, an E1B gene-attenuated adenovirus, causes tumor-specific cy-tolysis and antitumoral efficacy that can be augmented by standard chemothera-peutic agents. Nat Med 1997; 3: 639–645.

86. Heise CC, Williams AM, Xue S, Propst M, Kirn DH. Intravenous administration of ONYX-015, a selectively replicating adenovirus, induces antitumoral efficacy. Cancer Res 1999; 59: 2623–2628.

87. Freytag SO, Rogulski KR, Paielli DL, Gilbert JD, Kim JH. A novel three-pronged approach to kill cancer cells selectively: concomitant viral, double suicide gene, and radiotherapy. Hum Gene Ther 1998; 9: 1323–1333.

88. Wildner O, Morris JC, Vahanian NN, Ford H Jr, Ramsey WJ, Blaese RM. Aden-oviral vectors capable of replication improve the efficacy of HSVtk/GCV suicide gene therapy of cancer. Gene Ther 1999; 6: 57–62.

89. Akao T, Kakehi Y, Itoh N, et al. High prevalence of functional inactivation by methylation modification of p16INK4A/CDKN2/MTS1 gene in primary urothelial cancers. Jpn J Cancer Res 1997; 88: 1078–1086.

90. Liu T-J, Zhang W-W, Taylor DL, Roth JA, Goepfert H Clayman GL. Growth sup-pression of human head and neck cancer cells by the introduction of a wild-type p53 gene via a recombinant adenovirus. Cancer Res 1994; 54: 3662–3667.

91. Fujiwara T, Cai DW, Georges RN, Mukhopadhyay T, Grimm EA, Roth JA. Thera-peutic effect of a retroviral wild-type p53 expression vector in an orthotopic lung cancer model. J Natl Cancer Inst 1994; 86: 1458–1462.

92. Wills KN, Maneval DC, Menzel P, et al. Development and characterization of recombinant adenoviruses encoding human p53 for gene therapy. Hum Gene Ther 1994; 5: 1079–1088.

93. Ko SC, Gotoh A, Thalmann GN, et al. Molecular therapy with recombinant p53 adenovirus in an androgen-independent, metastatic human prostate cancer model. Hum Gene Ther 1996; 7: 1683–1691.

94. Nielsen LL, Dell J, Maxwell E, Armstrong L, Maneval D, Catino JJ. Efficacy of p53 adenovirus-mediated gene therapy against human breast cancer xenografts. Cancer Gene Ther 1997; 4: 129–138.

95. Xu M, Kumar D, Srinivas S, et al. Parental gene therapy with p53 inhibits human breast tumors in vivo through a bystander mechanism without evidence of toxicity. Hum Gene Ther 1997; 8: 177–185.

96. Roth JA, Nguyen D, Lawrence DD, et al. Retrovirus-mediated wild-type p53 gene transfer to tumors of patients with lung cancer. Natl Med 1996; 2: 985–991.

97. Swisher SG, Roth JA, Nemunaitis J, et al. Adenovirus-mediated p53 gene transfer in advanced non-small cell lung cancer. J Natl Cancer Inst 1999; 91: 763–771.

98. Werthman PE, Drazan KE, Rosenthal JT, Khalili R, Shaked A. Adenoviral-p53 gene transfer to orthotopic and peritoneal murine bladder cancer. J Urol 1996; 155: 753–756.

99. Engler H, Anderson SC, Machemer TR, Philopena JM, Connor RJ, Wen SF, Maneval DC. Ethanol improves adenovirus-mediated gene transfer and expression to bladder epthelium of rodents. Urology 1999; 53: 1049–1053.

100. Xu H-J, Zhou Y, Seigne J, Perng G-S, Mixon M, Zhang C, et al. Enhanced tumor suppressor gene therapy via replication-deficient adenovirus vectors expressing an N-terminal truncated retinoblastoma. Cancer Res 1996; 56: 2245–2249.

101. Demers GW, Harris MP, Wen SF, Engler H, Nielsen LL, Maneval DC. A recombinant adenoviral vector expressing full-length human retinoblastoma gene inhibits human tumor cell growth. Cancer Gene Ther 1998; 5: 207–214.

102. Grim J, D'Amico A, Frizelle S, Zhou J, Kratzke RA, Curiel DT. Adenovirus-mediated delivery of p16 to p16-deficient human bladder cancer cells confers chemoresistance to cisplatin and paclitaxel. Clin Cancer Res 1997; 3: 2415–2423.

103. Sandig V, Brand K, Herwig S, Kukas J, Bartek J, Strauss M. Adenovirally transferred p16 and p53 genes cooperate to induce apoptotic tumor cell death. Nat Med 1997; 3: 313–319.

104. Lowe SW, Bodis S, McClatchey A, Remington L, Ruley HE, Fisher DE, et al. p53 status and the efficacy of cancer therapy in vivo. Science 1994; 266: 807–810.

105. Brachman DG, Beckett M, Graves D, Haraf D, Vokes E, Weichselbaum RR. p53 mutation does not correlate with radiosensitivity in 24 head and neck cancer cell lines. Cancer Res 1993; 53: 3667–3669.

106. Chiarugi V, Magnelli L, Cinelli M. Role of p53 mutations in the radiosensitivity status of tumor cell. Tumori 1998; 84: 517–520.

107. Gjerset RA, Turla ST, Sobol RE, Scalise JJ, Mercola D, Collins H, Hopkins PJ. Use of wild-type p53 to achieve complete treatment sensitization of tumor cells expressing endogenous mutant p53. Molecular Carcinogenesis 1995; 14: 275–285.

108. Spitz FR, Nguyen D, Skibber JM, Meyn RE, Cristiano RJ, Roth JA. Adenoviral-mediated wild-type p53 gene expression sensitizes colorectal cancer cells to ionizing radiation. Clin Cancer Res 1996; 2: 1665–1671.

109. Xu GW, Sun ZT, Forrester K, Wang XW, Coursen J, Harris CC. Tissue-specific growth suppression and chemosensitivity promotion in human hepatocellular carcinoma by retroviral-mediated transfer of the wild-type p53 gene. Gastroenterology 1996; 24: 1264–1268.

110. Nguyen DM, Spitz FR, Yen N, Cristiano RJ, Roth JA. Gene therapy for lung cancer: enhancement of tumor suppression by a combination of sequential systemic

cisplatin and adenovirus-mediated p53 gene transfer. J Thor Cardiovas Surg 1996; 112: 1372–1377.

111. Lesoon-Wood LA, Kim WH, Kleinman HK, Weintraub BD, Mixson AJ. Systemic gene therapy with p53 reduces growth and metastases of a malignant human breast cancer in nude mice. Hum Gene Ther 1995; 6: 395–405.

112. Nishizaki M, Fujiwara T, Tanida T, Hizuta A, Nishimori H, Tokino T, et al. Recombinant adenovirus expressing wild-type p53 is antiangiogenic: a proposed mechanism for bystander effect. Clin Cancer Res 1999; 5: 1015–1023.

113. Moolten FL. Tumor chemosensitivity conferred by inserted herpes thymidine kinase genes: paradigm for a prospective cancer control strategy. Cancer Res 1986; 46: 5276–5281.

114. Bi WL, Parysek LM, Warnick R, Stambrook PJ. In vitro evidence that metabolic cooperation is responsible for the bystander effect observed with HSV-tk retroviral gene therapy. Hum Gene Ther 1993; 4: 725–731.

115. Vile RG, Nelson JA, Castleden S, Chong H, Hart IR. Systemic gene therapy of murine melanoma using tissue specific expression of the HSV-tk gene involves an immune component. Cancer Res 1994; 54: 6226–6234.

116. Elshami AA, Saavedra A, Zhang H, Kucharczuk JC, Spray DC, Fishman GI, et al. Gap junctions play a role in the "bystander effect" of the herpes simplex virus thymidine kinase/ganciclovir system in vitro. Gene Ther 1996; 3: 85–92.

117. Mesnil M, Piccoli C, Tirabi G, Willecke K, Yamasaki H. Bystander killing of cancer cells by herpes simplex virus thymidine kinase gene is mediated by connexins. Proc Natl Acad Sci USA 1996; 93: 1831–1835.

118. Hamel W, Magnelli L, Chiarugi VP, Israel MA. Herpes simplex virus thymidine kinase/ganciclovir-mediated apoptotic death of bystander cells. Cancer Res 1996; 56: 2697–2702.

119. Sutton M, Berkman S, Chen S-H, Block A, Troung DD, Kattan MW, et al. Adenovirus-mediated suicide gene therapy for experimental bladder cancer. Urology 1997; 49: 173–180.

120. Herman JR, Lerner SP. Current status of gene therapy for prostate and bladder cancer. Int J Urol 1997; 4: 435–440.

121. Barba D, Hardin J, Sadelain M, Gage FH. Development of anti-tumor immunity following thymidine kinase-mediated killing of experimental brain tumors. Proc Natl Acad Sci USA 1994; 91: 4348–4352.

122. Bi W, Kim YG, Feliciano ES, Pavelic L, Wilson KM, Pavelic ZP, Stambrook PJ. An HSVtk-mediated local and distant antitumor bystander effect in tumors of head and neck origin in athymic mice. Cancer Gene Ther 1997; 4: 246–252.

123. Kuriyama S, Sakamoto T, Masui K, Nakatani T, Tominga K, Kikikawa M, et al. Tissue-specific expression of HSV-tk gene can induce efficient antitumor effect and protective immunity to wildtype hepatocellular tumor. Int J Cancer 1997; 71: 470–475.

124. Gagandeep S, Brew R, Green B. Christmas SE, Klatzmann D, Poston GJ, Kinsella AR. Prodrug-activated gene therapy: involvement of an immunological component in the bystander effect. Cancer Gene Ther 1996; 3: 83–88.

125. Yamamto S, Suzuki S, Hoshino A, Akimoto M, Shimada T. Herpes simplex virus thymidine kinase/ganciclovir-mediated killing of tumor cells induces tumor-specific cytotoxic T cells in mice. Cancer Gene Ther 1997; 4: 91–96.

126. Kianmanesh AR, Perrin H, Panis Y, Fabre M, Nagy HJ, Houssin D, Klatzmann D. A distant bystander effect of suicide gene therapy: regression of non transduced tumors together with a distant transduced tumor. Hum Gene Ther 1997; 8: 1807–1814.

127. Hall SJ, Sanford MA, Atkinson G, Chen S-H. Induction of potent anti-tumor natural killer cell activity by HSV-tk and ganciclovir therapy in an orthotopic mouse model of prostate cancer. Cancer Res 1998; 58: 3221–3225.

128. Connor J, Bannerji R, Saito S, Heston W, Fair W, Gilboa E. Regression of bladder tumors in mice treated with interleukin-2 gene modified tumor cells. J Exp Med 1993; 177: 1127–1134.

129. Saito S, Bannerji R, Gansbacher B, Rosenthal FM, Romanenko P, Heston WDW, et al. Immunotherapy of bladder cancer with cytokine gene-modified tumor vaccines. Cancer Res 1994; 54: 3516–3520.

130. Simons JW, Mikhak B. Ex vivo gene therapy using cytokine-transduced tumor vaccines: molecular and clinical pharmacology. Semin Oncol 1998; 25: 661–676.

131. Greten TF, Jaffee EM. Cancer vaccines. J Clin Oncol 1999; 17: 1047–1060.

132. Porgador A, Tzehoval E, Vadai E, Feldman M, Eisenbach L. Combined vaccination with major histocompatability class I and interleukin 2 gene-transduced melanoma cells synergizes the cure of postsurgical established lung metastases. Cancer Res 1995; 55: 4941–4949.

133. Salvadori S, Gansbacher B, Wernick I, Tirelli S, Zier K. B7–1 amplifies the response to interleukin-2-secreting tumor vaccines in vivo, but fails to induce a response by naive cells in vitro. Hum Gene Ther 1995; 6: 1299–1306.

134. Cao X, Chen G, Zhang W, Tao Q, Yu Y, Ye T. Enhanced efficacy of combination of IL-2 gene and IL–6 gene-transfected tumor cells in the treatment of established metastatic tumors. Gene Ther 1996;3: 421–426.

135. Gaken JA, Hollingsworth SJ, Hirst WJR, Buggins AGS, Galea-Lauri J, Peakman M, et al. Irradiated NC adenocarcinoma cells transduced with both B7.1 and interleukin-2 induce CD4+-mediated rejection of established tumors. Hum Gene Ther 1997; 8: 477–488.

136. Sanda MG, Smith DC, Charles LG, Hwang C, Pienta KJ, Schlom J, et al. Recombinant vaccinia-PSA (PROSTVAC) can induce a prostate-specific immune response in androgen-modulated human prostate cancer. Urology 1999; 53: 260–266.

137. Murphy GP, Tjoa BA, Simmons SJ, Ragde H, Rogers M, Elgamal A, et al. Phase II prostate cancer vaccine trial: report of a study involving 37 patientswith disease recurrence following primary treatment. Prostate 1999; 39: 54–59.

138. Gilboa E, Nair SK, Lyerly HK. Immunotherapy of cancer with dendritic-cell-based vaccines. Cancer Immunol Immunother 1998; 46: 82–87.

139. Cordier L, Duffour MT, Sabourin JC, Lee MG, Cabannes J, Ragot T, et al. Complete recovery of mice from a pre-established tumor by direct intra-tumoral delivery of an adenovirus vector harboring the murine IL-2 gene. Gene Ther 1995; 2: 16–21.

140. Addison CL, Braciak T, Ralston R, Muller WJ, Gauldie J, Graham FL. Intratumoral injection of an adenovirus expressing interleukin 2 induces regression and immunity in a murine breast cancer model. Proc Natl Acad Sci USA 1995; 92: 8522–8526.

141. Meko JB, Yim JH, Tsung K, Norton JA. High cytokine production and effective antitumor activity of a recombinant vaccina virus encoding murine interleukin 12. Cancer Res 1995; 55: 4765–4770.

142. Chen SH, Kosai K, Xu B, Pham-Nguyen K, Contant C, Finegold MJ, Woo SL. Combination suicide and cytokine gene therapy for hepatic metastases of colon carcinoma: sustained antitumor immunity prolongs animal survival. Cancer Res 1996; 56: 3758–3762.

143. Hayashi S, Emi N, Yokoyama I, Namii Y, Uchida K, Takagi H. Inhibition of establishment of hepatic metastasis in mice by combination gene therapy using both

herpes simplex virus-thymidine kinase and granulocyte macrophage-colony stimu-
lating factor genes in murine colon cancer. Cancer Gene Ther 1997; 4: 339–344.

144. Castleden SA, Chong H, Garcia-Ribas I, Melcher AA, Hutchinson G, Roberts B,
et al. A family of bicistronic vectors to enhance both local and systemic antitumor
effects of HSVtk or cytokine expression in a murine melanoma model. Hum Gene
Ther 1997; 8: 2087–2102.

145. Kong HL, Hecht D, Song W, Kovesdi I, Hackett NR, Yayon A, Crystal RG.
Regional suppression of tumor growth by in vivo transfer of a cDNA encoding a
secreted form of the extracellular domain of the flt-1 vascular endothelial growth
factor receptor. Hum Gene Ther 1998; 9: 823–833.

146. Goldman CK, Kendall RL, Cabrera G, Soroceanu L, Heike Y, Gillespie GY, et al.
Paracrine expression of a native soluble vascular endothelial growth factor receptor inhibits tumor growth, metastasis, and mortality rate. Proc Natl Acad Sci USA
1998; 95: 8795–8800.

147. O'Reilly MS, Holmgren L, Shing Y, Chen C, Rosenthal RA, Moses M, et al.
Angiostatin: a novel angiogenesis inhibitor that mediates the suppression of metastases by a Lewis lung carcinoma. Cell 1994; 79: 315–328.

148. O'Reilly MS, Boehm T, Shing Y, Fukai N, Vasios G, Lane WS, et al. Endostatin:
an endogenous inhibitor of angiogenesis and tumor growth. Cell 1997; 88: 277–
285.

149. Cao Y, O'Reilly MS, Marshall B, Flynn E, Ji RW, Folkman J. Expression of angiostatin cDNA in a murine fibrosarcoma suppresses primary tumor growth and produces long-term dormancy of metastases. J Clin Invest 1998; 101: 1055–1063.

150. Tanaka T, Cao Y, Folkman J, Fine HA. Viral vector-targeted anti-angiogenic gene
therapy utlizing an angiostatin complementary DNA. Cancer Res 1998; 58: 3362–
3369.

151. Blezinger P, Wang J, Gondo M, Quezada A, Mehrens D, French M, et al. Systemic
inhibition of tumor growth and tumor metastases by intramuscular administration
of the endostatin gene. Nat Biotech 1999; 17: 343–348.

17

Statistical Considerations in the Phase II Evaluation of New Therapies

Randall Millikan, MD, PHD
and Peter F. Thall, PHD

CONTENTS

INTRODUCTION

As discussed in Chapter 16, there are many new therapies for urothelial cancer currently being developed and evaluated. Within the classical phase II paradigm for identifying promising new therapies, an estimate of the efficacy of each of these would be obtained in a single-arm trial, ideally conducted in a population of previously untreated patients. Although at first glance this seems straightforward, in fact there are multiple challenges, both ethical and scientific, in the conduct and interpretation of phase II trials. In this chapter we explore some aspects of the "phase II problem" and some of the tools available for investigating new therapies.

SCIENCE AND ETHICS IN PHASE II

The basic statistical rationale underlying a single-arm phase II trial of an experimental treatment, E, is that one wishes to estimate the efficacy of E and compare that estimate to the corresponding value for "standard" therapy, S. In practice, S represents the treatment that the patients in the

From: *Current Clinical Urology: Bladder Cancer: Current Diagnosis and Treatment*
Edited by: M. J. Droller © Humana Press Inc., Totowa, NJ

trial would have been given as standard therapy if they were not enrolled in the trial of E. If there are two or more current standards, then S is a composite of these. For example, if treatment efficacy is determined by whether the patient has a particular outcome, "response," having probabilities p_E under E and p_S under S, then the phase II goal is to estimate p_E . Whether or not it is explicitly stated in the trial design, however, phase II always involves comparison of E to S, either in terms of the difference $p_E - p_S$, or an analogous, more complicated collection of such effects including differences in toxicity probabilities. The comparison may be part of formal tests of hypotheses to address such questions as "Is E more efficacious than S?" or "Is E more toxic than S?" *(1–5)*. Alternatively, the comparison may be in the context of one or more Bayesian safety monitoring rules that do not test hypotheses but are in place only to shut down the trial if E is found to be unsafe or inefficacious compared to S *(6–11)*. Such comparisons are scientifically problematic, however, due to the fact that the estimates corresponding to E and S arise from different trials. In the simplest case of a binary response outcome noted above, the estimated difference $p_E - p_S$ is confounded by trial effects. Specifically, the thing being estimated is not $(p_E - p_S)$ but rather is $(p_E - p_S) + (t_E - t_S)$, where t_E and t_S are the respective effects associated with the separate trials of E and S. Thus, when trial-to-trial variability $(t_E - t_S)$ is large relative to $(p_E - p_S)$, the statistical comparison may be very misleading. Although this confounding can be mitigated to some extent by fitting a statistical regression model that adjusts for observed patient covariates, of course such methods cannot account for unobserved "latent" effects that cause between-trial variability. The only valid way to avoid such confounding is to conduct a randomized trial including both E and S in the first place.

The common practice of conducting single-arm phase II trials originated in settings where no effective agent existed, the so-called "phase IIA" setting. Here, $p_S = 0$ and thus a single-arm trial of E is a sensible way to obtain an estimate of p_E and decide whether p_E is sufficiently large, e.g., at least 15–20%, to warrant further study *(10,12,13)*. The underlying idea is that the early outcome, such as 50% tumor shrinkage or a particular biomarker response, is sufficiently predictive of improved survival that its occurrence, even at such a low rate, might warrant further study of E as part of a combination therapy in a later phase II trial or in a large randomized trial of E versus S. In the "phase IIB" setting, where a standard therapy with antidisease activity in the particular patient–disease group being studied already exists, there still may be practical motivations for conducting a single-arm trial. These include limited accrual, the need to evaluate multiple new treatments that become available sequentially over time, and possible ethical considerations that preclude the equipose between E and S necessary to ethically randomize.

If the potential confounding of treatment and trial effects is kept in mind, and if appropriate early stopping rules are used, then a single-arm phase II trial of E may provide information useful for estimating a wide variety of quantities, including p_E, probabilities of toxicity, and early mortality, and the average values of surrogate biomarkers. One may then decide, on the basis of these estimates, how next to proceed.

Perhaps the most important consideration in any clinical trial conducted with human patients is that it be ethically sound. In phase II trials, the ethical problems are generally related to both safety and assessment of benefit. Early stopping rules in statistical designs for phase II are usually formulated in terms of tests of hypotheses or Bayesian decision rules, and hence they have scientific meaning. Such rules also reflect the ethical imperative to stop a trial because, based on the experience gained thus far in the trial, it is unethical to continue treating patients with E. Although not always explicitly acknowledged, safety is in fact a primary issue in phase II trials. This is inevitably the case because either the treatment being studied has only limited prior use in humans, or, at the very least, has very limited use in the particular population being studied.

In phase I dose-finding trials *(14)*, it is well recognized that some problems do not come to light until there is wider or longer term experience with the treatment. For example, most of the designs in use for phase I evaluation focus on acute toxicity observed in only the first or second cycle. Thus, long-term toxicity that appears only with more prolonged exposure is not even part of a typical phase I analysis. Recent methods for dealing with late onset toxicities have been proposed by Thall, Lee, Tseng, and Estey *(15)* and Cheung and Chappell *(16)*. Another problem with conventional dose-finding methods is that they reduce toxicity to a binary "yes/no" variable. A new method that accounts for grade of toxicity has been proposed by Simon et al. *(17)*. An entirely different complication arises in the evaluation of many of the newer "biologic" agents coming into the clinic. Many of these agents must be taken chronically, making low-grade, but sustained, toxicity "dose limiting" in a sense that is not recognized in the traditional design and analysis of classic cytotoxics. Beyond these issues of accounting for toxicity, the optimal dose and schedule for a new drug or new combination are often not well characterized by current phase I designs. A "phase I/II" method that determines a best dose based on both response and toxicity has been proposed by Thall and Russell *(18)* and extended by Thall, Estey, and Sung

(19). In particular, this method may be used in settings, as with biologic agents, where the probability of "response" is not a continuously increasing function of dose but rather increases to a plateau with no increase in efficacy despite further increases in dose.

Another well-known issue is that the dose emerging from a phase I trial may be heavily influenced by the selection factors at work in the patient group studied. If the overall prognostic level of phase II patients is higher than that of the phase I patients, then the "maximum tolerated dose" obtained in phase I may be lower than what should be used ideally in phase II. Together, these limitations require that learning to characterize and manage both acute and chronic toxicity, and refinement of dose and schedule are commonly part of phase II trials. Unfortunately, these important issues do not usually receive much attention in the formal trial design and analysis. It is somewhat ironic but true that usually the "real" goal of a phase I trial is to look for hints of clinical activity, and the "real" goal of a phase II trial is to refine emerging information about dose and toxicity in the setting of a clinically promising therapy. That is, every phase I trial has at least some phase II goals, and conversely. The hybrid phase I/II designs noted previously address this issue directly and explicitly. Extensions to accommodate multiple treatment courses, adjust for patient covariates, and allow late onset toxicities scored on an ordinal rather than a binary scale are all still areas of active research, and practical statistical dose-finding designs that deal with these issues are in development. In any case, an ethically acceptable phase II trial must offer patients new therapies in the context of appropriate safety monitoring for both acute and delayed adverse events.

Many phase II trials are formulated strictly in terms of a binary response, with statements in portions of the trial protocol separate from the statistical design that describe adverse outcomes and assure that "safety monitoring" will be done. When explicit early stopping rules in terms of adverse events are not formulated and included as part of the trial design, such "safety monitoring" can only be done using informal, subjective, ad hoc criteria. The actual properties of such informal decision rules are often very different from what those making the decisions may imagine. That is, the informal "algorithm" may be unlikely to stop the trial in circumstances where one would in fact very much want to stop or, conversely, such considerations may stop the trial when one would not want to stop. The point is that formal rules are needed, and a statistician should evaluate the rules and modify them as appropriate so that they reflect the clinician's actual safety standards. Thus, although it is certainly more work for both the statisticians and physicians involved, it is very important that safety monitoring rules be formalized and their properties studied and confirmed before starting the trial.

A more subtle ethical issue, of particular relevance in trials targeting patients with metastatic urothelial cancer, is the problem of how to introduce treatments of unknown efficacy into a clinical research setting in which multiple active therapies already exist. Currently, front-line therapy for metastatic bladder cancer more than *triples* the median survival expected from the natural history of the disease, and is curative for a small percentage. Thus, despite the fact that nearly all such patients will eventually die of their disease, it is clearly ethically problematic to forego therapy known to significantly prolong survival in order to test a therapy of unknown efficacy in a population of untreated patients. At all times, there is an ethical obligation to offer all patients a therapeutic intervention that can be reasonably construed to be as good as whatever the current "standard" therapy happens to be. A trial involving a new therapy of unknown efficacy can, however, be ethically acceptable in some circumstances, such as when there is confidence of effective "salvage" treatment, or the case of testing a close analog of a known treatment that could reasonably be expected to perform as well as the standard, but, for example, is likely to have a more favorable toxicity profile. In general, little attention has been paid to the issue of how to design trials that introduce newer agents or treatment paradigms in a way that ensures that patients also get the full benefit of available therapy. In the specific context of metastatic urothelial cancer, this means that for practical purposes we will need to study new therapies in cohorts of patients already treated with standard therapy, or look at combination studies with conventional cytotoxics from the outset. As discussed in Chapter 16, we are particularly drawn to the study of new agents as a "consolidation" after maximal benefit from conventional therapy.

The general ethical problem in phase II evaluation of new therapies ultimately comes down to the desire to offer patients the "best" available therapy. The question then becomes what is meant by "best," and here uncertainty with regard to the probabilities of efficacy and adverse events with available and experimental treatments comes into play. Consequently, the problem of constructing designs that are both ethically and scientifically sound must involve both medicine and statistics, as the latter provides probability models that quantify uncertainty. The phase II problem becomes much more complex when multiple experimental treatments are available. Statistical methods for dealing with this setting include both randomization and algorithms for selecting one or more treatments. This scientific problem must be addressed while also dealing with the physician's problem of selecting the "best" for an individual patient. Thus, the ethical concerns that drive therapy evaluation are fully congruent with the scientific concerns.

This being the case, it is all the more disappointing that the status 0quo for phase II evaluation is very likely the worst situation imaginable. Currently, there are a plethora of small studies, each enrolling 20 to 30 patients, often reported without accounting for prognostic features and often from referral centers with substantial, but uncharacterized, patient selection factors at work. This guarantees that it will be impossible to place the reported results into a larger context. One needs only casual acquaintance with the abstracts from the annual American Society of Clinical Oncology meeting to appreciate that we have a lot of data, but little information. In the remainder of this chapter, we describe some methods for improving the information yield from a phase II trial.

REGRESSION:
ADJUSTING FOR PATIENT HETEROGENEITY

It is well known that patient selection can easily obscure effects of therapy. In biostatistical terms, measures of efficacy may be confounded by the prognostic covariates of the patients being studied. A simple example is a single-arm phase II trial of E in which the patients have, on average, much better prognostic characteristics than those of typical patients. In this case, a large observed improvement in response rate compared with that seen historically with S may be due entirely to the superior patient prognostic effects in the trial of E rather than any actual superiority of E over S. Simply put, you can get whatever "response rate" you like depending on how you pick the patients. Despite the fact that this a very well known phenomenon, in practice it may be difficult to determine which covariates are most important, to say nothing of the prospective collection and reporting of this information. Nonetheless, it is beyond question that prognostic features should be sought, refined, and reported, in order that hypothesis generating comparisons with historical expectation can be made, and that results from different institutions can be ordered—even if only in a preliminary way.

Given appropriate patient covariate data, statistical regression analysis may be used to adjust for varying patient prognosis. However, as noted earlier, when comparing the results of nonrandomized trials, standard regression methods such as Cox or logistic model analysis cannot eliminate latent trial effects. In this context, the recent report of Bajorin et al. *(20)*, at Memorial Sloan-Kettering Cancer Center, is especially timely and important. They examined their experience treating 203 patients

with unresectable or metastatic bladder cancer with cisplatin, methotrexate, vinblastine, and adriamycin (M-VAC) chemotherapy. The availability of a databank of patients treated on consecutive clinical trials
with similar eligibility criteria allowed them to develop a prognostic
model that could be reasonably validated by "bootstrapping" multiple
data samples from the larger dataset. In the final model, two clinical
features were found to be highly predictive of survival: compromised
performance status (i.e., Karnofsky performance status <80%) and visceral metastases. Bajorin et al. *(21)* found that cohorts with 0, 1, or 2
of these two risk factors demonstrated median survivals of 33, 13.4, and
9.4 mo, respectively. Thus, the expected survival of a group of patients
treated with M-VAC could easily vary by up to 2 yr, depending on the
prognostic makeup of the cohort. The important implication of this work
is that results obtained with newer therapies can be compared to what
one might have reasonably "expected" on the basis of the model, thus
placing the results in a more informative context. Indeed, the group at
Sloan-Kettering has done this in relation to the development of potential
M-VAC successors. The current results with their ifosamide, paclitaxel,
and cisplatin (ITP) regimen do, in fact, appear to be better than historical
expectation *(21)*, and this provides a substantial rationale for the further
development of this regimen.

We also have considerable experience with the M-VAC regimen over
a series of consecutive trials at MD Anderson Cancer Center. Most recently,
81 patients were treated on the standard therapy arm of a phase III trial.
There were 62 deaths with overall median survival of 13.7 mo (95%
confidence interval 11.4–18.9 mo), well within historical expectation
for M-VAC. We performed a Cox model survival analysis to assess the
prognostic significance of the covariates: age, pretreatment hemoglobin, performance status, lung metastases, liver metastases, and bone
involvement.

After a preliminary assessment of the martingale residuals of each
quantitative predictor to determine whether a transformation was needed
to achieve appropriate fit under the proportional hazards assumption *(22)*,
we performed a backward elimination using p-value cutoff 0.05, starting
with all variables. The final model, summarized in Table 1, includes only
the binary indicators of performance status = 3 (PS3 in Table 1) and bone
involvement (BONE). A Grambsch-Therneau *(23)* goodness-of-fit test
with identity transformation of the model had global p-value 0.89, indicating that the Cox model assumption was well met. Neither the presence of 1 nor 2 of the risk factors identified in the Memorial Sloan-
Kettering model were individually significant in our data. However, note
that the features we found most informative are simply extremes of a

Table 1
Final Parameter Estimates of the Fitted Cox Model

Variable	Coefficient	SE	Relative risk	p-value
PS3	1.648	0.543	5.2	0.002
BONE	0.996	0.345	2.7	0.004

SE = standard error of the coefficient estimate.

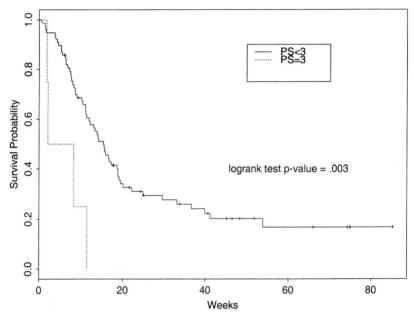

Fig. 1. Kaplan-Maier estimate of overall survival by Zubrod performance status (PS) in a cohort of 81 patients with metastatic urothelial cancer treated with M-VAC.

compromised performance status and "visceral" metastases, and thus our findings are very similar to the risk factors in the Memorial Sloan-Kettering model. The Kaplan-Meier estimates of survival according to performance status, and for the presence or absence of bone metastases are shown in Figs. 1 and 2, respectively.

The importance of accounting for significant prognostic covariates is illustrated by the confidence interval estimates of median survival in each of the patient subgroups determined by PS3 and BONE (*see* Table 2). Note that the overall 95% confidence interval (11.4, 18.9), considered alone and ignoring the prognostic covariates, would be overly optimistic for patients having either of these two unfavorable characteristics.

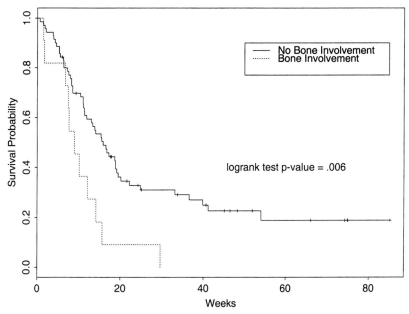

Fig. 2. Kaplan-Maier estimate of overall survival according to the presence or absence of bone involvement in a cohort of 81 patients with metastatic urothelial cancer treated with M-VAC.

Table 2
Median Survival Estimates in Three Patient
Prognostic Subgroups, Based on the Fitted Cox Model

PS = 3	Bone involvement	No. patients	Estimated median survival (95% confidence interval)
Yes	No	4	6.3 (3.8, —)
No	Yes	11	8.3 (6.4, 15.9)
No	No	66	16.6 (13.9, 24.9)

(A "Yes, Yes" row representing patients with both PS = 3 and bone involvement is not included because there were no such patients in this data set, although the fitted model would extrapolate to predict a 2.1-mo median survival with 95% lower confidence bound 1.5 mo.

SELECTION

As discussed earlier, one of the challenges emerging in this era of multiple, active combination therapies available for metastatic bladder cancer is the problem of selecting promising regimens for further development. Moreover, as most patients are, in fact, eventually treated with more than one regimen, there is the additional complexity of identifying particularly attractive combinations of regimens, including their sequence of administration. This problem represents the next logical step in phase II evaluation of regimens in bladder cancer. It is undoubtedly true that selecting from the myriad of phase II studies being reported is really a more formidable problem than developing additional novel combinations. Clearly, it is not possible to do pairwise phase III comparisons on even a fraction of the novel combinations being reported. The pressing issue, therefore, is to apply some "screening method" that will identify the most promising regimens, or sequences of regimens, over multiple courses of therapy.

In clinical practice involving multiple courses of therapy, medical oncologists commonly use an informal, intuitive approach to this problem that is actually fairly powerful. When many treatment options are available, the usual clinical paradigm is (1) try something; (2) evaluate the benefit of that intervention; (3) if benefit is apparent, give more of the same therapy until some threshold of "success" is achieved or, (4) if no early benefit is apparent, then switch to some alternative therapy. Treatments that look promising initially, but that ultimately fail to produce an overall therapeutic "success," are said to produce "low-quality" response. Conversely, treatments that look promising initially and then go on, after subsequent courses of treatment, to produce an overall "successful therapy" are said to produce "high-quality" responses. Treatments that produce a favorable response after failure with some other treatment are said to be "non-cross-resistant." Thus, there is an informal, mental calculus by which oncologists "score" treatments. Treatments that produce more overall patient successes than expected on the basis of prior experience, and especially those that are beneficial despite the prejudice of prior failure with some other treatment, are "promoted," whereas failure to achieve these thresholds is accounted negatively. Such intuitive accounting is really the basis for "expert consensus" that remains the most commonly applied method for choosing the experimental arm for large comparative trials.

We have recently formalized this familiar paradigm, by providing a probability model and statistical rules for decision making in order to provide a scientific basis for clinical investigation that reflects physicians' actual clinical practice. The methodology provides an algorithm for efficient selection among a pool of contending therapies *(24)*. Figure 3 illustrates the algorithm for an ongoing prostate cancer trial evaluating four different treatments given in various possible combinations over two to four courses of treatment. Note that in this formalized version of usual clinical practice we have added the device of randomization. This

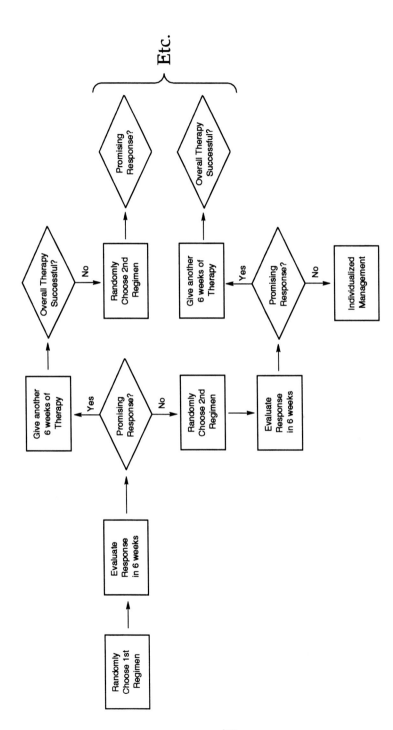

Fig. 3. Algorithm for treatment assignment in a clinical trial based on the "play the winner, drop the loser" selection paradigm.

provides a basis for unbiased treatment comparison. We have also taken explicit account of the fact that overall success for a given patient's therapy is a compound event that in general requires first meeting some modest threshold that serves to justify further treatment, and subsequently meeting a higher threshold of response that is sufficient to declare the overall therapy "successful." This algorithm has several interesting properties. First, patients are evaluated early on, and thus a patient is quickly switched from a treatment that is not producing an appropriate initial response. Second, the design is "adaptive" in that all treatment choices after the first are based on the particular patient's history thus far in the trial, using what might be called a "play the winner and drop the loser" strategy. In this way, each patient "finds" the optimal therapy for his/her cancer. Third, in the face of even modest salvage activity (i.e., non-cross-resistance) the outcome for a cohort treated by this algorithm can be superior to the outcome obtained if all patients had been treated with the arm showing the highest initial response rate.

Systemic chemotherapy for urothelial cancer presents an ideal application for such a selection algorithm, as the following features characterize the current situation: (1) there are multiple regimens of apparently comparable activity available; (2) one can typically make some assessment of response within 6 wk of initiating treatment; (3) it is already established that many patients failing with one treatment can demonstrate response to another.

Although a trial conducted according to the algorithm shown in Fig. 3 is intuitive and operationally simple, the statistical analysis is somewhat complex. In a trial of four regimens in which each patient may have up to two different treatments, using a "two failures and out" rule, there are actually 12 different treatment strategies under investigation—corresponding to each of the four treatments given initially, followed by each of the remaining three if the first fails to achieve overall patient "success." This leads to a probability structure that, although complex, can be written down explicitly. Thus, trial results can be used to estimate the relevant probabilities of success directly. In addition, the underlying probability model characterizes the response quality and cross-resistance between all treatment pairs in the trial. In the model, the parameters are estimated using the pooled experience of multiple patients, maximizing the information gain from the trial, and making powerful treatment strategy selection possible from a relatively small number of patients. A computer simulation study of this design under a wide variety of possible clinical scenarios showed that the design is surprisingly likely to select the best among the 12 possible strategies. Intuitively, this is due to the fact that statistical estimates of the probabilities of patient

Regimen	Scenario 1				Scenario 2			
	A	B	C	D	A	B	C	D
Probability of initial "Response"	0.5	0.5	0.5	0.6	0.5	0.5	0.5	0.5
Probability of "Successful" Therapy Overall after Initial "Response"	0.4	0.4	0.4	0.5	0.4	0.4	0.4	0.4
Probability of "Response" after Failure with a Previous Therapy	0.3	0.3	0.3	0.45	0.2	0.2	0.2	0.4

Fig. 4. Two scenarios used to evaluate the properties of the multicourse selection algorithm.

success under each treatment strategy "borrow strength" across common treatments in the earlier courses.

Two of the scenarios used for the computer simulations are illustrated in Fig. 4. In this figure, four hypothetical regimens, A–D, are characterized by three key probabilities: (1) the probability of meeting some initial threshold of benefit that will justify additional treatment (e.g., a "partial response" for a chemosensitive disease such as bladder cancer); (2) the probability that a patient having some initial success will go on to be an "overall success" (e.g., a clinical "complete response"); and (3) the probability that a treatment will produce a response after failure with some other regimen. For the hypothetical treatments shown, a traditional "one-stage" randomized phase II trial *(25)* evaluating only the overall response rate to the initially assigned regimen would require 240 patients to have 80% probability of correctly selecting regimen D. Under the new multicourse selection paradigm, however, only 136 patients are required to achieve an 80% correct selection probability.

A more subtle case is shown in scenario 2 in Fig. 4. Here, the four regimens have identical probabilities of initial response and "overall success," but regimen D is less cross-resistant after failure with treatments A, B, or C. A single-stage trial would never even consider the information required to detect this difference, as in that setting patients would go "off-study" before such an effect could be observed. Under the multicourse selection design, which aims to select the optimal 2-treatment strategy out of the 12 that are possible, a sample size of 204 patients would ensure an 80% probability that one of the optimal strategies (A, D), (B, D), or (C, D) will be selected from the 12 possible, compared to the probability 3/12 (25%) of correctly guessing one of the three to be best.

Another ongoing trial at MD Anderson utilizes this design to compare four regimens in bladder cancer based on an extension of this multicourse design. In this case, we have included two regimens based on intermediate-dose ifosfamide and two based on gemcitabine. The protocol mandates that if a patient fails one of the ifosfamide regimens, then he or she is randomized to one of the gemcitabine regimens, and vice versa. Thus, the treatments are grouped such that no patient may receive two consecutive ifosfamide-based or two consecutive gemcitabine-based regimens. A clinical "complete response" is the threshold for "overall success." It is anticipated that this trial will provide information about the cross-resistance among these regimens. In addition, we hope that this approach will provide a much more objective basis for choosing regimens for phase III evaluation, and that the explicit investigation of cross-resistance will provide clues for future investigations of novel regimen combinations.

The selection paradigm and trial design just outlined is but one attempt to maximize information from clinical experience and to have some basis other than anecdote to address the central problem of selection. Doubtless there are refinements that can be made to our analysis, and doubtless other paradigms will be invented.

The rapid advances in identifying prognostic features, surrogate endpoints, and standardized toxicity assessment make multidimensional analysis of clinical trials more plausible now than ever before. By use of expanded clinical characterization of patient factors, disease factors, and outcome, much more refined notions of "response" can be obtained, and such results can be meaningfully compared in order to rank advances and generate hypotheses for larger trials of definitive statistical power. These aspects of clinical trial design and analysis remain substantial challenges, both in constructing the appropriate statistical models and methods, and in bringing these new methodologies to application in the clinic. It seems likely that greater interaction between clinicians and biostatisticians will be required to meet these challenges. The authors continue to find such collaboration richly rewarding, and recommend the experience to our colleagues.

REFERENCES

1. Fleming TR. One sample multiple testing procedure for phase II clinical trials. Biometrics 1982; 38: 143–151.
2. Bryant J, Day R. Incorporating toxicity considerations into the design of two-stage phase II clinical trials. Biometrics 1995; 51: 1372–1383.
3. Chang M, Wieand HS, Therneau T. Designs for group-sequential phase II clinical trials. Biometrics 1987; 43: 865–874.
4. Simon R. Optimal two-stage designs for phase II clinical trials. Control Clin Trials 1989; 10: 1–10.
5. Thall PF, Simon R. Incorporating historical control data in planning Phase II clinical trials. Stat Med 1990; 9: 215–228.

6. Thall PF, Simon R. Practical Bayesian guidelines for phase IIB clinical trials. Biometrics 1994; 50: 337–349.

7. Thall PF, Simon R. A Bayesian approach to establishing sample size and monitoring criteria for phase II clinical trials. Control Clin Trials 1994; 15: 463–481.

8. Thall PF, Simon R, Estey EH. Bayesian sequential monitoring designs for single-arm clinical trials with multiple outcomes. Stat Med 1995; 14: 357–379.

9. Thall PF, Simon RM, Estey EH. New statistical strategy for monitoring safety and efficacy in single-arm clinical trials. J Clin Oncol 1996; 14: 296–303.

10. Thall PF, Sung HG. Some extensions and applications of a Bayesian strategy for monitoring multiple outcomes in clinical trials. Stat Med 1998; 17: 1563–1580.

11. Stallard N, Thall PF, Whitehead J. Decision theoretic designs for phase II clinical trials with multiple outcomes. Biometrics 1999; 55: 971–977.

12. Gehan EA. The determination of the number of patients required in a follow up trial of a new therapeutic agent. J Chronic Dis 1961; 13: 346–353.

13. Thall PF, Simon R. Recent developments in the design of phase II clinical trials. In: *Recent Advances in the Design and Analysis of Clinical Trials* (Thall P, ed.). Kluwer, Norwell, MA, 1995, pp. 49–71.

14. O'Quigley J, Pepe M, Fisher, L. Continual reassessment method: a practical design for Phase I clinical trials in cancer. Biometrics 1990; 46: 33–38.

15. Thall PF, Lee JJ, Tseng C-H, Estey E. Accrual strategies for phase I trials with delayed patient outcome. Stat Med 1999; 18: 1155–1169.

16. Cheung YK, Chappell R. Sequential designs for phase I clinical trials with late-onset toxicities. Biometrics 2000; 56: 1177–1182.

17. Simon R, Freidlin B, Rubinstein L, Arbuck SG, Collins J, Christian MC. Accelerated titration designs for phase I clinical trials in oncology. J Natl Cancer Inst 1997; 89: 1138–1147.

18. Thall PF, Russell KT. A strategy for dose-finding and safety monitoring based on efficacy and adverse outcomes in phase I/II clinical trials. Biometrics 1998; 54: 251–264.

19. Thall PF, Estey EH, Sung H-G. A new statistical method for dose-finding based on efficacy and toxicity in early phase clinical trials. Invest New Drugs 1999; 17: 155–167.

20. Bajorin DF, Dodd PM, Mazuumdar M, McCaffrey JA, Scher HI, Herr H, et al. Long-term survival in metastatic transitional-cell carcinoma and prognostic factors predicting outcome of therapy. J Clin Oncol 1999; 17: 3173–3181.

21. Bajorin DF, McCaffrey JA, Dodd PM, Hilton S, Mazumdar M, Kelly WK, et al. Ifosfamide, paclitaxel, cisplatin for patients with advanced transitional cell carcinoma of the urothelial tract: final report of a phase II trial evaluating two dosing schedules. Cancer 2000; 88: 1671–1678.

22. Therneau TM, Grambsch PM, Fleming TR. Martingale based residuals for survival models. Biometrika 1990; 77: 147–160.

23. Grambsch PA, Therneau TM. Proportional hazards tests and diagnostics based on weighted residuals. Biometrika 1994; 81: 515–526.

24. Thall PF, Millikan R, Sung H-G. Evaluating multiple treatment courses in clinical trials. Stat Med 2000; 19: 1011–1028.

25. Simon R, Wittes RE, Ellenberg SS. Randomized phase II clinical trials. Cancer Treat Rep 1985; 69, 1375–1381.

Index